Brain Tumor Microenvironment

Brain Tumor Microenvironment

Guest Editors

Annunziato Mangiola
Gianluca Trevisi

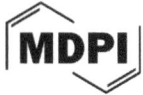

Basel • Beijing • Wuhan • Barcelona • Belgrade • Novi Sad • Cluj • Manchester

Guest Editors

Annunziato Mangiola
Department of Neurosciences
G. D'Annunzio University
Chieti-Pescara
Chieti
Italy

Gianluca Trevisi
Department of Neurosciences
G. D'Annunzio University
Chieti-Pescara
Chieti
Italy

Editorial Office
MDPI AG
Grosspeteranlage 5
4052 Basel, Switzerland

This is a reprint of the Special Issue, published open access by the journal *Cancers* (ISSN 2072-6694), freely accessible at: www.mdpi.com/journal/cancers/special_issues/brain_TME.

For citation purposes, cite each article independently as indicated on the article page online and using the guide below:

Lastname, A.A.; Lastname, B.B. Article Title. *Journal Name* **Year**, *Volume Number*, Page Range.

ISBN 978-3-7258-2924-8 (Hbk)
ISBN 978-3-7258-2923-1 (PDF)
https://doi.org/10.3390/books978-3-7258-2923-1

© 2025 by the authors. Articles in this book are Open Access and distributed under the Creative Commons Attribution (CC BY) license. The book as a whole is distributed by MDPI under the terms and conditions of the Creative Commons Attribution-NonCommercial-NoDerivs (CC BY-NC-ND) license (https://creativecommons.org/licenses/by-nc-nd/4.0/).

Contents

About the Editors vii

Preface ix

Gianluca Trevisi and Annunziato Mangiola
Editorial for Special Issue "Brain Tumor Microenvironment"
Reprinted from: *Cancers* **2024**, *16*, 3864, https://doi.org/10.3390/cancers16223864 1

Philippa K. Brosch, Tessa Korsa, Danush Taban, Patrick Eiring, Philipp Kreisz and Sascha Hildebrand et al.
Glucose and Inositol Transporters, SLC5A1 and SLC5A3, in Glioblastoma Cell Migration
Reprinted from: *Cancers* **2022**, *14*, 5794, https://doi.org/10.3390/cancers14235794 3

Ashok Panigrahy, Regina I. Jakacki, Ian F. Pollack, Rafael Ceschin, Hideho Okada and Marvin D. Nelson et al.
Magnetic Resonance Spectroscopy Metabolites as Biomarkers of Disease Status in Pediatric Diffuse Intrinsic Pontine Gliomas (DIPG) Treated with Glioma-Associated Antigen Peptide Vaccines
Reprinted from: *Cancers* **2022**, *14*, 5995, https://doi.org/10.3390/cancers14235995 20

Nazik Alturki, Muhammad Umer, Abid Ishaq, Nihal Abuzinadah, Khaled Alnowaiser and Abdullah Mohamed et al.
Combining CNN Features with Voting Classifiers for Optimizing Performance of Brain Tumor Classification
Reprinted from: *Cancers* **2023**, *15*, 1767, https://doi.org/10.3390/cancers15061767 31

Salvatore Marino, Grazia Menna, Rina Di Bonaventura, Lucia Lisi, Pierpaolo Mattogno and Federica Figà et al.
The Extracellular Matrix in Glioblastomas: A Glance at Its Structural Modifications in Shaping the Tumoral Microenvironment—A Systematic Review
Reprinted from: *Cancers* **2023**, *15*, 1879, https://doi.org/10.3390/cancers15061879 46

Hannah K. Jackson, Christine Mitoko, Franziska Linke, Donald Macarthur, Ian D. Kerr and Beth Coyle
Extracellular Vesicles Potentiate Medulloblastoma Metastasis in an EMMPRIN and MMP-2 Dependent Manner
Reprinted from: *Cancers* **2023**, *15*, 2601, https://doi.org/10.3390/cancers15092601 66

Tingyu Shi, Jun Zhu, Xiang Zhang and Xinggang Mao
The Role of Hypoxia and Cancer Stem Cells in Development of Glioblastoma
Reprinted from: *Cancers* **2023**, *15*, 2613, https://doi.org/10.3390/cancers15092613 86

Vera Nickl, Juliana Eck, Nicolas Goedert, Julian Hübner, Thomas Nerreter and Carsten Hagemann et al.
Characterization and Optimization of the Tumor Microenvironment in Patient-Derived Organotypic Slices and Organoid Models of Glioblastoma
Reprinted from: *Cancers* **2023**, *15*, 2698, https://doi.org/10.3390/cancers15102698 108

Xiong Xiao, Xiaoou Li, Yi Wang, Changcun Pan, Peng Zhang and Guocan Gu et al.
Classification of Brainstem Gliomas Based on Tumor Microenvironment Status
Reprinted from: *Cancers* **2023**, *15*, 4224, https://doi.org/10.3390/cancers15174224 126

Gianluca Trevisi and Annunziato Mangiola
Current Knowledge about the Peritumoral Microenvironment in Glioblastoma
Reprinted from: *Cancers* **2023**, *15*, 5460, https://doi.org/10.3390/cancers15225460 . . . . **142**

Vassilis Genoud, Ben Kinnersley, Nicholas F. Brown, Diego Ottaviani and Paul Mulholland
Therapeutic Targeting of Glioblastoma and the Interactions with Its Microenvironment
Reprinted from: *Cancers* **2023**, *15*, 5790, https://doi.org/10.3390/cancers15245790 . . . . **164**

About the Editors

Annunziato Mangiola

Annunziato Mangiola has a degree in medicine and surgery and a specialization in neurosurgery. From 2000 to 2017 he held the role of researcher at the Catholic University of the Sacred Heart of Rome, Fondazione Policlinico Gemelli. He is currently an associate professor at the University of Chieti-Pescara and has obtained the qualification as a full professor. He has always been interested in neuro-oncological pathology (along with Italian and foreign multidisciplinary collaborations), with particular attention to the mechanisms underlying tumor recurrence from both a biological and physical point of view. His further fields of interest include pituitary tumors, hydrocephalus, and cranial traumatology. He has obtained funding from the Italian Ministry of Research for his research activities. The obtained results from his recent studies highlight the possibility of accurately detecting the tumor lesion boundary with a completely non-invasive, contactless, and portable technology, revealing thermal IR imaging as a very promising tool for neurosurgeons.

Gianluca Trevisi

Dr. Gianluca Trevisi is an associate professor of neurosurgery within the Department of Neurosciences, Imaging, and Clinical Sciences at G. d'Annunzio University of Chieti-Pescara. He concurrently serves as a practicing neurosurgeon at the Ospedale Santo Spirito in Pescara, Italy.

Dr. Trevisi's clinical and research endeavors are primarily focused on the field of neuro-oncology, with a particular emphasis on applying the principles of functional neuro-oncology to the treatment of brain tumors. His expertise in neuroanatomy and brain mapping contributes to optimized surgical precision and minimizes neurological complications.

Furthermore, Dr. Trevisi is actively involved in translational research aimed at developing novel therapies and improving patient outcomes in neuro-oncology. He actively participates in national and international research collaborations and has authored numerous publications in peer-reviewed scientific journals.

Preface

This Special Issue explores the brain tumor microenvironment, a complex interplay crucial for tumor behavior. We aim to achieve the following: characterize tumor microenvironment features; investigate cell–environment interactions; identify novel therapeutic targets; understand the role of extracellular vesicles; develop and validate preclinical models; and integrate advanced imaging. Gliomas, like glioblastoma, pose significant challenges due to their aggressive nature and resistance to therapies. By understanding the microenvironment, we can develop more effective treatments, improve patient outcomes, and advance our understanding of tumor biology.

This Special Issue is for neuroscientists, oncologists, radiologists, immunologists, pharmacologists, and researchers. This work builds upon research emphasizing the heterogeneity of the brain tumor microenvironment, the importance of patient-derived models, the role of extracellular vesicles in tumor progression, and the potential of artificial intelligence. By exploring these intricate interactions, we can unlock new avenues for therapeutic intervention and ultimately improve patient outcomes.

This Special Issue aims to serve as a valuable resource for advancing our understanding of this critical aspect of brain tumor biology.

Annunziato Mangiola and Gianluca Trevisi
Guest Editors

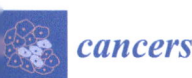

Editorial

Editorial for Special Issue "Brain Tumor Microenvironment"

Gianluca Trevisi [1,2,*] and Annunziato Mangiola [1]

1. Department of Neurosciences, Imaging and Clinical Sciences, G. D'Annunzio University Chieti-Pescara, 66100 Chieti, Italy
2. Neurosurgical Unit, Ospedale Spirito Santo, 65122 Pescara, Italy
* Correspondence: gianluca.trevisi@unich.it

The tumor microenvironment (TME) is a complex interplay of cells, extracellular matrix, and signaling molecules that significantly influences tumor growth, invasion, and resistance to therapy. This Special Issue delves into the intricate relationship between brain tumors and their surrounding microenvironment, shedding light on critical factors that drive tumor progression and resistance to treatment.

A comprehensive understanding of the TME is crucial for developing effective therapeutic strategies. Xiao et al. [1] highlight the heterogeneity of the TME in brainstem gliomas, a particularly challenging type of brain tumor. By classifying these tumors based on their TME characteristics, this study provides valuable insights for developing targeted therapies that can exploit the specific vulnerabilities of each TME subtype.

Glioblastoma, the most aggressive primary brain tumor, is one of the main focuses of this issue. Nickl et al. [2] explore the use of patient-derived tumor models to study the TME. These models offer a unique opportunity to understand the complex interplay between tumor cells and their microenvironment, including the role of immune cells, stromal cells, and extracellular matrix components. By studying these interactions, researchers can identify potential therapeutic targets and develop novel strategies to overcome treatment resistance.

Extracellular vesicles (EVs) are emerging as key players in cancer progression [3]. Jackson et al. [4] demonstrate how EVs secreted by medulloblastoma cells can promote tumor metastasis by activating specific proteins on their surface, such as matrix metalloproteinases. Targeting these EVs may offer a promising approach to prevent tumor spread and improve patient outcomes.

Artificial intelligence is revolutionizing cancer research. Alturki et al. [5] present a novel method for classifying brain tumors using deep learning techniques. By analyzing large datasets of imaging and genomic data, this approach can identify subtle patterns that may be missed by traditional methods, leading to a more accurate and earlier diagnosis of brain tumors.

Panigrahy et al. [6] explore the use of magnetic resonance spectroscopy (MRS) to monitor treatment response in pediatric diffuse intrinsic pontine gliomas (DIPG). By measuring metabolic changes within the tumor, MRS may provide valuable insights into tumor progression and treatment effectiveness. This non-invasive technique can help clinicians assess treatment response and adjust treatment plans accordingly.

Brosch et al. [7] investigate the role of sugar transporters in glioblastoma cell migration. By understanding how these transporters fuel tumor cell movement, we may be able to develop novel strategies to inhibit tumor invasion and metastasis. Targeting these transporters may offer a promising approach to limit tumor spread and improve patient survival.

Genoud et al. [8] provide a comprehensive review of current therapeutic strategies for glioblastoma, emphasizing the importance of targeting the TME. By understanding the complex interactions between tumor cells and their microenvironment, we can develop more effective treatments. This review highlights the potential of targeting immune cells, stromal cells, and signaling pathways within the TME to improve treatment outcomes.

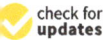

Citation: Trevisi, G.; Mangiola, A. Editorial for Special Issue "Brain Tumor Microenvironment". *Cancers* **2024**, *16*, 3864. https://doi.org/10.3390/cancers16223864

Received: 12 November 2024
Accepted: 15 November 2024
Published: 18 November 2024

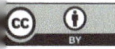

Copyright: © 2024 by the authors. Licensee MDPI, Basel, Switzerland. This article is an open access article distributed under the terms and conditions of the Creative Commons Attribution (CC BY) license (https://creativecommons.org/licenses/by/4.0/).

The peritumoral brain zone (PBZ) is a critical region surrounding the tumor core that plays a significant role in tumor recurrence. Trevisi and Mangiola [9] review the biology of the PBZ, highlighting its unique microenvironment and its impact on tumor progression. Targeting the PBZ may offer a promising strategy to prevent tumor recurrence and improve patient survival.

Hypoxia, a condition characterized by low oxygen levels, is a common feature of solid tumors, including brain tumors. Shi et al. [10] review the role of hypoxia and cancer stem cells in glioblastoma development. Hypoxia can promote the survival and self-renewal of cancer stem cells, which are thought to be resistant to treatment and contribute to tumor recurrence. Targeting hypoxia and cancer stem cells may offer a novel approach to improve treatment outcomes.

The extracellular matrix (ECM) provides structural support and regulates cell behavior. Marino et al. [11] review the role of the ECM in glioblastoma, highlighting its modifications in the tumor microenvironment and its impact on tumor progression. Targeting the ECM may offer a promising strategy to inhibit tumor invasion and metastasis.

In conclusion, this Special Issue highlights the critical role of the TME in brain tumor progression. By understanding the complex interactions between tumor cells and their microenvironment, we can develop more effective therapies to improve patient outcomes. Future research should continue to investigate the TME and identify novel therapeutic targets to combat brain tumors.

Conflicts of Interest: The authors declare no conflicts of interest.

References

1. Xiao, X.; Li, X.; Wang, Y.; Pan, C.; Zhang, P.; Gu, G.; Li, T.; Jiang, Z.; Zhang, Y.; Zhang, L. Classification of Brainstem Gliomas Based on Tumor Microenvironment Status. *Cancers* **2023**, *15*, 4224. [CrossRef] [PubMed]
2. Nickl, V.; Eck, J.; Goedert, N.; Hübner, J.; Nerreter, T.; Hagemann, C.; Ernestus, R.-I.; Schulz, T.; Nickl, R.C.; Keßler, A.F.; et al. Characterization and Optimization of the Tumor Microenvironment in Patient-Derived Organotypic Slices and Organoid Models of Glioblastoma. *Cancers* **2023**, *15*, 2698. [CrossRef] [PubMed]
3. Cela, I.; Capone, E.; Trevisi, G.; Sala, G. Extracellular Vesicles in Glioblastoma: Biomarkers and Therapeutic Tools. *Semin. Cancer Biol.* **2024**, *101*, 25–43. [CrossRef] [PubMed]
4. Jackson, H.K.; Mitoko, C.; Linke, F.; Macarthur, D.; Kerr, I.D.; Coyle, B. Extracellular Vesicles Potentiate Medulloblastoma Metastasis in an EMMPRIN and MMP-2 Dependent Manner. *Cancers* **2023**, *15*, 2601. [CrossRef] [PubMed]
5. Alturki, N.; Umer, M.; Ishaq, A.; Abuzinadah, N.; Alnowaiser, K.; Mohamed, A.; Saidani, O.; Ashraf, I. Combining CNN Features with Voting Classifiers for Optimizing Performance of Brain Tumor Classification. *Cancers* **2023**, *15*, 1767. [CrossRef] [PubMed]
6. Panigrahy, A.; Jakacki, R.I.; Pollack, I.F.; Ceschin, R.; Okada, H.; Nelson, M.D.; Kohanbash, G.; Dhall, G.; Bluml, S. Magnetic Resonance Spectroscopy Metabolites as Biomarkers of Disease Status in Pediatric Diffuse Intrinsic Pontine Gliomas (DIPG) Treated with Glioma-Associated Antigen Peptide Vaccines. *Cancers* **2022**, *14*, 5995. [CrossRef] [PubMed]
7. Brosch, P.K.; Korsa, T.; Taban, D.; Eiring, P.; Kreisz, P.; Hildebrand, S.; Neubauer, J.; Zimmermann, H.; Sauer, M.; Shirakashi, R.; et al. Glucose and Inositol Transporters, SLC5A1 and SLC5A3, in Glioblastoma Cell Migration. *Cancers* **2022**, *14*, 5794; Erratum in *Cancers* **2023**, *15*, 5139. [CrossRef] [PubMed]
8. Genoud, V.; Kinnersley, B.; Brown, N.F.; Ottaviani, D.; Mulholland, P. Therapeutic Targeting of Glioblastoma and the Interactions with Its Microenvironment. *Cancers* **2023**, *15*, 5790. [CrossRef] [PubMed]
9. Trevisi, G.; Mangiola, A. Current Knowledge about the Peritumoral Microenvironment in Glioblastoma. *Cancers* **2023**, *15*, 5460. [CrossRef] [PubMed]
10. Shi, T.; Zhu, J.; Zhang, X.; Mao, X. The Role of Hypoxia and Cancer Stem Cells in Development of Glioblastoma. *Cancers* **2023**, *15*, 2613. [CrossRef] [PubMed]
11. Marino, S.; Menna, G.; Di Bonaventura, R.; Lisi, L.; Mattogno, P.; Figà, F.; Bilgin, L.; D'Alessandris, Q.G.; Olivi, A.; Della Pepa, G.M. The Extracellular Matrix in Glioblastomas: A Glance at Its Structural Modifications in Shaping the Tumoral Microenvironment—A Systematic Review. *Cancers* **2023**, *15*, 1879. [CrossRef] [PubMed]

Disclaimer/Publisher's Note: The statements, opinions and data contained in all publications are solely those of the individual author(s) and contributor(s) and not of MDPI and/or the editor(s). MDPI and/or the editor(s) disclaim responsibility for any injury to people or property resulting from any ideas, methods, instructions or products referred to in the content.

Glucose and Inositol Transporters, SLC5A1 and SLC5A3, in Glioblastoma Cell Migration

Philippa K. Brosch [1,†], Tessa Korsa [1,2,†], Danush Taban [1], Patrick Eiring [1], Philipp Kreisz [3], Sascha Hildebrand [1], Julia Neubauer [2], Heiko Zimmermann [2,4,5], Markus Sauer [1], Ryo Shirakashi [6], Cholpon S. Djuzenova [7], Dmitri Sisario [1,*,‡] and Vladimir L. Sukhorukov [1,*,‡]

1. Department of Biotechnology & Biophysics, Biocenter, University of Würzburg, 97074 Würzburg, Germany; philippa.brosch@uni-wuerzburg.de (P.K.B.); tessa.korsa@ibmt.fraunhofer.de (T.K.); danush.taban@uni-wuerzburg.de (D.T.); patrick.eiring@uni-wuerzburg.de (P.E.); sascha.hildebrand@stud-mail.uni-wuerzburg.de (S.H.); m.sauer@uni-wuerzburg.de (M.S.)
2. Fraunhofer Institute for Biomedical Engineering (IBMT), 66280 Sulzbach, Germany; julia.neubauer@ibmt.fraunhofer.de (J.N.); heiko.zimmermann@ibmt.fraunhofer.de (H.Z.)
3. Julius-von-Sachs Institute, University of Würzburg, 97082 Würzburg, Germany; philipp.kreisz@uni-wuerzburg.de
4. Department of Molecular and Cellular Biotechnology, Saarland University, 66123 Saarbrücken, Germany
5. Faculty of Marine Science, Universidad Católica del Norte, Coquimbo 1281, Chile
6. Institute of Industrial Science, The University of Tokyo, Tokyo 153-8505, Japan
7. Department of Radiation Oncology, University Hospital of Würzburg, 97080 Würzburg, Germany; djuzenova_t@ukw.de
* Correspondence: dmitri.sisario@uni-wuerzburg.de (D.S.); sukhorukov@biozentrum.uni-wuerzburg.de (V.L.S.); Tel.: +49-931-31-84511 (V.L.S.); Fax: +49-931-31-84529 (V.L.S.)
† These authors contributed equally to this work.
‡ These authors contributed equally to this work as senior authors.

Simple Summary: Cell migration is the main obstacle to the treatment of highly invasive brain cancer glioblastoma multiforme (GBM). We investigated in vitro the potential role of two solute carrier proteins (SLCs), SLC5A1 and SLC5A3, and their respective substrates, glucose and inositol, in GBM cell migration. We found that GBM cell motility was increased by medium supplementation with glucose and inositol and was strongly impaired by inhibition of SLC5A1/3 proteins. Using conventional and super-resolution fluorescence microscopy, we showed that both SLCs were not only highly expressed in migrating GBM cells, but they also localized to the lamellipodia, i.e., the migration-governing cell protrusions. Taken together, our data suggest that SLC5A1 and SLC5A3 are involved in GBM cell migration, presumably by mediating solute transport, osmotic water fluxes and thus local volume regulation in the lamellipodium.

Abstract: (1) Background: The recurrence of glioblastoma multiforme (GBM) is mainly due to invasion of the surrounding brain tissue, where organic solutes, including glucose and inositol, are abundant. Invasive cell migration has been linked to the aberrant expression of transmembrane solute-linked carriers (SLC). Here, we explore the role of glucose (SLC5A1) and inositol transporters (SLC5A3) in GBM cell migration. (2) Methods: Using immunofluorescence microscopy, we visualized the subcellular localization of SLC5A1 and SLC5A3 in two highly motile human GBM cell lines. We also employed wound-healing assays to examine the effect of SLC inhibition on GBM cell migration and examined the chemotactic potential of inositol. (3) Results: While GBM cell migration was significantly increased by extracellular inositol and glucose, it was strongly impaired by SLC transporter inhibition. In the GBM cell monolayers, both SLCs were exclusively detected in the migrating cells at the monolayer edge. In single GBM cells, both transporters were primarily localized at the leading edge of the lamellipodium. Interestingly, in GBM cells migrating via blebbing, SLC5A1 and SLC5A3 were predominantly detected in nascent and mature blebs, respectively. (4) Conclusion: We provide several lines of evidence for the involvement of SLC5A1 and SLC5A3 in GBM cell migration, thereby complementing the migration-associated transportome. Our findings suggest that SLC inhibition is a promising approach to GBM treatment.

Keywords: volume regulation; transportome; phlorizin

1. Introduction

Glioblastoma multiforme (GBM) is a high-grade astrocytoma with a dismal prognosis. Even after surgical resection and radiochemotherapy, the median survival time for patients does not exceed 15 months [1,2]. Recurrence is mainly due to the diffuse invasion of tumor cells into the surrounding brain tissue [3,4]. Thus, considerable efforts have been made to inhibit GBM cell migration [5–7], with many studies focusing on cytoskeletal dynamics at the leading edge of lamellipodium [8–12].

In addition to lamellipodia and ruffles [13], the leading edge of migrating cancer cells frequently displays transient spherical protrusions of the plasma membrane, known as "blebs" [5,14]. Preceding bleb nucleation, the actin cortex underlying the membrane becomes locally ruptured or detached, allowing the formation of membrane protrusion. Blebs, initially devoid of filamentous actin, then rapidly inflate and eventually, upon reconstruction of the actin cortex, contract and disappear [15,16].

According to the osmotic engine migration model [17], a variety of membrane transporters and channels enable a net water/solute-exchange at the anterior and posterior end of the cell. Interestingly, an increasing number of studies on highly motile cancer cells have reported a polarized distribution of water and ion channels, collectively known as the migration-associated transportome [17,18].

In addition to inorganic ions, various small organic osmolytes (SOOs) are also involved in the cell volume regulation of mammalian cells [19]. Among the most abundant SOOs in the human brain are glucose [20,21] and inositol [22–25]. Aberrant inositol levels have been linked to glial proliferation, high-grade astrocytoma and glioblastoma multiforme [26,27] and the increased glucose uptake of cancer cells has been studied extensively [28].

Cellular glucose and inositol uptake occur via specific transporters belonging to the solute carrier (SLC) 5-gene family [29,30]. SLC5A1, also known as sodium/glucose cotransporter 1 (SGLT1), mediates the cellular uptake of glucose, whereas inositol transport through cell membranes is achieved by SLC5A3, also known as sodium/myo-inositol cotransporter (SMIT1). Increasing evidence points to the involvement of SLCs in cancer progression. Not only are many SLC-transporters upregulated in tumor cells [31,32], but recently, they have come into focus as a marker of cancer phenotype [33,34]. Interestingly both SLC5A1 and SLC5A3 are highly expressed in various types of cancer [35].

While glucose is the main metabolic substrate required for cancer cell survival and proliferation [36], inositol serves as an important osmolyte in cell volume regulation and fluid homeostasis, particularly in the brain [37]. Inositol is also the precursor of phosphatidylinositol 4,5-bisphosphate (PIP2), known as a key signaling lipid in cancer cell migration [38].

However, little is known about the subcellular expression of the glucose and inositol transporters SLC5A1 and SLC5A3 and their possible involvement in GBM cell migration. In this study, we thus examined the impact of glucose and inositol, as well as SLC inhibition on the migration of two highly motile glioblastoma cell lines, DK-MG and SNB19. We also visualized, using immunostaining and fluorescence microscopy, the intracellular localization of both transporters in migrating and non-motile GBM cells.

2. Materials and Methods

2.1. Cell Culture

Both human glioblastoma (GBM) cell lines, DK-MG and SNB19, were acquired from DSMZ (Braunschweig, Germany) and routinely cultured under standard conditions (5% CO_2, 37 °C) in complete growth medium (CGM), consisting of Dulbecco's modified Eagle's medium (DMEM, Sigma, Deisenhofen, Germany) supplemented with 10% FBS. Cells were used at low (<15) passages after thawing. In addition, they were authenticated on the basis of morphology, expression of PTEN and p53, and growth curve analysis and were regularly tested for Mycoplasma (MycoAlert; Lonza, Rockland, ME, USA).

2.2. Immunostaining

DK-MG or SNB19 cells were seeded at either 5×10^4 or 5×10^3 cells per well, respectively, on eight-well chambered cover glasses (Sarstaedt, Nümbrecht, Germany) and then washed in pre-warmed (37 °C) phosphate-buffered saline (PBS). Cells were fixed using a PBS solution containing 0.25% glutaraldehyde and 4% paraformaldehyde (methanol-free) for 10 min at room temperature. Cells were then washed thrice in PBS for 5 min. Permeabilization was performed with 0.1% Triton X-100 in PBS for 10 min, followed by three washing steps with PBS for 5 min. Thereafter, the samples were incubated with blocking buffer containing 5% bovine serum albumin (BSA; Sigma Aldrich, St. Louis, MO, USA) in PBS for one hour. Following the blocking phase, cells were incubated for one hour with either rabbit SMIT1 antibodies (Abcam, Cambridge, UK) or goat SGLT1 antibodies (Everest Biotech, Bicester, UK) diluted 1:400 in blocking buffer. After incubation with primary antibodies, the samples were washed 3 times in PBS for 5 min. The cells were stained by incubating them in blocking buffer with 1:200-diluted Alexa Fluor (AF) 532-conjugated goat anti-rabbit IgG (Thermo Fisher Scientific, Waltham, MA, USA), AF488-conjugated rabbit anti-goat IgG (Thermo Fisher Scientific, Waltham, MA, USA), AF647 AffiniPure F(ab')$_2$ fragment donkey anti-rabbit IgG (Jackson ImmunoResearch, Ely, UK) or AF647-conjugated donkey anti-goat IgG (Invitrogen, Waltham, MA, USA) for 1 h, respectively. Finally, the cells were washed 3 times with PBS. For actin-staining experiments, cells were additionally incubated overnight with phalloidin-conjugated AF647 or AF532 (Thermo Fisher Scientific, Waltham, MA, USA) diluted 1:200 in PBS at 4 °C and washed with PBS prior to measurement. For microtubule staining, following SLC staining, the cells were incubated for 1 h in mouse anti-β-tubulin antibodies (Sigma Aldrich, St. Louis, MO, USA) diluted 1:200 in blocking buffer.

Immunostaining of wounded cell monolayers was performed by seeding 5×10^5 (DK-MG) or 2×10^5 (SNB19) cells per well on eight-well chambered cover glasses and incubated under standard conditions. Upon reaching confluence, the monolayer was scratched with a pipette tip and the culture medium was replaced to remove the detached cell debris. The cells were then incubated for 3 h under standard conditions until staining was performed, as described above.

2.3. Cell Volumetry

Volumetric measurements were performed to analyze cell volume regulation upon exposure to inositol, glucose, mannitol and sucrose, as described previously. [19,39] Briefly, detached cells were placed in an observation chamber and allowed to adhere to a poly-D-lysine-coated glass slide for 10 min prior to observation. Images were taken at 10-s intervals for 20 min. During measurement, the medium was replaced using a syringe pump with a perfusion speed set to 20 µL/s. Cell volume changes were induced by applying SOO solutions of 150 mOsm. Perfusion media (pH 7.4) contained 4.6 mOsm of K$_2$HPO$_4$/KH$_2$PO$_4$, 0.1 mM CaAc$_2$ and 0.02 mM MgAc$_2$, yielding ~5 mOsm of inorganic electrolytes. Each experiment was carried out at least 3 times. Starting 30 s into video recording, 0.5 mL SOO solution was pumped through the chamber. Frames 1–3 served as a reference for isotonic cell volume (V_0). Cell volume was determined by assuming spherical geometry and measuring the cross-section area with a custom-made ImageJ plugin [19]. From these volumetric data, we used the following equation to calculate the SOO-dependent regulatory volume decrease (RVD) inhibition index [40]:

$$IC_{RVD} = \left(\frac{v_{20} - v_0}{v_5 - v_0} \right) * 100\% \qquad (1)$$

with $v_0 = 1$ as normalized isotonic cell volume and v_5 and v_{20} as the normalized cell volumes after 5- and 20-min exposure to hypotonic medium, respectively. As pointed out elsewhere [40], an $IC_{RVD} \approx 0$ means complete recovery of initial cell volume, while $IC_{RVD} = 100\%$ shows that RVD was abolished and the cells remained swollen. An IC_{RVD} larger than 100% indicates continuous secondary swelling.

2.4. Confocal Laser Scanning Microscopy (CLSM)

Confocal fluorescence images were acquired with a Zeiss confocal LSM 700 microscope using a Plan-Apochromat 63×/1.40 oil immersion objective (Zeiss, Jena, Germany) and argon laser light excitations at 488, 555 and 639 nm. Image processing was carried out with ImageJ software.

2.5. dSTORM (Direct Stochastic Optical Reconstruction Microscopy)

Reversible photoswitching of the dyes AlexaFluor 647 and AlexaFluor 532 was performed in a photoswitching buffer containing 100 mM mercaptoethylamine (Sigma) in PBS at pH ~7.4. A detailed experimental setup for dSTORM was described previously [41]. Measurements were performed in 8-well chambered cover glasses (Sarstaedt, Nümbrecht, Germany). For localization data processing and image reconstruction, the open access software rapidSTORM 3.2 was used, as previously described [42,43]. Image processing was performed with ImageJ. Localization densities were determined via an in-house developed Python-based DBSCAN ("Density Based Spatial Clustering of Applications with Noise") algorithm.

2.6. Gene Expression Profiling Interactive Analysis of SLC5A1 and SLC5A3 in GBM

The bioinformatics tool Gene Expression Profiling Interactive Analysis (GEPIA2 [44] http://gepia.cancer-pku.cn/index.html (accessed on 24 February 2021)) was used to analyze patient survival data and tumor-vs.-normal differential expression data from the freely accessible data banks Genotype-Tissue Expression project (GTEx) and The Cancer Genome Atlas (TCGA) regarding SLC5A1- and SLC5A3-expression in GBM cells.

2.7. Wound Healing Assay

Cell migration rates were analyzed via a scratch assay. One day prior to measurements, 4×10^5 cells/mL were seeded in a Petri dish (diameter 35 mm) in 2 mL of CGM supplemented with 30 mM glucose (GLU) or inositol (INO). CGM supplemented with 30 mM of metabolically inert mannitol (MAN) served as a tonicity control. Before starting the video microscopy experiments, several wounds were introduced into the confluent cell monolayer by gentle scratching with a pipette tip, followed by removal of culture media, a washing step with PBS and addition of the respective SOO-supplemented media. Afterwards, the cells were placed for 18 h in an incubator (37 °C, 5% CO_2, 20% O_2) with an integrated camera (Biostation IM-Q, Nikon, Melville, NY, USA). For the inhibition experiments, 50 nM of phlorizin was present 3 h prior to and during the video recording. Phlorizin is a competitive inhibitor of SLC5A1 [45] and inhibits SLC5A3 [46]. For each experimental condition, ~10 regions of interest (ROI) were recorded for 18 h. Images of each ROI were acquired every 10 min with an image resolution of 1600 × 1200 and a pixel size of 0.44 µm²/pixel. The wound closure rate (µm²/min) for each condition was then determined as previously described [5,7].

2.8. Statistical Analysis

Data are presented as mean ± SE unless otherwise noted. A Student's unpaired t-test was performed when statistical comparisons were made between two sets of data. A p-Value of <0.05 was considered significant and indicated by "*" where applicable.

3. Results

Increasingly, aberrant expression of the SLC5 sub-family members has been linked to cancer cell invasion and metastasis [33]. Biopsy analysis of GBM also revealed expression of the proteins SLC5A1 and SLC5A3 in brain tumors (Supplementary Materials Figure S1A,B).

Moreover, glucose and *myo*-inositol, the substrates of these transporters, are abundant in brain tissue, with inositol even serving as an NMR biomarker in GBM diagnostics [27,47]. However, little is known about the role of these solutes' transport in GBM cell invasion and migration. We therefore examined in two highly motile GBM cell lines, DK-MG and SNB19, (1) the impact of elevated concentrations of glucose and inositol on the migratory activity by wound healing assays, (2) the subcellular expression patterns of SLC5A1 and SLC5A3 proteins by fluorescent immunostaining and (3) the GBM membrane permeability for glucose and inositol by osmotic swelling assay.

3.1. Wound-Healing and Chemotaxis Assays

Using time-lapse video-microscopy, we first examined the wound closure rates in DK-MG and SNB19 cell monolayers exposed to slightly hypertonic growth media supplemented with 30 mM glucose or inositol. In the hypertonic control experiments, the medium was instead supplemented with 30 mM of metabolically inert mannitol (Figure 1A,B). The data for the wound healing assay on both cell lines are statistically summarized in Figure 1C,D.

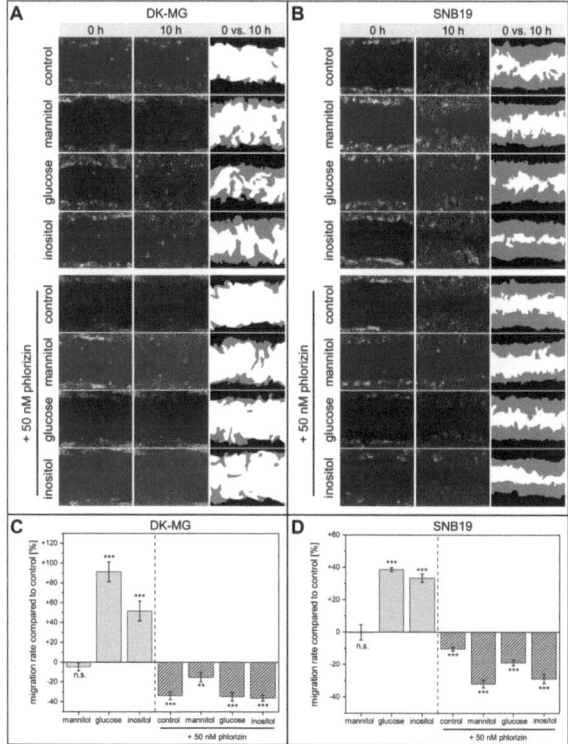

Figure 1. Wound healing assays of DK-MG and SNB19 cells incubated in culture medium supplemented with either mannitol, glucose or inositol or treated with phlorizin. Representative phase contrast images of wounded DK-MG (**A**) and SNB19 (**B**) cell monolayers shown in the left and middle columns were acquired at 0 and 10 h. The white color in the RHS column of A and B represents the cell-free area, and the black and gray colors denote cell-covered areas at 0 and 10 h, respectively. (**C,D**) Bar graphs summarizing the impact of organic solute-supplemented medium or phlorizin on the wound closure rate of DK-MG (**C**) and SNB19 cells (**D**), expressed in percentage difference to control. Each bar represents the mean ± SE of at least three independent experiments conducted in quadruplicate. "**" and "***" denote $p < 0.01$ and $p < 0.001$, respectively; "n.s." means "not significant".

We found that glucose significantly accelerated the wound closure in both DK-MG and SNB19 cell monolayers by 91% and 39%, respectively, as compared to isotonic controls. Likewise, inositol also increased the wound closure rate in DK-MG and SNB19 monolayers by 52% and 33%, respectively.

In contrast, although some studies have reported that medium tonicity impacts cell migration [17,48], we found that increasing extracellular osmolarity via metabolically inert mannitol did not affect GBM migration rates (Figure 1C,D). The increased migration speed in cells incubated in inositol- and glucose-supplemented medium thus cannot be attributed to higher medium osmolarity but stems from the specific osmolyte used as supplement.

Medium supplementation with 50 nM phlorizin, an inhibitor of both SLC5A1 [45] and SLC5A3 [46], significantly impaired the migration of both cell lines (Figure 1). Thus, phlorizin-treated DK-MG (Figure 1C) and SNB19 cells (Figure 1D) exhibited 34% and 10% decreased wound healing rates, respectively, as compared to drug-free controls. The inhibitory effect of phlorizin on the wound closure of both cell lines persisted even in the presence of supplemental solutes, including mannitol, glucose or inositol.

The faster cell migration in the presence of inositol revealed by the wound-healing assay prompted us to explore whether inositol can act as a chemoattractant. To this end, we conducted a chemotaxis assay of individual DK-MG cells (Figure 2A) in a microfluidic channel, along which an inositol gradient of 30 mM/100 μm was maintained. Because of their directionally persistent migration [5], DK-MG cells appeared most suitable for chemotaxis experiments. Single-cell migration was examined with the in-house modified software Time Lapse Analyzer, which yields individual cell trajectories (Figure 2B,C) along with data on migration speed and directionality (Figure 2E). In agreement with our previous study [5], individual DK-MG cells display a single large lamellipodium with multiple transient blebs, easily identified in phase contrast microscopy as dark spherical protrusions at the leading edge (Figure 2A).

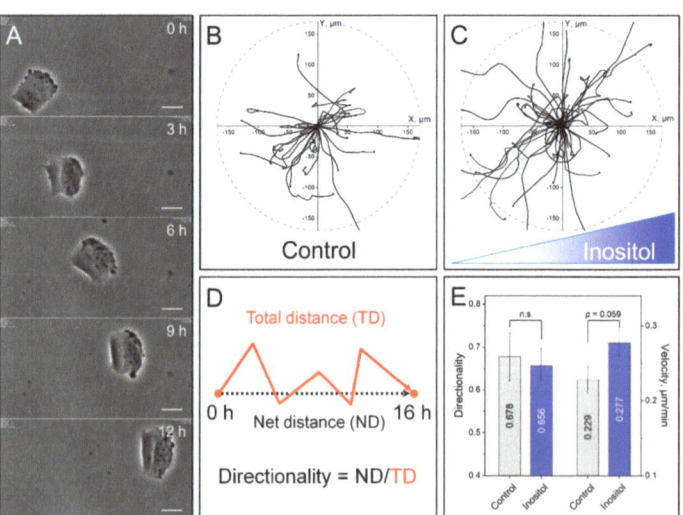

Figure 2. Chemotaxis experiments via μ-slide assays. (A) DK-MG cells were automatically tracked by the software TLA, which is able to consistently detect the cells center. Scale bar: 10 μm. (B,C) Plotting of the single tracks in a coordinate system shows directional movement, but without favoring the movement along the gradient, which increased from left to right in the x-axis. $N_{control}$ = 24 $N_{inositol}$ = 42. Endpoints were only partially marked for better visibility of tracks at the center (D) Definition of directionality. (E) Cell directionality and total velocity were calculated. Differences in directionality were not significant, while the presence of SOOs slightly increased cell velocity (±SD). However, Student's t-test showed p-values of >0.05, making the differences insignificant.

As is evident from the tracking diagrams in Figure 2C, which show no preferential migration along the applied inositol gradient, this solute does not exert any chemotactic effect on DK-MG cells. However, consistent with the strongly polarized morphology of DK-MG cells, cell tracking (Figure 2B,C) reveals a relatively high degree of migration directionality (>0.65, Figure 2E), defined as the net distance from the starting position divided by the length of the total distance (Figure 2D). While the directionality of DK-MG cells exposed to inositol showed no significant difference from controls (Figure 2E), the final positions of a large portion of inositol-treated DK-MG cells were more distant from the starting point (Figure 2B,C, respectively). These findings, statistically summarized in Figure 2E, imply a higher migration speed of individual DK-MG cells in the presence of inositol, which is in line with the results of wound healing in DK-MG cell monolayers (Figure 1).

3.2. SLC5A1 and SLC5A3 Preferentially Localize to the Leading Edge of GBM Cells

Confocal laser-scanning microscopy of immuno-stained wounded DK-MG cell monolayers revealed that both transporter proteins were predominantly expressed in cells constituting the edge of the monolayer facing the wound area (Figure 3A). In contrast, cell-covered areas within the cell monolayer, consisting of non-motile cells, were virtually devoid of both transporters (bottom half of Figure 3A). This is even more evident from the intensity profiles (Figure 3B) of the boxed areas in Figure 3A, which shows that the fluorescence signals of both transporters reach their peak values at ~5 µm from the wound border. Thereafter, SLC5A1 fluorescence gradually decreases up to the distance of ~10 µm and finally falls to background level at ~35 µm, which roughly matches the lateral dimension of a single adherent DK-MG cell (see below Figure 5A). In contrast, the SLC5A3 signal already vanished ~10 µm from the wound border, indicating that expression of this transporter is confined to the leading cell edge. Qualitatively similar fluorescence distributions of both transporter proteins were found in the wounded SNB19 cell monolayers (Figure 3C,D).

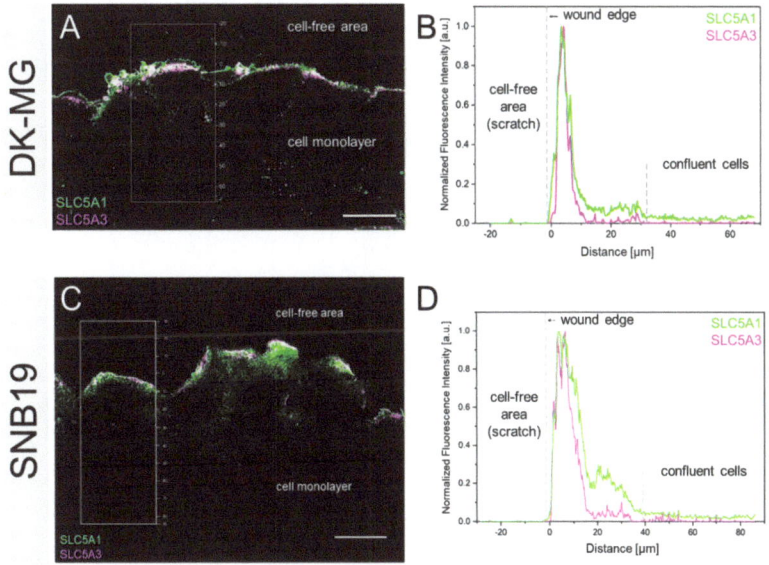

Figure 3. Representative LSM images of a DK-MG (**A**) and a SNB19 (**C**) cell monolayer, stained for SLC5A1 and SLC5A3 3 h after wounding. (**B,D**) Intensity profiles of the boxed area in A and C. Cells at the wound edge (0–~35 µm) display marked fluorescence signal peaks facing the cell-free area. In contrast, confluent cells were almost devoid of SLC5A1 and SLC5A3 signals. Scale bar in (**A,C**): 30 µm.

Prompted by the above findings in multicellular monolayers, we further analyzed the subcellular distribution of SLC5A1 and SLC5A3 in single migrating DK-MG and SNB19 cells. In a previous study [5], we found that the two cell lines differed greatly in morphology and migration behavior. DK-MG cells maintained a unipolar morphology with a single lamellipodium, leading to directionally persistent migration. In contrast, the randomly migrating SNB19 cells displayed multiple lamellipodia.

In the following single cell immunofluorescence experiments, in addition to SLC protein, we also stained actin filaments in order to visualize the morphological details of the leading cell edge, such as lamellipodia, ruffles and blebs. In particular, actin staining in DK-MG cells, exhibiting high blebbing activity at the leading edge of the lamellipodium [5], allowed us to infer the stage of the bleb life cycle from the thickness of its actin cortex [15,49]. To visualize in real time the formation of the actin cortex in the blebs of DK-MG cells, we performed dual live-cell fluorescence labeling of the cell membrane and actin (Figure 4). Judging from the membrane staining (green signal in Figure 4A), the bleb indicated by the arrow increases rapidly in size (Figure 4A, 5 s) and reaches its maximum diameter 25 s after the onset of bleb expansion. During the expansion phase (Figure 4A, time < 25 s), the bleb did not display any significant actin fluorescence. Only during the following retraction phase, i.e., between 25 and 90 s (Figure 4A), the actin cortex becomes visible and its thickness increases as bleb retraction progresses (Figure 4A, 130 s). The biphasic kinetics of bleb growth to the maximum volume of 120 fL at ~30 s and retraction during the following ~2 min are statistically (N = 8) summarized in Figure 4B, while Figure 4C shows the time courses of the actin and membrane signal densities within the bleb area. Interestingly, the kinetics of the membrane signal density (green symbols in Figure 4C) matches well the bleb volume kinetics (Figure 4B). In sharp contrast, actin signal density gradually increases during both the growth and retraction phases, which is consistent with the role of acto-myosin contraction in bleb shrinkage [49,50].

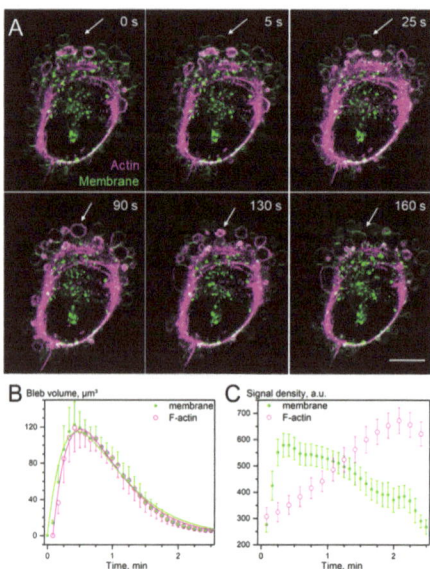

Figure 4. Membrane blebs in DK-MG cells. (**A**) Live-cell imaging of a representative blebbing DK-MG cell stained for F-actin (magenta) and plasma membrane (green) reveals individual bleb dynamics over time (white arrow). Scale bar: 10 μm. (**B**) Statistically summarized biphasic kinetics of membrane and F-actin formation shows a temporal shift in bleb growth. (**C**) Plotting of fluorescence intensity of plasma membrane and F-actin signals in individual blebs over time reveals a lag in F-actin signal build-up compared to the plasma membrane.

In light of the above live-cell observations (Figure 4) and data reported elsewhere [15,49], the absence of cortical actin in the fixed immunostained cells shown below signifies nascent blebs in the growth phase, whereas a thicker actin cortex indicates matured retracting blebs. We found that in DK-MG cells, SLC5A1 frequently localized to nascent expanding blebs, readily identifiable by the absence of cortical actin (Figure 5A,a). In contrast, SLC5A3 exclusively localized to mature, retracting blebs, evident from their thick actin cortex (Figure 5C,c), whereas nascent blebs were virtually devoid of SLC5A3. This is particularly evident from the samples co-stained for both transporter proteins (Figure 5E). Interestingly, SLC5A1 and SLC5A3 co-localized only in smaller, retracting blebs, but not in the large anterior nascent blebs (Figure 5e).

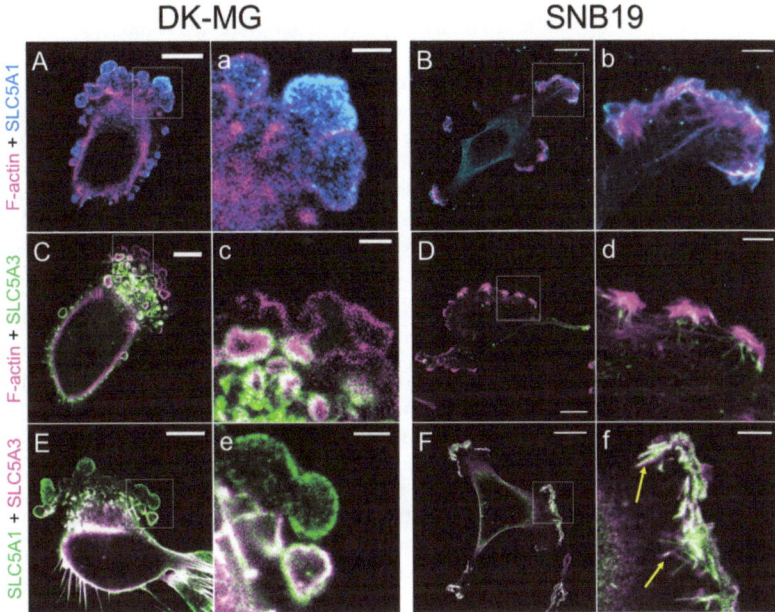

Figure 5. Confocal fluorescence images of DK-MG and SNB19 cells co-stained for F-actin and SLC5A1 (**A**,**B**), F-actin and SLC5A3 (**C**,**D**) or SLC5A1 and SLC5A3 (**E**,**F**). Co-localization of SLC5A1 and SLC5A3 is depicted in white. SLC5A1 predominantly localized to the cell compartments involved in migration, i.e., lamellipodia (**B–F**) and blebs (**A**,**C**,**E**). Lowercase letters show magnifications of the boxed regions in (**A–F**). Both transporter proteins display colocalization in lamellipodial tips of SNB19 cells (arrows in **f**). Scale bars: 15 µm in (**B–F**), 10 µm in (**A**,**C**,**E**), 5 µm in (**d**), 2.5 µm in (**a–c,e,f**).

In agreement with our previous study [5], single SNB19 cells displayed a multipolar morphology with numerous lamellipodia (Figure 5B,D). In addition to the diffuse fluorescence of actin-rich membrane ruffles (magenta in Figure 5B,D), the tips of lamellipodia exhibited marked expression of both transporter proteins SLC5A1 and SLC5A3 (Figure 5B,D, respectively). Co-staining of SLC5A1 with SLC5A3 reveals multiple spike-like membrane protrusions, most likely representing filopodia extending upward from the lamellipodial tip (arrows in Figure 5f). In contrast to the differential localization of SLC5A1 and SLC5A3 in DK-MG cell blebs (Figure 5e), the two transporter proteins strongly co-localized in the lamellipodial tips of SNB19 cells (Figure 5F).

Irrespective of the supplementing solute (mannitol, glucose or inositol), cultivation in slightly hypertonic (+30 mOsm) growth medium did not noticeably affect the intracellular distribution patterns of the two transporter proteins in both DK-MG and SNB19 cell lines, as seen, respectively, in Supplementary Materials Figures S2 and S3. Thus, similar to isotonic controls, hypertonically cultured DK-MG cells expressed SLC5A1 throughout the entire lamellipodium, including the membrane of the anterior-most nascent blebs, which however, were completely devoid of SLC5A3. Interestingly, even slight hypertonicity seems to affect the morphological appearance of the leading edge of DK-MG cells, where one or a few giant blebs of irregular shape are evident (yellow arrows in Figure S2), formed, most likely, by fusion of several regular-sized blebs, as seen in isotonic cells (Figure 5 and white arrows in Figure S2).

Interestingly, LSM images of DK-MG cells exposed to 50 nM phlorizin 16 h prior to fixation displayed barely any SLC5A1 and SLC5A3 signal at the leading edge of the cell compared to untreated controls (Supplementary Materials Figure S2). Furthermore, phlorizin-treated DK-MG cells showed virtually no migratory blebs. In contrast, phlorizin treated SNB19 cells showed both SLC5A1 and SLC5A3 signals throughout their multiple lamellipodia (Supplementary Materials Figure S3). However, phlorizin apparently impairs the formation of filopodia (Supplementary Materials Figure S3, inset).

Fluorescence staining of the microtubule protein β-tubulin, involved, among other functions, in intracellular vesicle trafficking [51,52], reveals the microtubular cytoskeleton as a pervasive cytosolic network in both DK-MG (Figure S4A,D) and SNB19 cell lines (Figure S4G,J). Interestingly, SLC5A1 strongly co-localizes with tubulin in large nascent blebs of DK-MG cells (yellow arrows, Figure S4B), whereas SLC5A3, confined to mature blebs, displays no such co-localization with tubulin (Figure S4D–F). In SNB19 cells, microtubules extend up to the lamellipodial tips, where they co-localize with both SLC5A1 (Figure S4G–I) and SLC5A3 (Figure S4J–L).

3.3. Super-Resolved (dSTORM) Images of SLC5A1, SLC5A3, F-Actin and Tubulin

In addition to conventional microscopy, we employed super-resolution microscopy to visualize, with molecular resolution, the localization of both transporter proteins in blebbing DK-MG cells along with actin and tubulin cytoskeleton, as shown in Figure 6. In agreement with our CLSM data (Figure 5), DK-MG cells display by far the highest localization density of SLC5A1 ($\sim$1.8 $\times$ 10^3 loc/μm^2) in the membrane of large expanding blebs devoid of actin cortex (Figure 6C,D). For comparison, the bulk cytosol and the bleb interior exhibit much lower SLC5A1 densities of $\sim$$10^2$ and $\sim$3 $\times$ 10^2 loc/μm^2, respectively (Figure 6D).

Unlike SLC5A1, SLC5A3 shows its highest localization density in the membrane of small, retracting blebs (Figure 6G; $\sim$2.0 $\times$ 10^4 loc/μm^2), exceeding by 1–2 orders of magnitude the density of SLC5A3 protein reported for the basal membrane of osmotically stressed HEK293 cells [19]. In contrast, blebs in the early stage of retraction, discernable by their newly formed thin actin cortex, exhibit barely any SLC5A3 signal ($\sim$3 $\times$ 10^2 loc/μm^2 Figure 6E,F). These results suggest that SLC5A3 expression in the bleb membrane increases during bleb retraction.

Although the bulk cytosol exhibits only sparse localization of SLC5A3 ($\sim$1.3 $\times$ 10^3 loc/μm^2) numerous spherical structures in the cytosol with a diameter of $\sim$0.5 μm (Figure 6I) contain large amounts of SLC5A3 (Figure 6H). The very high SLC5A3 density of $\sim$2.3 $\times$ 10^4 loc/μm^2 found in the cytosolic spherical structures is strikingly similar to that observed in the membrane of mature retracted blebs (Figure 6H), which suggests that these SLC5A3-rich structures represent endocytic vesicles involved in SLC5A3 recycling. This notion is further reinforced by the close localization of SLC5A3 vesicles to microtubules (Figure 6J), a well known component of vesicle trafficking [51,52]. Finally, in agreement with our LSM images (Supplementary Materials Figures S2 and S3), dSTORM revealed a dense intertwined meshwork of microtubules, most notable in the lamellae of DK-MG cells, with individual microtubules even extending to the anterior-most blebs. The pronounced microtubular network is indicative of high vesicular trafficking activity in the lamellipodium, which is also evident from phase-contrast live-cell imaging (Supplementary Materials Video S1).

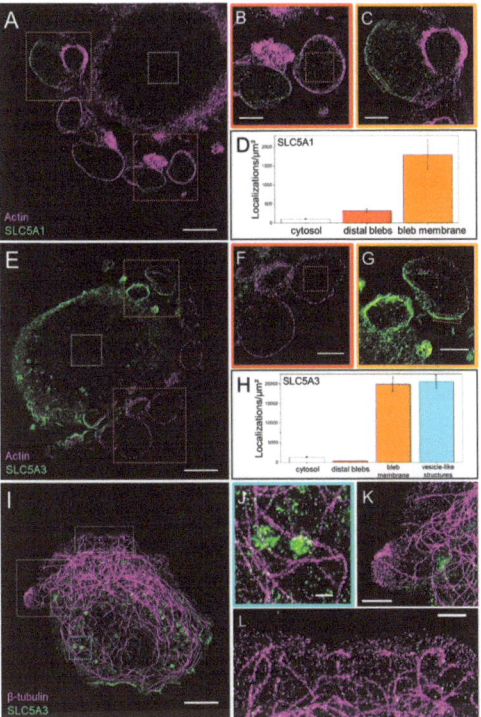

Figure 6. Two-color *d*STORM analyses of SLC5A1 and SLC5A3 in DK-MG cells. (**A**) Representative *d*STORM image of a DK-MG cell co-stained for SLC5A1 and F-actin. (**B,C**) Magnifications of the boxed regions in (**A**), depicting blebs with (**B**) or lacking (**C**) an actin cortex. (**D**) SLC5A1-localizations per µm² in different cell compartments corresponding to the boxed regions in (**A**). The highest localization densities were found in the membrane of blebs most distant from the main cell body. (**E**) Representative *d*STORM image of a DK-MG cell co-stained for SLC5A3 and F-actin. (**F,G**) Magnifications of the boxed regions in (**E**), depicting distal blebs lacking SLC5A3 signal (**F**) and blebs in various life cycle stages (**G**). (**H**) SLC5A3-localizations per µm² in different cell compartments corresponding to the boxed regions in (**E**). The highest localization densities were found in the membrane of blebs closest to the main cell body (**F**), as well as in vesicle-like structures close to the cell periphery (**J**). (**I**) Representative *d*STORM image of a DK-MG cell co-stained for SLC5A3 and β-tubulin. (**J**) Vesicle-like SLC5A3 structures localized in close vicinity to microtubules. (**K,L**) Microtubules extending into the outermost leading edge, virtually devoid of SLC5A3. Scale bars: 5 µm in (**A,E,I**); 2 µm in (**B,C,F,G**), 1 µm in (**K,L**); 500 nm in (**J**).

3.4. Osmotic Swelling Assay for Glucose and Inositol

The high expression of both transporter proteins SLC5A1 and SLC5A3 in the membranes of GBM cells (Figure 5) is likely associated with substantial membrane permeability to the respective transporter substrates. To probe the solute permeability of the cell membrane, we performed osmotic cell swelling experiments in hypotonic solutions containing either glucose, inositol, mannitol or sucrose as the major solute.

Cell volume changes were monitored by video microscopy following the rapid transfer of cells from isotonic CGM (~300 mOsm) to a hypotonic sugar solution. Figure S5 shows the mean volumetric response of the two cell lines to various sugar solutions with the same osmolality of 150 mOsm. Independent of the sugar used, the sudden exposure to hypotonicity caused both GBM cell lines to swell rapidly within the first 3–5 min from their original isotonic volume V_0 to the V_{max} level due to the fast water influx driven by the applied osmotic gradient. Hypotonic solutions of all tested sugars gave rise to qualitatively similar rates and magnitudes (~20%) of initial swelling in both cell lines.

The data in Figure S5A,B reveal striking differences between the disaccharide sucrose and the monomeric sugars and sugar-alcohols, including glucose, inositol and mannitol in respect to their effects on the secondary cell volume changes. After the fast initial swelling in hypotonic sucrose solution, both cell lines underwent a regulatory volume decrease (RVD), during which they shrank gradually, fully recovering their original isotonic volume (V_0) within ~15–20 min despite persisting hypotonicity. RVD relies on the release of cytosolic solutes through swelling-activated membrane pathways accompanied by osmotically obligated water efflux, which allows cells to recover their original isotonic volume [19,53]. In agreement with our findings for DK-MG and SNB19 cells presented here (Figure S5) and elsewhere [54], other cell lines, including glioma cells, are able to quickly readjust their volume in anisotonic media via several mechanisms, including chloride pathways and aquaporins [55–57], only in the presence of membrane impermeable solutes such as dimeric sugars, sucrose or trehalose [39].

In sharp contrast to the disaccharide sucrose, the monomeric sugars partially (mannitol) or completely abolished the RVD (glucose and inositol) in DK-MG cells (Figure S5A). In SNB19 cells, glucose, mannitol and inositol not only abolished RVD, but even induced secondary swelling (Figure S5B). As shown elsewhere [58], RVD inhibition is based on the uptake of extracellular monomeric sugars into the cytosol through swelling-activated membrane pathways. The influx of permeable extracellular solutes compensates for the loss of cytosolic osmolytes, thus preventing RVD. As expressed by Equation (1) (see Materials and Methods), the extent of RVD inhibition by various solutes is indicative of their membrane permeabilities [40]. Accordingly, an $IC_{RVD} \approx 0$ means complete recovery of initial cell volume by RVD, i.e., in the presence of the impermeable sucrose. The range $0 < IC_{RVD} < 100\%$ indicates partial-to-complete RVD inhibition. Highly permeable solutes such as glucose, mannitol and inositol in SNB19 cells, cause secondary cell swelling and thus exhibit $IC_{RVD} \gg 100\%$ (200–222%).

The values of IC_{RVD} [%] calculated with Equation (1) from the data in Figure S5A yield the following descending rank order of solute permeability in DK-MG cells: *inositol* (90%) $\approx$ *glucose* (78%) > *mannitol* (41%) > *sucrose* (0%). In contrast to DK-MG cells, glucose displayed by far the highest permeability among the tested solutes in SNB19 cells: *glucose* (222%) > *inositol* (209%) > *mannitol* (~200%) $\gg$ *sucrose* (~0%). Taken together, the data in Figure S5 suggest that even a slight cell volume increase of ~25% rendered the GBM cell membranes highly permeable to glucose and inositol. Similar to the hypotonic activation of SLC5A3 in HEK293 cells [19], swelling-activated pathways for glucose and inositol in GBM cells reported here might also include SLC5A1 and SLC5A3 transporters.

4. Discussion

Our findings, briefly summarized below, suggest that SLC5A1 and SLC5A3 are involved in GBM cell migration. Medium supplementation with glucose and inositol increased migration rates in both cell lines by 33–91% above the respective controls (Figure 1C,D). The significant increase in wound healing rate displayed by DK-MG and SNB19 cells (+52% and +33%, respectively) in the presence of inositol (Figure 1C,D) is likely connected to inositol serving as a precursor of phosphatidylinositol 4,5-bisphosphate (PIP2), a key signaling lipid in cancer cell migration [38]. The observed increased migration rate of GBM cells exposed to glucose (+91% in DK-MG cells; +39% in SNB19 cells) can be explained by the metabolic promotion of invasive cancer cell behavior by this solute. Indeed, elevated glucose levels are known to promote cancer cell migration [59–61]. In contrast, the SLC inhibitor phlorizin [45,46] decreased migration rates by 10–36% (Figure 1C,D). As shown in Supplementary Materials Figures S2 and S3, phlorizin altered the expression of SLC5A1 and SLC5A3 at the leading edge of both tested cell lines compared to the respective untreated controls. In agreement with our findings, Gao et al. (2019) [62] also reported that phlorizin decreased the expression of SLC proteins in cancer cells. In terestingly, the highly invasive [6] SNB19 cells exposed only to phlorizin displayed the lowest reduction in motility (−10%) of all experimental conditions involving inhibition. This corroborates our previous finding that SNB19 cells react only moderately to pharmacological inhibition of migration [5,7]. Our immunostaining of wounded GBM cell monolayers (Figure 3A,C) revealed that both SLC5A1 and SLC5A3 are highly expressed only in migrating cells at the monolayer edge but not in the non-motile cells within the confluent monolayer (Figure 3B,D). Interestingly, a variety of studies have demonstrated that such extensive remodeling of membrane solute channel expression, as seen in edge cells, is also observed during epithelial-mesenchymal transition (EMT) [63], a crucial factor in cancer cell metastasis and wound healing [64,65].

Our immuno-staining experiments on single, actively migrating DK-MG and SNB19 cells lend further support to the involvement of SLC transporters in GBM cell migration. As seen in Figures 5 and S2–S4, both SLC5A1 and SLC5A3 are predominantly expressed in the lamellipodia (Figure 5B,D,F) and blebs (Figure 5A,C,E), i.e., the expanding cell protrusions known for driving cell migration [18,50,66].

Interestingly, lamellipodia expansion by local volume increase can be achieved by the import of solutes and osmotically obliged water influx [66]. Furthermore, SLC5A1 has been shown to be involved in glucose-driven modulation of membrane protrusions [67]. As we have shown in Supplementary Materials Figure S5, both DK-MG and SNB19 cell membranes are highly permeable to glucose and inositol. The presence of SLC5A1 and SCL5A3 in the lamellipodial tips of SNB19 cells (Figure 5b,f) thus points to the possible involvement of these transporters in the local volume increase required for lamellipodium protrusion during cell migration.

As pointed out elsewhere [18], cell migration requires the concerted activity of various channels and transporters belonging to diverse protein families. Efficient cell migration thus necessitates not the isolated function of a single channel or transporter but the interdependent activity of a transport protein network.

The involvement of aquaporins in bleb formation and blebbing activity [68–70] suggests that water flux through the bleb membrane may also play a key role in migratory cell blebbing. Since SLC5A1 was detected in nascent blebs devoid of actin cortex (Figure 5a), we can infer that this glucose transporter present in the bleb membrane during bleb expansion enabled the uptake of extracellular glucose, leading to the osmotically obligated water influx (facilitated by aquaporins), i.e., local volume increase. The high SLC5A1 levels in nascent blebs were confirmed by our nanoscale imaging (Figure 6A), in which only expanding blebs displayed a marked SLC5A1 signal (Figure 6C). Additionally, the cytosol in expanding blebs displayed significantly higher amounts of SLC5A1 compared to the cytosol of the main cell body (Figure 6D), possibly due to the dissociation of SLC5A1 from the bleb membrane.

In contrast to SLC5A1, the inositol transporter SLC5A3 was found only in smaller *retracting* blebs with a reestablished actin cortex (Figures 5c,e and 6G), while the anteriormost blebs were virtually devoid of the SLC5A3 signal (Figure 6F). We therefore conclude that SLC5A3 can contribute to bleb retraction via an osmotic bleb volume decrease due to inositol/water efflux. Consistent with this assumption, SLC5A3 was previously shown to be involved in the regulatory volume decrease in HEK293 cells [19]. This notion is further supported by our finding that the SLC5A3 signal increased with increasing bleb maturity (Figure 6G). In larger blebs (upper right in Figure 6G), SLC5A3 was detected only at the bleb membrane hemisphere facing the cell body, if at all (Figure 6F).

Previous studies have demonstrated that SLCs are inserted into the plasma membrane from cytosolic vesicles during swelling-activated exocytosis [19,71]. Interestingly, our super-resolution *d*STORM imaging revealed sub-μm-sized vesicle-like clusters of SLC5A3 located in close proximity to microtubules (Figure 6I,J), suggesting that SLC protein trafficking occurs via vesicles moving along the microtubular network. Indeed, co-localization of tubulin and the taurine transporter SLC6A6 was already reported elsewhere [72]. Furthermore, SLC6A12, a transporter of SOO betaine, was found to relocate from the cytosol to the plasma membrane upon hypertonic stimulation [73]. This points to the membrane incorporation of SLC transporters via exocytosis, i.e., vesicular fusion, as a common phenomenon for proteins of the SLC family, as was also demonstrated for various other SLCs [74,75]. Accordingly, we frequently observed that in large blebs, SLC5A3 appeared at the bleb side facing the main cell body (Figure 6G, upper right corner), consistent with insertion via vesicular fusion.

Furthermore, our finding that microtubule structures extend into the anterior-most blebs virtually devoid of SLC5A3 (Figures 6K,L and S4E) suggests that other SLC transporters might also be incorporated into blebs via vesicle transport along microtubules (Figure S4B). Thus, our findings provide an additional rationale for targeting microtubules in the context of inhibiting cell migration and invasion [76–78].

5. Conclusions

Taken together, the high expression of SLC5A1 and SLC5A3 transporters in the lamellipodia of GBM cells and the impaired cell motility upon SLC inhibition point to the transporters' involvement in GBM cell migration. We thus propose to include SLC5A1 and SLC5A3 in the migration-associated transportome. The revealed SLC-related cell motility might offer therapeutic potential in GBM treatment, especially given the abundance of inositol and glucose in the human brain.

Supplementary Materials: The following supporting information can be downloaded at: https://www.mdpi.com/article/10.3390/cancers14235794/s1, Figure S1: Kaplan-Meier plots of overall survival and expression of SLC5A1 and SLC5A3 in GBM patients; Figure S2: Confocal images of SLC5A1/A3 in DK-MG cells treated with mannitol, glucose or inositol; Figure S3: Confocal images of SLC5A1/A3 in SNB19 cells treated with mannitol, glucose or inositol; Figure S4: Confocal images of β-tubulin, SLC5A1 and SLC5A3 in DK-MG and SNB19 cells; Figure S5: Volumetric measurements of DK-MG and SNB19 cells treated with sucrose, mannitol, glucose or inositol; Video S1: Vesicle trafficking in the lamellipodium of GBM cells.

Author Contributions: V.L.S., C.S.D., J.N., M.S. and H.Z. conceived the project. P.K.B., D.S., V.L.S. and C.S.D. designed the experiments. P.K.B., D.S., T.K. and S.H. performed the experiments. D.T. and P.K.B. performed the volumetric experiments. P.K. performed the chemotaxis experiments. P.K.B. D.S., T.K., R.S. and V.L.S. carried out data analysis with input from P.E. All authors have read and agreed to the published version of the manuscript.

Funding: This research received no external funding.

Institutional Review Board Statement: Not applicable.

Informed Consent Statement: Not applicable.

Data Availability Statement: Not applicable.

Conflicts of Interest: The authors declare no conflict of interest.

References

1. Stupp, R.; Mason, W.P.; van den Bent, M.J.; Weller, M.; Fisher, B.; Taphoorn, M.J.B.; Belanger, K.; Brandes, A.A.; Marosi, C.; Bogdahn, U.; et al. Radiotherapy plus Concomitant and Adjuvant Temozolomide for Glioblastoma. *N. Engl. J. Med.* **2005**, *352*, 987–996. [CrossRef] [PubMed]
2. Nakada, M.; Nakada, S.; Demuth, T.; Tran, N.L.; Hoelzinger, D.B.; Berens, M.E. Molecular Targets of Glioma Invasion. *Cell. Mol. Life Sci.* **2007**, *64*, 458. [CrossRef] [PubMed]
3. Ulrich, T.A.; de Juan Pardo, E.M.; Kumar, S. The Mechanical Rigidity of the Extracellular Matrix Regulates the Structure, Motility and Proliferation of Glioma Cells. *Cancer Res.* **2009**, *69*, 4167–4174. [CrossRef] [PubMed]
4. Vollmann-Zwerenz, A.; Leidgens, V.; Feliciello, G.; Klein, C.A.; Hau, P. Tumor Cell Invasion in Glioblastoma. *Int. J. Mol. Sci.* **2020**, *21*, 1932. [CrossRef] [PubMed]
5. Memmel, S.; Sisario, D.; Zöller, C.; Fiedler, V.; Katzer, A.; Heiden, R.; Becker, N.; Eing, L.; Ferreira, F.L.R.; Zimmermann, H.; et al. Migration Pattern, Actin Cytoskeleton Organization and Response to PI3K-, MTOR-, and Hsp90-Inhibition of Glioblastoma Cells with Different Invasive Capacities. *Oncotarget* **2017**, *8*, 45298–45310. [CrossRef]

6. Djuzenova, C.S.; Fiedler, V.; Memmel, S.; Katzer, A.; Hartmann, S.; Krohne, G.; Zimmermann, H.; Scholz, C.-J.; Polat, B.; Flentje, M.; et al. Actin Cytoskeleton Organization, Cell Surface Modification and Invasion Rate of 5 Glioblastoma Cell Lines Differing in PTEN and P53 Status. *Exp. Cell Res.* **2015**, *330*, 346–357. [CrossRef]
7. Djuzenova, C.S.; Fiedler, V.; Memmel, S.; Katzer, A.; Sisario, D.; Brosch, P.K.; Göhrung, A.; Frister, S.; Zimmermann, H.; Flentje, M.; et al. Differential Effects of the Akt Inhibitor MK-2206 on Migration and Radiation Sensitivity of Glioblastoma Cells. *BMC Cancer* **2019**, *19*, 299. [CrossRef] [PubMed]
8. Parsons, J.T.; Horwitz, A.R.; Schwartz, M.A. Cell Adhesion: Integrating Cytoskeletal Dynamics and Cellular Tension. *Nat. Rev. Mol. Cell Biol.* **2010**, *11*, 633–643. [CrossRef]
9. Cramer, L.P. Forming the Cell Rear First: Breaking Cell Symmetry to Trigger Directed Cell Migration. *Nat. Cell Biol.* **2010**, *12*, 628–632. [CrossRef]
10. Le Clainche, C.; Carlier, M.-F. Regulation of Actin Assembly Associated with Protrusion and Adhesion in Cell Migration. *Physiol. Rev.* **2008**, *88*, 489–513. [CrossRef]
11. Carlier, M.-F.; Clainche, C.L.; Wiesner, S.; Pantaloni, D. Actin-Based Motility: From Molecules to Movement. *BioEssays* **2003**, *25*, 336–345. [CrossRef] [PubMed]
12. Pantaloni, D.; Clainche, C.L.; Carlier, M.-F. Mechanism of Actin-Based Motility. *Science* **2001**, *292*, 1502–1506. [CrossRef] [PubMed]
13. Borm, B.; Requardt, R.P.; Herzog, V.; Kirfel, G. Membrane Ruffles in Cell Migration: Indicators of Inefficient Lamellipodia Adhesion and Compartments of Actin Filament Reorganization. *Exp. Cell Res.* **2005**, *302*, 83–95. [CrossRef]
14. Charras, G.; Paluch, E. Blebs Lead the Way: How to Migrate without Lamellipodia. *Nat. Rev. Mol. Cell Biol.* **2008**, *9*, 730–736. [CrossRef] [PubMed]
15. Charras, G.T.; Coughlin, M.; Mitchison, T.J.; Mahadevan, L. Life and Times of a Cellular Bleb. *Biophys. J.* **2008**, *94*, 1836–1853. [CrossRef] [PubMed]
16. Paluch, E.K.; Raz, E. The Role and Regulation of Blebs in Cell Migration. *Curr. Opin. Cell Biol.* **2013**, *25*, 582–590. [CrossRef] [PubMed]
17. Stroka, K.M.; Jiang, H.; Chen, S.-H.; Tong, Z.; Wirtz, D.; Sun, S.X.; Konstantopoulos, K. Water Permeation Drives Tumor Cell Migration in Confined Microenvironments. *Cell* **2014**, *157*, 611–623. [CrossRef]
18. Schwab, A.; Fabian, A.; Hanley, P.J.; Stock, C. Role of Ion Channels and Transporters in Cell Migration. *Physiol. Rev.* **2012**, *92*, 1865–1913. [CrossRef]
19. Andronic, J.; Shirakashi, R.; Pickel, S.U.; Westerling, K.M.; Klein, T.; Holm, T.; Sauer, M.; Sukhorukov, V.L. Hypotonic Activation of the Myo-Inositol Transporter SLC5A3 in HEK293 Cells Probed by Cell Volumetry, Confocal and Super-Resolution Microscopy. *PLoS ONE* **2015**, *10*, e0119990. [CrossRef]
20. Shestov, A.A.; Emir, U.E.; Kumar, A.; Henry, P.-G.; Seaquist, E.R.; Öz, G. Simultaneous Measurement of Glucose Transport and Utilization in the Human Brain. *Am. J. Physiol. Endocrinol. Metab.* **2011**, *301*, E1040–E1049. [CrossRef] [PubMed]
21. Duelli, R.; Kuschinsky, W. Brain Glucose Transporters: Relationship to Local Energy Demand. *News Physiol. Sci.* **2001**, *16*, 71–76. [CrossRef] [PubMed]
22. Heilig, C.W.; Stromski, M.E.; Blumenfeld, J.D.; Lee, J.P.; Gullans, S.R. Characterization of the Major Brain Osmolytes That Accumulate in Salt-Loaded Rats. *Am. J. Physiol.* **1989**, *257*, F1108–F1116. [CrossRef] [PubMed]
23. Michaelis, T.; Merboldt, K.D.; Bruhn, H.; Hänicke, W.; Frahm, J. Absolute Concentrations of Metabolites in the Adult Human Brain in Vivo: Quantification of Localized Proton MR Spectra. *Radiology* **1993**, *187*, 219–227. [CrossRef]
24. Haris, M.; Cai, K.; Singh, A.; Hariharan, H.; Reddy, R. In Vivo Mapping of Brain Myo-Inositol. *Neuroimage* **2011**, *54*, 2079–2085. [CrossRef]
25. Soupart, A.; Silver, S.; Schroöeder, B.; Sterns, R.; Decaux, G. Rapid (24-Hour) Reaccumulation of Brain Organic Osmolytes (Particularly Myo-Inositol) in Azotemic Rats after Correction of Chronic Hyponatremia. *J. Am. Soc. Nephrol.* **2002**, *13*, 1433–1441. [CrossRef]
26. Brand, A.; Richter-Landsberg, C.; Leibfritz, D. Multinuclear NMR Studies on the Energy Metabolism of Glial and Neuronal Cells. *Dev. Neurosci.* **1993**, *15*, 289–298. [CrossRef]
27. Castillo, M.; Smith, J.K.; Kwock, L. Correlation of Myo-Inositol Levels and Grading of Cerebral Astrocytomas. *AJNR Am. J. Neuroradiol.* **2000**, *21*, 1645–1649.
28. Kim, J.; Dang, C.V. Cancer's Molecular Sweet Tooth and the Warburg Effect. *Cancer Res.* **2006**, *66*, 8927–8930. [CrossRef]
29. El-Gebali, S.; Bentz, S.; Hediger, M.A.; Anderle, P. Solute Carriers (SLCs) in Cancer. *Mol. Asp. Med.* **2013**, *34*, 719–734. [CrossRef]
30. Wright, E.M. Glucose Transport Families SLC5 and SLC50. *Mol. Asp. Med.* **2013**, *34*, 183–196. [CrossRef]
31. Nakanishi, T.; Tamai, I. Putative Roles of Organic Anion Transporting Polypeptides (OATPs) in Cell Survival and Progression of Human Cancers. *Biopharm. Drug Dispos.* **2014**, *35*, 463–484. [CrossRef] [PubMed]
32. Guo, G.F.; Cai, Y.C.; Zhang, B.; Xu, R.H.; Qiu, H.J.; Xia, L.P.; Jiang, W.Q.; Hu, P.L.; Chen, X.X.; Zhou, F.F.; et al. Overexpression of SGLT1 and EGFR in Colorectal Cancer Showing a Correlation with the Prognosis. *Med. Oncol.* **2011**, *28*, 197–203. [CrossRef]
33. Casneuf, V.F.; Fonteyne, P.; Van Damme, N.; Demetter, P.; Pauwels, P.; de Hemptinne, B.; De Vos, M.; Van de Wiele, C.; Peeters, M. Expression of SGLT1, Bcl-2 and P53 in Primary Pancreatic Cancer Related to Survival. *Cancer Investig.* **2008**, *26*, 852–859. [CrossRef] [PubMed]
34. Shorthouse, D.; Riedel, A.; Kerr, E.; Pedro, L.; Bihary, D.; Samarajiwa, S.; Martins, C.P.; Shields, J.; Hall, B.A. Exploring the Role of Stromal Osmoregulation in Cancer and Disease Using Executable Modelling. *Nat. Commun.* **2018**, *9*, 3011. [CrossRef] [PubMed]

35. Cao, X.; Fang, L.; Gibbs, S.; Huang, Y.; Dai, Z.; Wen, P.; Zheng, X.; Sadee, W.; Sun, D. Glucose Uptake Inhibitor Sensitizes Cancer Cells to Daunorubicin and Overcomes Drug Resistance in Hypoxia. *Cancer Chemother. Pharmacol.* **2007**, *59*, 495–505. [CrossRef]
36. Scafoglio, C.; Hirayama, B.A.; Kepe, V.; Liu, J.; Ghezzi, C.; Satyamurthy, N.; Moatamed, N.A.; Huang, J.; Koepsell, H.; Barrio, J.R.; et al. Functional Expression of Sodium-Glucose Transporters in Cancer. *Proc. Natl. Acad. Sci. USA* **2015**, *112*, E4111–E4119. [CrossRef]
37. Dai, G.; Yu, H.; Kruse, M.; Traynor-Kaplan, A.; Hille, B. Osmoregulatory Inositol Transporter SMIT1 Modulates Electrical Activity by Adjusting PI(4,5)P2 Levels. *Proc. Natl. Acad. Sci. USA* **2016**, *113*, E3290–E3299. [CrossRef]
38. Leslie, N.R.; Batty, I.H.; Maccario, H.; Davidson, L.; Downes, C.P. Understanding PTEN Regulation: PIP2, Polarity and Protein Stability. *Oncogene* **2008**, *27*, 5464–5476. [CrossRef]
39. Kiesel, M.; Reuss, R.; Endter, J.; Zimmermann, D.; Zimmermann, H.; Shirakashi, R.; Bamberg, E.; Zimmermann, U.; Sukhorukov, V.L. Swelling-Activated Pathways in Human T-Lymphocytes Studied by Cell Volumetry and Electrorotation. *Biophys. J.* **2006**, *90*, 4720–4729. [CrossRef]
40. Bobak, N.; Bittner, S.; Andronic, J.; Hartmann, S.; Mühlpfordt, F.; Schneider-Hohendorf, T.; Wolf, K.; Schmelter, C.; Göbel, K.; Meuth, P.; et al. Volume Regulation of Murine T Lymphocytes Relies on Voltage-Dependent and Two-Pore Domain Potassium Channels. *Biochim. Et Biophys. Acta (BBA)-Biomembr.* **2011**, *1808*, 2036–2044. [CrossRef]
41. van de Linde, S.; Löschberger, A.; Klein, T.; Heidbreder, M.; Wolter, S.; Heilemann, M.; Sauer, M. Direct Stochastic Optical Reconstruction Microscopy with Standard Fluorescent Probes. *Nat. Protoc.* **2011**, *6*, 991–1009. [CrossRef]
42. Sisario, D.; Memmel, S.; Doose, S.; Neubauer, J.; Zimmermann, H.; Flentje, M.; Djuzenova, C.S.; Sauer, M.; Sukhorukov, V.L. Nanostructure of DNA Repair Foci Revealed by Superresolution Microscopy. *FASEB J.* **2018**, *32*, 6469–6477. [CrossRef]
43. Wolter, S.; Löschberger, A.; Holm, T.; Aufmkolk, S.; Dabauvalle, M.-C.; van de Linde, S.; Sauer, M. RapidSTORM: Accurate, Fast Open-Source Software for Localization Microscopy. *Nat. Methods* **2012**, *9*, 1040–1041. [CrossRef]
44. Tang, Z.; Kang, B.; Li, C.; Chen, T.; Zhang, Z. GEPIA2: An Enhanced Web Server for Large-Scale Expression Profiling and Interactive Analysis. *Nucleic Acids Res.* **2019**, *47*, W556–W560. [CrossRef]
45. Ikeda, T.S.; Hwang, E.S.; Coady, M.J.; Hirayama, B.A.; Hediger, M.A.; Wright, E.M. Characterization of a Na+/Glucose Cotransporter Cloned from Rabbit Small Intestine. *J. Membr. Biol.* **1989**, *110*, 87–95. [CrossRef] [PubMed]
46. Kwon, H.M.; Yamauchi, A.; Uchida, S.; Preston, A.S.; Garcia-Perez, A.; Burg, M.B.; Handler, J.S. Cloning of the CDNa for a Na+/Myo-Inositol Cotransporter, a Hypertonicity Stress Protein. *J. Biol. Chem.* **1992**, *267*, 6297–6301. [CrossRef]
47. Steidl, E.; Pilatus, U.; Hattingen, E.; Steinbach, J.P.; Zanella, F.; Ronellenfitsch, M.W.; Bähr, O. Myoinositol as a Biomarker in Recurrent Glioblastoma Treated with Bevacizumab: A 1H-Magnetic Resonance Spectroscopy Study. *PLoS ONE* **2016**, *11*, e0168113. [CrossRef]
48. Rosengren, S.; Henson, P.M.; Worthen, G.S. Migration-Associated Volume Changes in Neutrophils Facilitate the Migratory Process in Vitro. *Am. J. Physiol.* **1994**, *267*, C1623–C1632. [CrossRef]
49. Charras, G.T.; Hu, C.-K.; Coughlin, M.; Mitchison, T.J. Reassembly of Contractile Actin Cortex in Cell Blebs. *J. Cell Biol.* **2006**, *175*, 477–490. [CrossRef]
50. Charras, G.T.; Yarrow, J.C.; Horton, M.A.; Mahadevan, L.; Mitchison, T.J. Non-Equilibration of Hydrostatic Pressure in Blebbing Cells. *Nature* **2005**, *435*, 365–369. [CrossRef]
51. Fletcher, L.M.; Welsh, G.I.; Oatey, P.B.; Tavaré, J.M. Role for the Microtubule Cytoskeleton in GLUT4 Vesicle Trafficking and in the Regulation of Insulin-Stimulated Glucose Uptake. *Biochem. J.* **2000**, *352 Pt 2*, 267–276. [CrossRef]
52. Caviston, J.P.; Holzbaur, E.L.F. Microtubule Motors at the Intersection of Trafficking and Transport. *Trends Cell Biol.* **2006**, *16*, 530–537. [CrossRef] [PubMed]
53. Andronic, J.; Bobak, N.; Bittner, S.; Ehling, P.; Kleinschnitz, C.; Herrmann, A.M.; Zimmermann, H.; Sauer, M.; Wiendl, H.; Budde, T.; et al. Identification of Two-Pore Domain Potassium Channels as Potent Modulators of Osmotic Volume Regulation in Human T Lymphocytes. *Biochim. Biophys. Acta* **2013**, *1828*, 699–707. [CrossRef] [PubMed]
54. Memmel, S.; Sukhorukov, V.L.; Höring, M.; Westerling, K.; Fiedler, V.; Katzer, A.; Krohne, G.; Flentje, M.; Djuzenova, C.S. Cell Surface Area and Membrane Folding in Glioblastoma Cell Lines Differing in PTEN and P53 Status. *PLoS ONE* **2014**, *9*, e87052. [CrossRef] [PubMed]
55. Djuzenova, C.S.; Krasnyanska, J.; Kiesel, M.; Stingl, L.; Zimmermann, U.; Flentje, M.; Sukhorukov, V.L. Intracellular Delivery of 2-Deoxy-D-Glucose into Tumor Cells by Long-Term Cultivation and through Swelling-Activated Pathways: Implications for Radiation Treatment. *Mol. Med. Rep.* **2009**, *2*, 633–640. [CrossRef]
56. McCoy, E.; Sontheimer, H. Expression and Function of Water Channels (Aquaporins) in Migrating Malignant Astrocytes. *Glia* **2007**, *55*, 1034–1043. [CrossRef]
57. Ernest, N.J.; Weaver, A.K.; Van Duyn, L.B.; Sontheimer, H.W. Relative Contribution of Chloride Channels and Transporters to Regulatory Volume Decrease in Human Glioma Cells. *Am. J. Physiol. Cell Physiol.* **2005**, *288*, C1451–C1460. [CrossRef]
58. Sukhorukov, V.L.; Imes, D.; Woellhaf, M.W.; Andronic, J.; Kiesel, M.; Shirakashi, R.; Zimmermann, U.; Zimmermann, H. Pore Size of Swelling-Activated Channels for Organic Osmolytes in Jurkat Lymphocytes, Probed by Differential Polymer Exclusion. *Biochim. Biophys. Acta* **2009**, *1788*, 1841–1850. [CrossRef]
59. Wu, J.; Chen, J.; Xi, Y.; Wang, F.; Sha, H.; Luo, L.; Zhu, Y.; Hong, X.; Bu, S. High Glucose Induces Epithelial-Mesenchymal Transition and Results in the Migration and Invasion of Colorectal Cancer Cells. *Exp. Ther. Med.* **2018**, *16*, 222–230. [CrossRef]

50. Lin, C.-Y.; Lee, C.-H.; Huang, C.-C.; Lee, S.-T.; Guo, H.-R.; Su, S.-B. Impact of High Glu-cose on Metastasis of Colon Cancer Cells. *World J. Gastroenterol.* **2015**, *21*, 2047–2057. [CrossRef]
51. Santos, J.M.; Hussain, F. Higher Glucose Enhances Breast Cancer Cell Aggressiveness. *Nutr. Cancer* **2020**, *72*, 734–746. [CrossRef] [PubMed]
52. Gao, H.-F.; Chen, L.-Y.; Cheng, C.-S.; Chen, H.; Meng, Z.-Q.; Chen, Z. SLC5A1 Promotes Growth and Proliferation of Pancreatic Carcinoma via Glucose-Dependent AMPK/MTOR Signaling. *Cancer Manag. Res.* **2019**, *11*, 3171–3185. [CrossRef] [PubMed]
53. Azimi, I.; Monteith, G.R. Plasma Membrane Ion Channels and Epithelial to Mesenchymal Transition in Cancer Cells. *Endocr.-Relat. Cancer* **2016**, *23*, R517–R525. [CrossRef] [PubMed]
54. Weber, C.E.; Li, N.Y.; Wai, P.Y.; Kuo, P.C. Epithelial-Mesenchymal Transition, TGF-β, and Osteopontin in Wound Healing and Tissue Remodeling After Injury. *J. Burn Care Res.* **2012**, *33*, 311–318. [CrossRef] [PubMed]
55. Dongre, A.; Weinberg, R.A. New Insights into the Mechanisms of Epithelial–Mesenchymal Transition and Implications for Cancer. *Nat. Rev. Mol. Cell Biol.* **2019**, *20*, 69–84. [CrossRef]
56. Schwab, A.; Stock, C. Ion Channels and Transporters in Tumour Cell Migration and Invasion. *Philos. Trans. R. Soc. B Biol. Sci.* **2014**, *369*, 20130102. [CrossRef]
57. Chen, X.-M.; O'Hara, S.P.; Huang, B.Q.; Splinter, P.L.; Nelson, J.B.; LaRusso, N.F. Localized Glucose and Water Influx Facilitates Cryptosporidium Parvum Cellular Invasion by Means of Modulation of Host-Cell Membrane Protrusion. *Proc. Natl. Acad. Sci. USA* **2005**, *102*, 6338–6343. [CrossRef]
58. Huebert, R.C.; Vasdev, M.M.; Shergill, U.; Das, A.; Huang, B.Q.; Charlton, M.R.; LaRusso, N.F.; Shah, V.H. Aquaporin-1 Facilitates Angiogenic Invasion in the Pathological Neovasculature That Accompanies Cirrhosis. *Hepatology* **2010**, *52*, 238–248. [CrossRef]
59. Taloni, A.; Kardash, E.; Salman, O.U.; Truskinovsky, L.; Zapperi, S.; La Porta, C.A.M. Volume Changes During Active Shape Fluctuations in Cells. *Phys. Rev. Lett.* **2015**, *114*, 208101. [CrossRef]
60. Paul, C.D.; Mistriotis, P.; Konstantopoulos, K. Cancer Cell Motility: Lessons from Migration in Confined Spaces. *Nat. Rev. Cancer* **2017**, *17*, 131–140. [CrossRef]
61. Kirk, K. Swelling-Activated Organic Osmolyte Channels. *J. Membr. Biol.* **1997**, *158*, 1–16. [CrossRef] [PubMed]
62. Voss, J.W.; Pedersen, S.F.; Christensen, S.T.; Lambert, I.H. Regulation of the Expression and Subcellular Localization of the Taurine Transporter TauT in Mouse NIH3T3 Fibroblasts. *Eur. J. Biochem.* **2004**, *271*, 4646–4658. [CrossRef] [PubMed]
63. Kempson, S.A.; Parikh, V.; Xi, L.; Chu, S.; Montrose, M.H. Subcellular Redistribution of the Renal Betaine Transporter during Hypertonic Stress. *Am. J. Physiol. -Cell Physiol.* **2003**, *285*, C1091–C1100. [CrossRef] [PubMed]
64. Uldry, M.; Thorens, B. The SLC2 Family of Facilitated Hexose and Polyol Transporters. *Pflug. Arch.–Eur. J. Physiol.* **2004**, *447*, 480–489. [CrossRef]
65. Eiden, L.E.; Schäfer, M.K.-H.; Weihe, E.; Schütz, B. The Vesicular Amine Transporter Family (SLC18): Amine/Proton Antiporters Required for Vesicular Accumulation and Regulated Exocytotic Secretion of Monoamines and Acetylcholine. *Pflug. Arch.-Eur. J. Physiol.* **2004**, *447*, 636–640. [CrossRef]
66. Etienne-Manneville, S. Microtubules in Cell Migration. *Annu. Rev. Cell Dev. Biol.* **2013**, *29*, 471–499. [CrossRef]
67. Watanabe, T.; Noritake, J.; Kaibuchi, K. Regulation of Microtubules in Cell Migration. *Trends Cell Biol.* **2005**, *15*, 76–83. [CrossRef]
68. Kaverina, I.; Straube, A. Regulation of Cell Migration by Dynamic Microtubules. *Semin. Cell Dev. Biol.* **2011**, *22*, 968–974. [CrossRef]

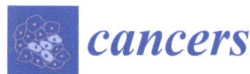

Article

Magnetic Resonance Spectroscopy Metabolites as Biomarkers of Disease Status in Pediatric Diffuse Intrinsic Pontine Gliomas (DIPG) Treated with Glioma-Associated Antigen Peptide Vaccines

Ashok Panigrahy [1,*], Regina I. Jakacki [2], Ian F. Pollack [3], Rafael Ceschin [1], Hideho Okada [4,5], Marvin D. Nelson [6,7], Gary Kohanbash [3], Girish Dhall [8] and Stefan Bluml [7]

1. Department of Radiology, UPMC Children's Hospital of Pittsburgh, 4401 Penn Ave Floor 2, Pittsburgh, PA 15224, USA
2. Department of Hematology Oncology, UPMC Children's Hospital of Pittsburgh, 4401 Penn Ave Floor 9, Pittsburgh, PA 15224, USA
3. Department of Neurosurgery, UPMC Children's Hospital of Pittsburgh, 4401 Penn Ave Floor 2, Pittsburgh, PA 15224, USA
4. Department of Neurological Surgery, Box 0112 505 Parnassus Ave, University of California San Francisco, Room M779, San Francisco, CA 94143, USA
5. Cancer Immunotherapy Program, Helen Diller Family Comprehensive Cancer Center, Box 0981 UCSF, San Francisco, CA 94143-0981, USA
6. Department of Radiology, Children's Hospital Los Angeles, 4650 Sunset Blvd, Los Angeles, CA 90027, USA
7. Keck School of Medicine, University of Southern California, 1441 Eastlake Ave # 2315, Los Angeles, CA 90089, USA
8. Department of Pediatrics, University of Alabama at Birmingham, 1600 7 th Ave S, Birmingham, AL 35233, USA
* Correspondence: ashok.panigrahy@chp.edu

Simple Summary: Diffuse intrinsic pontine gliomas in children are rare, highly malignant infiltrating tumors in a location precluding surgical resection. The absence of non-invasive correlates of response and disease progression in these tumors invites the exploration of imaging biomarkers. Magnetic resonance spectroscopy is an advanced imaging technique for measuring cell metabolites. This study evaluated whether measurements of in vivo cell metabolites using magnetic resonance spectroscopy may serve as biomarkers of response to therapy, including progression. Single-voxel magnetic resonance spectra were serially acquired in two cohorts of patients with these tumors treated with radiation therapy with or without concurrent chemotherapy and prior to progression: 14 participants were enrolled in a clinical trial of adjuvant glioma-associated antigen peptide vaccines and 32 patients were enrolled who did not receive adjuvant vaccine therapy. In the vaccine cohort, an elevated myo-inositol/choline ratio after 2–3 doses was associated with longer survival. Scans performed up to 6 months before death showed a terminal decline in the myo-inositol/choline ratio. Higher myo-inositol/choline ratios following radiation therapy, consistent with less proliferate tumors and decreased cell turnover, were associated with longer survival, suggesting that this ratio can serve as a biomarker of prognosis following radiation therapy.

Abstract: Purpose: Diffuse intrinsic pontine gliomas (DIPG) are highly aggressive tumors with no currently available curative therapy. This study evaluated whether measurements of in vivo cell metabolites using magnetic resonance spectroscopy (MRS) may serve as biomarkers of response to therapy, including progression. Methods: Single-voxel MR spectra were serially acquired in two cohorts of patients with DIPG treated with radiation therapy (RT) with or without concurrent chemotherapy and prior to progression: 14 participants were enrolled in a clinical trial of adjuvant glioma-associated antigen peptide vaccines and 32 patients were enrolled who did not receive adjuvant vaccine therapy. Spearman correlations measured overall survival associations with absolute metabolite concentrations of myo-inositol (mI), creatine (Cr), and n-acetyl-aspartate (NAA) and their ratios relative to choline (Cho) during three specified time periods following completion of RT. Linear

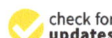

Citation: Panigrahy, A.; Jakacki, R.I.; Pollack, I.F.; Ceschin, R.; Okada, H.; Nelson, M.D.; Kohanbash, G.; Dhall, G.; Bluml, S. Magnetic Resonance Spectroscopy Metabolites as Biomarkers of Disease Status in Pediatric Diffuse Intrinsic Pontine Gliomas (DIPG) Treated with Glioma-Associated Antigen Peptide Vaccines. *Cancers* 2022, 14, 5995. https://doi.org/10.3390/cancers14235995

Academic Editors: Antonio Randazzo, Gianluca Trevisi and Annunziato Mangiola

Received: 6 September 2022
Accepted: 25 November 2022
Published: 5 December 2022

Publisher's Note: MDPI stays neutral with regard to jurisdictional claims in published maps and institutional affiliations.

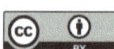

Copyright: © 2022 by the authors. Licensee MDPI, Basel, Switzerland. This article is an open access article distributed under the terms and conditions of the Creative Commons Attribution (CC BY) license (https://creativecommons.org/licenses/by/4.0/).

mixed-effects regression models evaluated the longitudinal associations between metabolite ratios and time from death (terminal decline). Results: Overall survival was not associated with metabolite ratios obtained shortly after RT (1.9–3.8 months post-diagnosis) in either cohort. In the vaccine cohort, an elevated mI/Cho ratio after 2–3 doses (3.9–5.2 months post-diagnosis) was associated with longer survival (rho = 0.92, 95% CI 0.67–0.98). Scans performed up to 6 months before death showed a terminal decline in the mI/Cho ratio, with an average of 0.37 ratio/month in vaccine patients (95% CI 0.11–0.63) and 0.26 (0.04–0.48) in the non-vaccine cohort. Conclusion: Higher mI/Cho ratios following RT, consistent with less proliferate tumors and decreased cell turnover, were associated with longer survival, suggesting that this ratio can serve as a biomarker of prognosis following RT. This finding was seen in both cohorts, although the association with OS was detected earlier in the vaccine cohort. Increased mI/Cho (possibly reflecting immune-effector cell influx into the tumor as a mechanism of tumor response) requires further study.

Keywords: brainstem glioma; MR spectroscopy; immunotherapy; pediatric brain tumor; vaccine therapy; myo-inositol; creatine; choline

1. Introduction

Diffuse intrinsic pontine gliomas (DIPG) in children are rare, highly malignant infiltrating tumors in a location precluding surgical resection. The median overall survival (OS) is less than one year, and no significant improvement in outcome has been achieved for decades [1]. Radiation therapy remains the only therapy with demonstrated short-term clinical benefit [2]. Although the overall prognosis is extremely poor, some patients have a longer reprieve after completing radiation therapy before the almost inevitable recurrence. Molecular biology studies have shown that certain patterns of gene mutations, most commonly involving histone H3 genes and other loci, may in part account for this variability [3,4], but this remains controversial.

The absence of non-invasive correlates of response and disease progression in DIPG invites the exploration of imaging biomarkers. Magnetic resonance spectroscopy (MRS) is an advanced imaging technique for measuring cell metabolites and can be readily integrated into standard clinical magnetic resonance (MR) imaging protocols. Cell metabolite profiles in newly diagnosed patients are often more characteristic of low-grade tumors, which may reflect that infiltrating tumor cells are interspersed with normal structures; as DIPG progresses after radiation therapy, metabolic profiles become increasingly consistent with higher-grade lesions, potentially reflecting the predominance of malignant cells in the tumor [5,6]. For example, increasing choline (Cho) typically indicates increasing membrane turnover and cell proliferation, which can be seen in fast-growing tumors as well as in inflammatory processes. Absolute or relative levels of other metabolites reflect the tumor physiology seen during malignant progression, e.g., decreased energy stores reflected by creatine (Cr), decreased astrocytic cell markers reflected by myo-inositol (mI), and decreased markers of healthy axons and neurons (n-acetyl aspartate, NAA) [7–12].

Our recently reported peptide vaccine study [13] targeted multiple glioma-associated antigen (GAA) epitopes as adjuvant therapy for children with malignant brain tumors, including a cohort of children with DIPG. Interferon-γ enzyme-linked immunosorbent spot (ELISPOT) assays identified immune responses to GAA epitopes with considerable between-patient variation in epitope response magnitude and duration. The therapy was generally well-tolerated, and the median OS (nominally superior to historical controls) in this highly selected cohort was encouraging. We performed MRS on a subset of patients with DIPG prior to and following the start of vaccine therapy. In a cohort of patients with DIPG from a separate institution who did not receive immunotherapy, MRS was performed prior to and following RT. Our hypothesis was that MRS indicators of progression would be slower or delayed in patients with longer overall survival, supporting further development of MRS as a non-invasive biomarker for DIPG treatment response and progression.

2. Materials and Methods

2.1. Patients and MR Spectroscopy

Informed consent was obtained for all patients enrolled in the peptide vaccine therapy clinical trial (ClinicalTrials.gov #NCT01130077), in accordance with institutional review board (IRB) policies. The MR spectroscopy was performed as part of the clinical MRI protocol. All patients completed irradiation (RT) with or without concurrent chemotherapy. Due to the detrimental impact of steroids on the effectiveness of immunotherapy, patients had to be off or on a very low dose of dexamethasone prior to trial enrollment. Additional details about trial inclusion and treatment may be found in the primary publication [13]. Parental consent was obtained for patients in the non-vaccine cohort who were enrolled in a number of prospective clinical trials, most of which involved irradiation with concurrent chemotherapy and adjuvant non-immunotherapy. An IRB waiver of consent was obtained to examine data acquired as part of the clinical care for patients who were not enrolled in a clinical trial. Thirteen of the thirty-two patients in the non-vaccine cohort were also included in a prior report [6].

For participants in the vaccine trial, vaccines were administered every 3 weeks x 8, and MRI scans were obtained at the baseline, weeks 6, 15, and 24, and then every 12 weeks or as clinically indicated. MRS studies were obtained between the pre- and post-contrast MR imaging. However, MRS studies were not obtained on every patient or at the time of each MRI. All studies were conducted on a clinical 1.5 T MR system (Signa LX, GE Healthcare Milwaukee, WI, USA). Single-voxel point-resolved spectroscopy (PRESS) with a short echo time (TE) of 35 ms, a repetition time (TR) of 1.5 s, and 128 signal averages was used for all acquisitions. Sizes and shapes of the ROIs were adjusted to lesion size and typically varied between 5 and 10 cm^3. The total acquisition time, including scanner adjustments, was less than five minutes per spectrum. Spectra were centrally processed with fully automated LCModel (Stephen Provencher Inc., Oakville, Ontario, Canada, LCModel Version 6.3–1 L software [14]. T2-weighted fast spin-echo, FLAIR, and T1-weighted FLAIR images were acquired in all cases, and the position of the region of interest (ROI) was documented on at least three MR images. All ROIs were a priori and independently reviewed to ensure that only spectra that were consistently positioned and representative of the tumor tissue were retained for subsequent processing and analysis.

Evaluation of MRS data was limited to metabolite concentrations and metabolite ratios deemed reliable as per previously published studies [5,6,9–12] (i.e., choline (Cho), creatine (Cr), myo-inositol (mI), n-acetyl-aspartate (NAA), and lactate (Lac)). Absolute metabolite levels were determined by using the unsuppressed water signal as the reference signal and the default water content set by the LCModel software (65% $\approx$ 36.1 mol/kg). The relative concentrations of mI/Cho, Cr/Cho, and NAA/Cho were the primary endpoints rather than absolute concentrations to reflect underlying processes involving multiple metabolites and to control for possible scan-level factors. Lipid intensities (with possible contributions from underlying macromolecules) at 1.3 ppm (from -CH$_2$ groups of lipid molecules, LipMM13 and at 0.9 ppm (terminal -CH$_3$, LipMM09) were analyzed as indicators of progressive disease [15].

2.2. Statistical Analysis

To identify MRS biomarkers associated with overall survival at predefined timepoints scans for both cohorts (vaccine and non-vaccine) were binned into comparable timepoints defined by the vaccine therapy schedule (vaccine cohort). Timepoint 0 (time of diagnosis pre-RT) scans were obtained only in the non-vaccine cohort. Timepoint 1 was post-RT and prior to vaccine therapy (1.9–3.8 months post-diagnosis) (vaccine cohort and non-vaccine cohort). Timepoint 2 included scans obtained after 2–3 vaccine doses (3.9–5.2 months post diagnosis) (vaccine cohort and non-vaccine cohort) and timepoint 3 scans were performed after 4–6 vaccine doses (5.3–7.6 months post-diagnosis) (vaccine cohort and non-vaccine cohort). Spearman rank-order correlations were used to measure associations between timepoint-specific metabolite ratios and overall survival, with confidence intervals esti mated using Fisher's r-to-z transformation. A single generalized estimating equations model for each ratio was considered instead of Spearman correlations, to adjust for multiple records from a single subject in the same timepoint and across time. The two cohorts were analyzed separately without direct comparison of associations between metabolites and survival due to limitations with the sample size and missing data points. The false discovery rate for groups of correlations was controlled at 0.05 through the method of Benjamini and Hochberg [16]. For a separate analysis summarizing longitudinal trends based on the time from death rather than the time from diagnosis, linear mixed-effects (random intercept) regression was used to evaluate the terminal decline in metabolite values and ratios. Statistical analyses were performed using SAS/STAT statistical software version 9.4 (SAS Institute, Cary, NC, USA) and R version 4.0.2 (R Foundation for Statistical Computing, Vienna, Austria).

3. Results

Fifty-eight MRS studies (1–8 scans per patient, median 4) were performed in 14 patients with DIPG enrolled in the peptide vaccine study. Eighty-two MRS studies (1–7 scans per patient, median 2.5) were performed on 32 patients in the non-vaccine cohort. Table 1 shows patient characteristics for the vaccine cohort (diagnosed between 2010 and 2012) and the non-vaccine cohort (diagnosed between 2001 and 2014). Patients were aged 2.2 to 17.9 years at diagnosis, with a median overall survival from diagnosis of 13.5 months (range 6.3–23.6 months) for the vaccine cohort and 11.2 months (range 3.7–37.6 months) for the non-vaccine cohort. The example spectra for patients with short survival and long survival are shown in Figure 1.

Table 1. Patient characteristics.

	Vaccine Cohort ($n = 14$)	Non-Vaccine Cohort ($n = 32$)
	Median (range)	Median (range)
Age at diagnosis, years	8.5 (2.2–17.9)	7 (3–15)
Number of MRS per patient	4 (1–8)	2.5 (1–7)
Survival from diagnosis, months	13.5 (6.3–23.6)	11.2 (3.7–37.6)
Sex		
Female	6 (43)	19 (59)
Male	8 (57)	13 (41)
Pre-vaccine therapy		
Radiotherapy only	10 (72)	6 (19)
Radiotherapy + bevacizumab	2 (14)	1 (3)
Radiotherapy + temozolomide	2 (14)	5 (16)
Radiotherapy + unknown/other *		20 (62)

MRS = magnetic resonance spectroscopy; * includes carboplatin + etoposide, gadolinium-texaphyrin, temozolomide + irinotecan.

Figure 2 shows associations in the vaccine cohort between metabolite ratio values within predefined time periods (defined above, timepoints 1–3) and survival duration. Figure 3 shows the same associations for the non-vaccine cohort, with an additional column for measurements obtained at the time of diagnosis (timepoint 0, pre-RT). At diagnosis, the ratios of interest (mI/Cho, Cr/Cho, and NAA/Cho) did not correlate with overall survival (first column of Figure 3). The ratios following RT (1.9–3.8 months post-diagnosis) also did not appear to be associated with overall survival in either cohort. By 3.9–5.2 months post-diagnosis (after 2–3 vaccine doses in the vaccine cohort), mI/Cho in the vaccine cohort was strongly associated with overall survival (rho = 0.92, 95% CI 0.67–0.98), even though the range of mI/Cho values was similar to the range at timepoint 1. The six patients scanned within the same timeframe in the non-vaccine cohort showed very little variation in mI/Cho values, precluding an association with overall survival. At 5.3–7.6 months post-diagnosis, the mI/Cho values in the vaccine cohort still showed a strong rank-order correlation with survival (rho = 0.95, 95% CI 0.81–0.99), a positive association that was also seen in the non-vaccine cohort (rho = 0.86, 95% CI 0.49–0.97). Descriptive displays of each patient's series of metabolite ratios and values relative to the time of diagnosis are shown in Figures S1–S4 to support the analyses presented above.

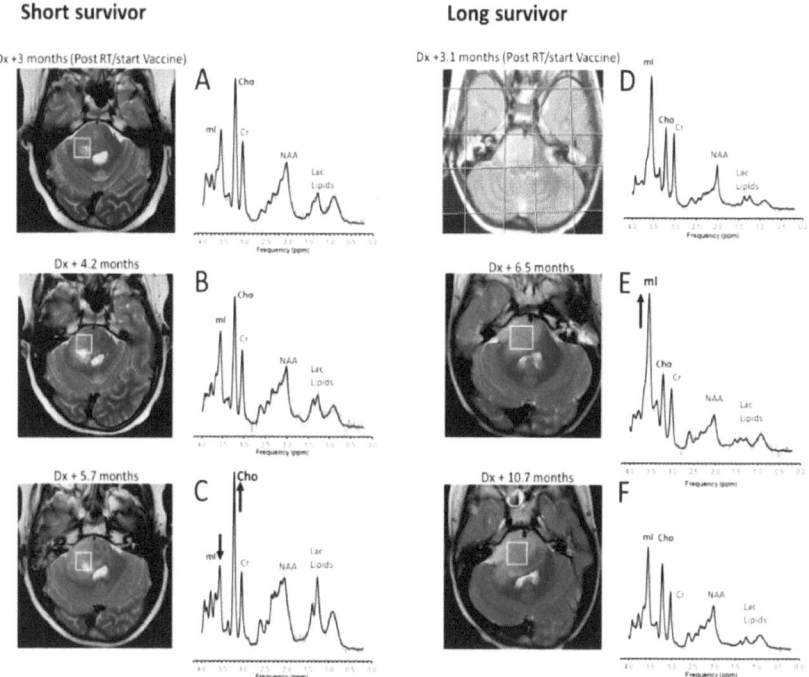

Figure 1. Transverse T2-weighted MRI and corresponding MR spectra. For a patient who survived 8.5 months after diagnosis (left column), metabolite levels at the start (**A**) and 1.5 months into vaccine therapy (**B**) are comparable. Soon before clinical and radiological deterioration (**C**), myo-inositol (mI) declined, and choline (Cho), lactate (Lac), and lipids all increased. For a patient who survived 23.6 months after diagnosis (**right column**), mI was prominent after completion of radiotherapy (**D**) and a further increase relative to Cho was noticeable 3 months after start of vaccine therapy (**E**). After another 4.2 months (and over a year before death) (**F**), a gradual decline of mI and a gradual increase in Cho were observed. Dx = diagnosis, RT = irradiation with or without concurrent chemotherapy mI = myo-inositol, Cho = choline, Cr = creatine, Lac = lactate. Shown are the unfiltered raw data (thin line) and the fit to the data used for quantitation (thick line).

These associations of mI/Cho with overall survival at timepoints 2 and 3 (3.9–7.6 months post-diagnosis) demonstrate promise for mI/Cho as a non-invasive biomarker for the prognosis at those timepoints. However, co-variation in metabolite values and survival at these timepoints may reflect the influence of treatment response or terminal decline, or potentially a combination of both. As an exploratory analysis, to isolate the effects of terminal change, we present a separate analysis counting time backward from death instead of forward from diagnosis. The MR spectra of vaccine cohort patients demonstrated a terminal decline of the three metabolite ratios, most clearly observed for mI/Cho (Figure S5). The rate of decline was estimated using random intercept linear mixed models of scans obtained within 6 months of death (Table 2). In the vaccine cohort, the mI/Cho ratio decreased an average of 0.37 units (95% CI 0.11–0.63)/month before death ($p = 0.01$). The average decrease in Cr/Cho was 0.12 units/month (95% CI 0.05–0.19, $p = 0.003$), and the average decrease in NAA/Cho was 0.06 units/month (95% CI −0.06–0.18, $p = 0.27$). No individual patient's data were unduly influential regarding the slope estimates; comparable slopes were obtained for models with both random slope and intercept and when analyzing scans within 12 months rather than within 6 months of death (Table 2). All three metabolite ratios also showed a pattern of terminal decline in the non-vaccine cohort, with attenuated slopes for mI/Cho and Cr/Cho compared to the vaccine cohort (Table 2). Terminal decline trajectories for individual metabolites are shown in Figure S6 (vaccine cohort) and Figure S7 (non-vaccine cohort). Myo-inositol showed a terminal decline for most patients in the vaccine cohort, with an average decrease of 0.92 i.u./month (95% CI 0.28–1.56, $p = 0.009$) in the last 6 months before death. High lactate and lipid levels were observed in some patients within months of death.

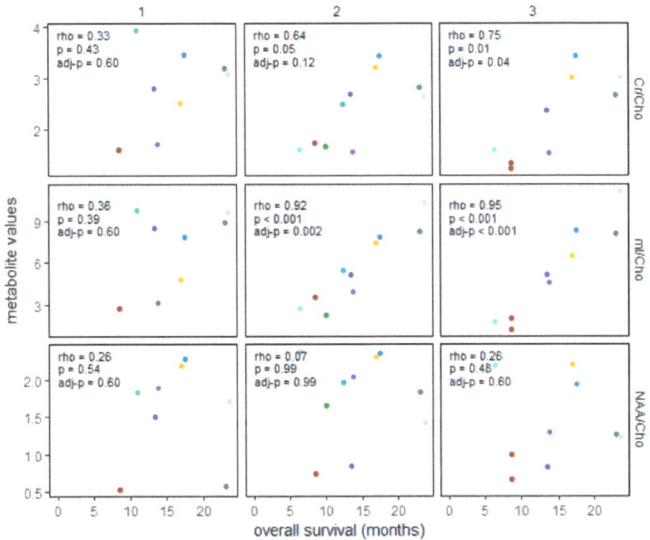

Figure 2. Association between metabolite ratios and overall survival in the vaccine cohort, grouped by timepoints relative to completion of RT (columns) (28 scans within 7.6 months of diagnosis in 12 patients). RT = irradiation with or without concurrent chemotherapy. Spearman rank-order correlations are shown for each panel, with Benjamini–Hochberg control of p-values to a false positive rate of 0.05 for all panels. Each color represents an individual patient. Timepoint 1 = post-RT and before vaccine therapy (1.9–3.8 months post-diagnosis); timepoint 2 = after 2–3 vaccine doses (3.9–5.2 months post-diagnosis); timepoint 3 = after 4–6 vaccine doses (5.3–7.6 months post-diagnosis).

Table 2. Monthly rate of terminal decline for key metabolite ratios, excluding scans at diagnosis. Linear mixed-effects (random intercept) models for each metabolite, fit separately for each study cohort.

	Within 6 Months of Death		Within 12 Months of Death	
	Vaccine Cohort (n = 22 Scans in 10 Patients)	Non-Vaccine Cohort (n = 37 Scans in 18 Patients)	Vaccine Cohort (n = 44 Scans in 13 Patients)	Non-Vaccine Cohort (n = 59 Scans in 23 Patients)
Metabolite ratio	Slope (95% CI)	Slope (95% CI)	Slope (95% CI)	Slope (95% CI)
mI/Cho	0.37 (0.11–0.63)	0.26 (0.04–0.48)	0.37 (0.21–0.54)	0.19 (0.05–0.34)
Cr/Cho	0.12 (0.05–0.19)	0.06 (-0.02–0.13)	0.11 (0.06–0.17)	0.06 (0.02–0.10)
NAA/Cho	0.06 (−0.06–0.18)	0.02 (−0.06–0.11)	0.07 (0.02–0.11)	0.08 (0.04–0.12)

mI = myo-inositol, Cho = choline, Cr = creatine.

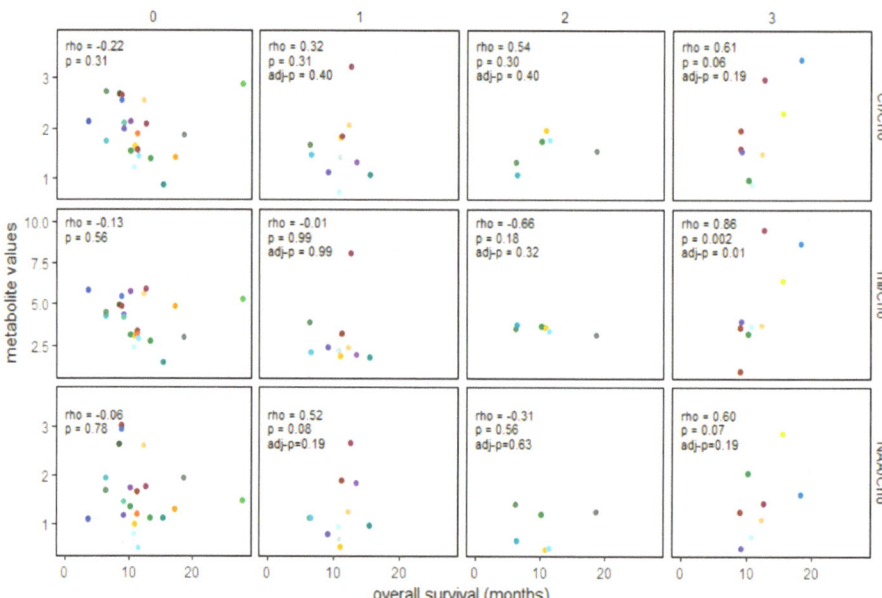

Figure 3. Association between metabolite ratios and overall survival in the non-vaccine cohort, at diagnosis (*n* = 23, left column), and at 3 timepoints defined relative to date of diagnosis to align with dosing categories for the vaccine cohort (28 scans within 7.6 months of diagnosis in 19 patients). RT = irradiation with or without concurrent chemotherapy. Spearman rank-order correlations are shown for each panel, with Benjamini–Hochberg control of *p*-values to a false positive rate of 0.05 for timepoints 1–3. Each color represents an individual patient. 0 = diagnosis, before RT; 1 = 1.9–3.8 months post-diagnosis (post-RT for most); 2 = 4.0–5.2 months post-diagnosis; 3 = 5.3–7.6 months post-diagnosis.

4. Discussion

Diffuse intrinsic pontine gliomas are incurable pediatric brain tumors, with most patients succumbing to their disease within a year of diagnosis. Recently, peptide vaccines and other immunotherapies have been developed as experimental treatments for these tumors [13,17]. Tumors in the pons cannot feasibly undergo serial biopsies to monitor their status; non-invasive means of monitoring response to treatment are needed. We reviewed the in vivo metabolic profiles of two cohorts of DIPG patients: participants in a clinical trial of peptide vaccine therapy (ClinicalTrials.gov #NCT01130077) and patients from a different institution who did not receive immunotherapy, to evaluate possible biomarkers of disease status. High mI/Cho ratios at 3.9–5.2 months following diagnosis, corresponding to the time frame when patients on the vaccine trial had received 2–3 vaccine doses, were associated with longer survival (Figures 2 and S1). This pattern was also seen in the non-vaccine cohort, although the association between higher mI/Cho ratios and longer overall survival was not observed until later (5.3–7.6 months post-diagnosis) (Figures 3 and S2).

Declines in mI/Cho, NAA/Cho, and Cr/Cho over time in both the vaccine cohort and non-vaccine cohort were observed (Table 2). First, we define benchmark timepoints for assessing MRS biomarkers to support their development for clinical use as a non-invasive prospective biomarker for disease status. Additionally, this study provides data to enhance the understanding of potential mechanisms of therapy response and disease progression by (a) presenting data from two separate cohorts: a clinical trial evaluating adjuvant immunotherapy and an independent cohort of patients treated with (chemo)radiation but not immunotherapy; and (b) examining MRS patterns forward from the time of diagnosis and backward from the time of death. Prior studies emphasized high or increasing Cho, low or decreasing NAA/Cho or Cr/Cho, and/or high lactate and lipids as indicators of poor prognosis [5,6,18–21]. While we found support for these findings in selected cohorts (Table 2) or patient trajectories (Figures S3 and S4), the pattern displayed most consistently across both cohorts was a terminal change in mI/Cho (Table 2, Figure S5).

Our study is one of the first to show a potentially useful non-invasive biomarker that can be evaluated after the post-RT MRI scan in patients with DIPG. Most DIPG neuroimaging biomarker studies have focused on the relationship between tumor volume and outcomes before radiation therapy [12,22]. These studies have demonstrated that the MRI response after completion of RT in comparison to the size pre-RT can be prognostic. For example, in patients receiving RT for DIPG, the largest decrease in tumor size was found at 2 weeks following completion of RT, with minimal subsequent changes observed in imaging at 6 to 8 weeks post-RT [23]. Other studies have shown that a >25% decrease in tumor volume following RT is significantly associated with better overall survival [24]. Further studies are needed to determine if there is an association between the mI/Cho ratio at this such timepoint and the change in the size of the tumor. Increased relative or absolute choline concentrations are believed to indicate increased cell membrane metabolism, and decreasing NAA is believed to reflect the replacement of residual axons/neurons by infiltrative tumor cells [10]. Lipids and lactate levels have been shown to increase as degenerating tumors outgrow their perfusion support and develop areas of necrosis [25].

Increasing mI in brain tumors is considered to reflect an increase in reactive astrocytes, microglia, and/or gliosis, either as an effect of radiation therapy or chronic inflammation. Similarly, low levels of choline can also reflect inactive glial cells. Other studies have suggested the converse, that decreasing mI and/or increasing choline in DIPG were consistent with progressive disease/reactivation of tumors [5,6,11], with the decrease in mI potentially a result of increasing tumoral edema and the increased choline reflective of increased cell turnover. The strong association of high mI/Cho ratios seen after 2–3 vaccines and sustained over a few months in patients with longer-term survival in vaccine therapy could be due to infiltration by vaccine-responsive immune cells with resultant inflammation and proliferation of microglia. In the non-vaccine cohort, the increase in mI/Cho occurred slightly later after the completion of RT, potentially reflecting a later onset of gliosis. This hypothesis is supported by consistently high mI in the enhancing brain lesions seen in multiple sclerosis [26–28] and the surrounding white matter [29,30], a disease primarily caused by T-lymphocyte infiltration with resultant activation and proliferation of microglia.

DIPG are relatively rare tumors, and the number of patients included in the early phase vaccine study is small, resulting in several study limitations. Because patients could complete initial RT before traveling to the vaccine trial study site, MRS data were not acquired at diagnosis or during RT for that cohort, so we were not able to evaluate previously reported prognostic factors at this timepoint [21]. While MRS measures describe a relevant range of tumor characteristics, targeted immune-imaging tracers [31,32] may also play a role in the development and selection of DIPG patients for immunotherapy trials. The small sample size also precluded the examination of MRS measures in patients with pseudoprogression (transient increased edema and/or contrast enhancement of the tumor, followed by stabilization/regression and symptomatic improvement), which was postulated to be an indicator of the vaccine treatment efficacy [13,33]. Finally, while steroids are relatively contra-indicated during vaccine therapy due to the suppression of an immune response, steroids are generally part of the initial management of symptoms as well as at the time of any neurologic worsening. It is unclear whether and to what extent steroids have an impact on metabolite concentrations and their measurement via MR spectroscopy. Although the imaging protocol was the same for both cohorts, differences in referral patterns to the sites, treatment regimens, small numbers of patients, and differences in scan timing introduce unmeasured confounders into treatment cohort comparisons, limiting direct comparisons.

5. Conclusions

In summary, long-term survivors were characterized by high mI/Cho ratios that developed following initial RT, suggesting that mI may constitute an in vivo, real-time surrogate indicator for the tumor microenvironment response to RT. The number of patients with serial MRS evaluations on the vaccine trial was too small to draw strong conclusions about the role of the vaccine in the observation of an increased mI/Cho ratio slightly earlier than in the non-immunotherapy cohort (Figures 2 and 3). The six-month terminal decline observed in 10 patients receiving peptide vaccine therapy and 18 patients in a non-vaccine cohort supports the hypothesis that progressive DIPG is characterized by increasing tumor membrane turnover (choline) accompanied by decreasing mI and creatine. Although it is possible that the more distinctive terminal decline slopes in the vaccine study (Table 2, Figure S5) are related to mechanisms of vaccine therapy resistance, the more likely explanation (beyond chance variation) is the uniformity of the vaccine therapy regimen compared to the non-vaccine cohort. These remain to be validated in other cohorts receiving RT with and without immunotherapy. Increased mI/Cho (possibly reflecting immune-effector cell influx into the tumor as a mechanism of tumor response) requires further study.

Supplementary Materials: The following supporting information can be downloaded at: https://www.mdpi.com/article/10.3390/cancers14235995/s1, Figure S1: Longitudinal trajectories (relative to date of diagnosis) for metabolite ratios of interest, Figure S2: Longitudinal trajectories (relative to date of diagnosis) for metabolite ratios of interest, Figure S3: Longitudinal trajectories (relative to date of diagnosis) for individual metabolites, Figure S4: Prospective change (relative to date of diagnosis) for individual metabolites, Figure S5: Terminal decline (relative to date of death, $X = 0$) for metabolite ratios of interest measured within 12 months of death, excluding scans at diagnosis myo-Inositol/choline (left column), creatine/choline (middle), NAA/choline (right column). Figure S6: Terminal change (relative to date of death) for individual metabolites (mmol/kg), Figure S7 Terminal change (relative to date of death) for individual metabolites (mmol/kg).

Author Contributions: Conceptualization, A.P., R.I.J., I.F.P. and R.C.; methodology, A.P., R.C.; validation, A.P., R.I.J., I.F.P. and R.C.; formal analysis, A.P., R.I.J., I.F.P. and R.C.; investigation, A.P. R.C. and G.D.; resources, A.P.; data curation, A.P. and R.C.; writing—original draft preparation A.P., R.I.J., I.F.P., R.C., H.O., M.D.N., G.K., G.D. and S.B.; writing—review and editing, A.P., R.I.J. I.F.P., R.C., H.O., M.D.N., G.K., G.D. and S.B.; visualization, A.P. and R.C.; supervision, A.P.; project administration, A.P.; funding acquisition, A.P. and I.F.P. All authors have read and agreed to the published version of the manuscript.

Funding: This clinical trial was supported by National Institutes of Health grants R21 CA149872, R01 CA187219, 1 R01 CA174858, and P01 NS40923, and the UPMC Hillman Cancer Center Immunological Monitoring Core and Biostatistics Shared Resource Facilities, supported in part by NIH award P30 CA47904; grants from the Pediatric Low-Grade Glioma Initiative via the National Brain Tumor Society and the Ellie Kavalieros Fund, the Translational Brain Tumor Research Fund, and the Connor's Cure Research Fund of the Children's Hospital of Pittsburgh Foundation; and the Pediatric Clinical and Translational Research Center, supported by the NIH through Grant Numbers UL1 RR024153 and UL1 TR000005. The imaging postprocessing was supported by the Ian's (Ian Yagoda) Friends Foundation Grant, Society of Pediatric Radiology Pilot Award, and NLM Grant 5 T15 LM007059-27.

Institutional Review Board Statement: The study was conducted in accordance with the Declaration of Helsinki, and approved by the Institutional Review Board of University of Pittsburgh (CR19050251 010, STUDY19050251, 13 September 2022).

Informed Consent Statement: Informed consent was obtained from all subjects involved in the study.

Data Availability Statement: Preliminary results have been presented at the 2015 Clinical Translation Pediatric Neurooncology symposium, in a 2017 publication describing advanced MR imaging in the peptide vaccine study [34], and at the 2019 International Society for Magnetic Resonance in Medicine annual meeting. The data presented in this study are available on request from the corresponding author. The data are not publicly available due to patient privacy.

Acknowledgments: UPMC Hillman Cancer Center Clinical Research Services for regulatory management, Andres Salazar, Oncovir, Inc., for provision of poly-ICLC, physicians who referred their patients, and the patients and families who participated in this trial. We thank Brenda Kurland and Shira R. Abberbock for support with statistical analysis. We also thank Angela K. Connelly, Sharon Dibridge, Fern Wasco, and Melanie Gieraltowski for research coordination.

Conflicts of Interest: Hideho Okada is an inventor in the U.S. Patent Application No. 60,611, 797 (Utility Patent Application) "Identification of An IL-13 Receptor Alpha2 Peptide Analogue Capable of Enhancing Stimulation of Glioma-Specific CTL Response". An exclusive licensing agreement has been completed on this application between University of Pittsburgh and Stemline, Inc. Due to the potential conflicts of interest, Hideho Okada did not participate in the interpretation of the data obtained for this study.

References

1. Clymer, J.; Kieran, M.W. The Integration of Biology Into the Treatment of Diffuse Intrinsic Pontine Glioma: A Review of the North American Clinical Trial Perspective. *Front. Oncol.* **2018**, *8*, 169. [CrossRef]
2. Hargrave, D.; Ute, B.; Eric, B. Diffuse brainstem glioma in children: Critical review of clinical trials. *Lancet. Oncol.* **2006**, *7*, 241–248. [CrossRef] [PubMed]
3. Khuong-Quang, D.-A.; Buczkowicz, P.; Rakopoulos, P.; Liu, X.-Y.; Fontebasso, A.M.; Bouffet, E.; Bartels, U.; Albrecht, S.; Schwartzentruber, J.; Letourneau, L. K27 M mutation in histone H3. 3 defines clinically and biologically distinct subgroups of pediatric diffuse intrinsic pontine gliomas. *Acta Neuropathol.* **2012**, *124*, 439–447. [CrossRef] [PubMed]
4. Castel, D.; Philippe, C.; Calmon, R.; Le Dret, L.; Truffaux, N.; Boddaert, N.; Taylor, K.R.; Saulnier, P.; Lacroix, L.; Mackay, A. Histone H3 F3 A and HIST1 H3 B K27 M mutations define two subgroups of diffuse intrinsic pontine gliomas with different prognosis and phenotypes. *Acta Neuropathol.* **2015**, *130*, 815–827. [CrossRef] [PubMed]
5. Laprie, A.; Pirzkall, A.; Haas-Kogan, D.A.; Cha, S.; Banerjee, A.; Le, T.P.; Lu, Y.; Nelson, S.; McKnight, T.R. Longitudinal multivoxel MR spectroscopy study of pediatric diffuse brainstem gliomas treated with radiotherapy. *Int. J. Radiat. Oncol. Biol. Phys.* **2005**, *62*, 20–31. [CrossRef]
6. Panigrahy, A.; Nelson, M.D., Jr.; Finlay, J.L.; Sposto, R.; Krieger, M.D.; Gilles, F.H.; Bluml, S. Metabolism of diffuse intrinsic brainstem gliomas in children. *Neuro. Oncol.* **2008**, *10*, 32–44. [CrossRef]
7. Negendank, W.G. Studies of human tumors by MRS: A review. *NMR Biomed.* **1992**, *5*, 303–324. [CrossRef]
8. Ross, B.D.; Bluml, S. Neurospectroscopy. In *Neuroimaging Second Edition; A Companion to Adams and Victor's Principles of Neurology*; Greenberg, J.O., Ed.; McGraw Hill: New York, NY, USA, 1999; pp. 727–773.
9. Curless, R.G.; Bowen, B.C.; Pattany, P.M.; Gonik, R.; Kramer, D.L. Magnetic resonance spectroscopy in childhood brainstem tumors. *Pediatr Neurol.* **2002**, *26*, 374–378. [CrossRef]
10. Astrakas, L.G.; Zurakowski, D.; Tzika, A.A.; Zarifi, M.K.; Anthony, D.C.; De Girolami, U.; Tarbell, N.J.; Black, P.M. Noninvasive magnetic resonance spectroscopic imaging biomarkers to predict the clinical grade of pediatric brain tumors. *Clin. Cancer Res.* **2004**, *10*, 8220–8228. [CrossRef]
11. Thakur, S.B.; Karimi, S.; Dunkel, I.J.; Koutcher, J.A.; Huang, W. Longitudinal MR spectroscopic imaging of pediatric diffuse pontine tumors to assess tumor aggression and progression. *AJNR Am. J. Neuroradiol.* **2006**, *27*, 806–809.
12. Lobel, U.; Hwang, S.; Edwards, A.; Li, Y.; Li, X.; Broniscer, A.; Patay, Z. Discrepant longitudinal volumetric and metabolic evolution of diffuse intrinsic Pontine gliomas during treatment: Implications for current response assessment strategies. *Neuroradiology* **2016**, *58*, 1027–1034. [CrossRef]
13. Pollack, I.F.; Jakacki, R.I.; Butterfield, L.H.; Hamilton, R.L.; Panigrahy, A.; Potter, D.M.; Connelly, A.K.; Dibridge, S.A.; Whiteside, T.L.; Okada, H. Antigen-specific immune responses and clinical outcome after vaccination with glioma-associated antigen peptides and polyinosinic-polycytidylic acid stabilized by lysine and carboxymethylcellulose in children with newly diagnosed malignant brainstem and nonbrainstem gliomas. *J. Clin. Oncol.* **2014**, *32*, 2050–2058. [CrossRef] [PubMed]
14. Provencher, S.W. Estimation of metabolite concentrations from localized in vivo proton NMR spectra. *Magn. Reson. Med.* **1993**, *30*, 672–679. [CrossRef] [PubMed]
15. Negendank, W.G.; Sauter, R.; Brown, T.R.; Evelhoch, J.L.; Falini, A.; Gotsis, E.D.; Heerschap, A.; Kamada, K.; Lee, B.C.; Mengeot, M.M.; et al. Proton magnetic resonance spectroscopy in patients with glial tumors: A multicenter study. *J. Neurosurg.* **1996**, *84*, 449–458. [CrossRef]
16. Benjamini, Y.; Hochberg, Y. Controlling the false discovery rate: A practical and powerful approach to multiple testing. *J. R. Stat. Soc. Ser. B* **1995**, *57*, 289–300. [CrossRef]
17. Sayour, E.; Grippin, A.; Mendez-Gomez, H.; De Leon, G.; Mitchell, D. Immu-63. Overcoming glioblastoma resistance to immune checkpoint blockade via RNA-loaded nanoparticles. *Neuro.-Oncol.* **2017**, *19*, vi126. [CrossRef]
18. Tedeschi, G.; Lundbom, N.; Raman, R.; Bonavita, S.; Duyn, J.H.; Alger, J.R.; Di Chiro, G. Increased choline signal coinciding with malignant degeneration of cerebral gliomas: A serial proton magnetic resonance spectroscopy imaging study. *J. Neurosurg.* **1997**, *87*, 516–524. [CrossRef]

19. Li, X.; Jin, H.; Lu, Y.; Oh, J.; Chang, S.; Nelson, S.J. Identification of MRI and 1 H MRSI parameters that may predict survival for patients with malignant gliomas. *NMR Biomed.* **2004**, *17*, 10–20. [CrossRef] [PubMed]
20. Stadlbauer, A.; Gruber, S.; Nimsky, C.; Fahlbusch, R.; Hammen, T.; Buslei, R.; Tomandl, B.; Moser, E.; Ganslandt, O. Preoperative grading of gliomas by using metabolite quantification with high-spatial-resolution proton MR spectroscopic imaging. *Radiology* **2006**, *238*, 958–969. [CrossRef]
21. Steffen-Smith, E.A.; Shih, J.H.; Hipp, S.J.; Bent, R.; Warren, K.E. Proton magnetic resonance spectroscopy predicts survival in children with diffuse intrinsic pontine glioma. *J. Neurooncol.* **2011**, *105*, 365–373. [CrossRef]
22. Yamasaki, F.; Kurisu, K.; Kajiwara, Y.; Watanabe, Y.; Takayasu, T.; Akiyama, Y.; Saito, T.; Hanaya, R.; Sugiyama, K. Magnetic resonance spectroscopic detection of lactate is predictive of a poor prognosis in patients with diffuse intrinsic pontine glioma. *Neuro.-Oncol.* **2011**, *13*, 791–801. [CrossRef] [PubMed]
23. Petanjek, Z.; Kostovic, I. Epigenetic regulation of fetal brain development and neurocognitive outcome. *Proc. Natl. Acad. Sci. USA* **2012**, *109*, 11062–11063. [CrossRef] [PubMed]
24. Poussaint, T.Y. MRI as a central component of clinical trials analysis in brainstem glioma: A report from the Pediatric Brain Tumor Consortium (PBTC). *Neuro.-Ldots.* **2011**, *13*, 417–427. [CrossRef] [PubMed]
25. Negendank, W.; Sauter, R. Intratumoral lipids in 1 H MRS in vivo in brain tumors: Experience of the Siemens cooperative clinical trial. *Anticancer. Res.* **1996**, *16*, 1533–1538. [PubMed]
26. Fernando, K.; McLean, M.; Chard, D.; MacManus, D.; Dalton, C.; Miszkiel, K.; Gordon, R.; Plant, G.; Thompson, A.; Miller, D. Elevated white matter myo-inositol in clinically isolated syndromes suggestive of multiple sclerosis. *Brain* **2004**, *127*, 1361–1369. [CrossRef]
27. Kirov, I.I.; Patil, V.; Babb, J.S.; Rusinek, H.; Herbert, J.; Gonen, O. MR spectroscopy indicates diffuse multiple sclerosis activity during remission. *J. Neurol. Neurosurg. Psychiatry.* **2009**, *80*, 1330–1336. [CrossRef]
28. Srinivasan, R.; Sailasuta, N.; Hurd, R.; Nelson, S.; Pelletier, D. Evidence of elevated glutamate in multiple sclerosis using magnetic resonance spectroscopy at 3 T. *Brain* **2005**, *128*, 1016–1025. [CrossRef]
29. Hannoun, S.; Bagory, M.; Durand-Dubief, F.; Ibarrola, D.; Comte, J.-C.; Confavreux, C.; Cotton, F.; Sappey-Marinier, D. Correlation of diffusion and metabolic alterations in different clinical forms of multiple sclerosis. *PLoS ONE* **2012**, *7*, e32525. [CrossRef]
30. Kirov, I.I.; Tal, A.; Babb, J.S.; Herbert, J.; Gonen, O. Serial proton MR spectroscopy of gray and white matter in relapsing-remitting MS. *Neurology* **2013**, *80*, 39–46. [CrossRef]
31. Mayer, A.T.; Gambhir, S.S. The Immunoimaging Toolbox. *J. Nucl. Med. Off. Publ. Soc. Nucl. Med.* **2018**, *59*, 1174–1182. [CrossRef]
32. Nigam, S.; McCarl, L.; Kumar, R.; Edinger, R.S.; Kurland, B.F.; Anderson, C.J.; Panigrahy, A.; Kohanbash, G.; Edwards, W.B. Preclinical ImmunoPET Imaging of Glioblastoma-Infiltrating Myeloid Cells Using Zirconium-89 Labeled Anti-CD11 b Antibody. *Mol. Imaging Biol. MIB Off. Publ. Acad. Mol. Imaging* **2019**, *22*, 685–694. [CrossRef] [PubMed]
33. Ceschin, R.; Kurland, B.F.; Abberbock, S.R.; Ellingson, B.M.; Okada, H.; Jakacki, R.I.; Pollack, I.F.; Panigrahy, A. Parametric Response Mapping of Apparent Diffusion Coefficient as an Imaging Biomarker to Distinguish Pseudoprogression from True Tumor Progression in Peptide-Based Vaccine Therapy for Pediatric Diffuse Intrinsic Pontine Glioma. *AJNR Am. J. Neuroradiol.* **2015**, *36*, 2170–2176. [CrossRef] [PubMed]
34. Furtado, A.D.; Ceschin, R.; Blüml, S.; Mason, G.; Jakacki, R.I.; Okada, H.; Pollack, I.F.; Panigrahy, A. Neuroimaging of peptide-based vaccine therapy in pediatric brain tumors: Initial experience. *Neuroimaging Clin.* **2017**, *27*, 155–166. [CrossRef] [PubMed]

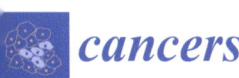

Article

Combining CNN Features with Voting Classifiers for Optimizing Performance of Brain Tumor Classification

Nazik Alturki [1], Muhammad Umer [2], Abid Ishaq [2], Nihal Abuzinadah [3], Khaled Alnowaiser [4], Abdullah Mohamed [5], Oumaima Saidani [1] and Imran Ashraf [6,*]

1 Department of Information Systems, College of Computer and Information Sciences, Princess Nourah bint Abdulrahman University, P.O. Box 84428, Riyadh 11671, Saudi Arabia
2 Department of Computer Science & Information Technology, The Islamia University of Bahawalpur, Bahawalpur 63100, Pakistan
3 Faculty of Computer Science and Information Technology, King Abdulaziz University, P.O. Box 80200, Jeddah 21589, Saudi Arabia
4 Department of Computer Engineering, College of Computer Engineering and Sciences, Prince Sattam Bin Abdulaziz University, Al-Kharj 11942, Saudi Arabia
5 Research Centre, Future University in Egypt, New Cairo 11745, Egypt
6 Department of Information and Communication Engineering, Yeungnam University, Gyeongsan 38541, Republic of Korea
* Correspondence: imranashraf@ynu.ac.kr

Simple Summary: This study presents a hybrid model for brain tumor detection. Contrary to manual featur extraction, features extracted from a convolutional neural network are used to train the model. Experimental results show the efficacy of CNN features over manually extracted features and model can detect brain tumor with a 99.9% accuracy.

Abstract: Brain tumors and other nervous system cancers are among the top ten leading fatal diseases. The effective treatment of brain tumors depends on their early detection. This research work makes use of 13 features with a voting classifier that combines logistic regression with stochastic gradient descent using features extracted by deep convolutional layers for the efficient classification of tumorous victims from the normal. From the first and second-order brain tumor features, deep convolutional features are extracted for model training. Using deep convolutional features helps to increase the precision of tumor and non-tumor patient classification. The proposed voting classifier along with convoluted features produces results that show the highest accuracy of 99.9%. Compared to cutting-edge methods, the proposed approach has demonstrated improved accuracy.

Keywords: brain tumor prediction; healthcare; deep convolutional features; ensemble learning

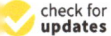

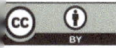

1. Introduction

Medical image analysis is a growing field that uses a variety of modern image processing techniques. As a result, a variety of diseases can now be detected in a timely manner. Early detection can help in the treatment of most life-threatening diseases such as tumors, eye disease, Alzheimer's, blood clots, and cancer [1]. Biopsies and images of the infected areas are used inr the diagnosis of these life-threatening diseases. Images of the affected areas are typically used to diagnosing diseases in the early stages. Biopsies on the other hand are used to confirm the presence of certain diseases [2]. In such cases, it is crucial that the modeling of infected areas is highly accurate and easily visualized.

The brain is a critical organ in the human body and plays a vital role in controlling the body and decision-making. Therefore, brain tumors are life-threatening conditions. Most malignancies involve the nervous system and thus it has important implications regarding diagnosis. The brain parenchyma, also referred to as metastases, is commonly involved [3]. The majority of brain tumors are brain metastases, which are estimated to have an incidence rate 10 times higher than primary brain tumors [4]. There are different types of gliomas and their malignancies also vary. In addition, they are different from most common primary brain tumors such as meningiomas and pituitary adenomas. The timely diagnosis and detection of primary brain tumors are essential as they are cancerous and life-threatening. The proper treatment of these cancerous tumors is critical, and different techniques are available to treat them. Treatment plans for brain tumors depend on how early the diagnosis is made and on the tumor type. Different diagnostic techniques are available tor efficiently diagnose brain tumors, such as magnetic resonance imaging (MRI) [5]. MRI provides vital information to classify the brain tumor and helps in treatment decisions [6].

The early detection of a brain tumors increases survival chances. Manual diagnosis and detection are laborious, time-consuming, and faulty. Expert radiologists are frequently required to gain a better understanding, identify the tumor, and compare tumor tissues to those in neighboring locations. For medical image analysis computer-aided imaging technology helps in the brain tumor early detection and categorization. The use of the latest technologies for the identification of brain tumors saves time and manpower as well. MRI is currently the most often used non-invasive technique for detecting brain tumors [7]. MRI scanning is the most commonly used technique for brain analysis. MRI can observe the difference in soft tissues which makes MRI advantageous over other techniques for brain tumor diagnosis. It has no side effects because it does not involve the application of ionizing radiation to brain areas [8]. MRI technique is extensively used by radiologists because it has the ability to diagnose the abnormal growth of cells. For brain tumor detection, a dual channel DC-BTD system was proposed by Zahoor et al. [9]. The authors used MRI images that show how minimal false negatives are. They used the static S-shaped features and for the discriminant dynamic features they used the D-channel. The study also included the use of techniques such as data normalization, augmentation, and four distinct machine learning classifiers. The findings of the study showed better results with 98.70% accuracy than existing studies. Similarly, ref. [10] used ensemble models to classify and diagnose brain tumors by enhancing MRI images with an average filter. Deep learning models are used for feature extraction such as ResNet-18 and AlexNet. SoftMax and SVM were used to classify these features. The proposed hybrid approach AlexNet+SVM achieved an accuracy score of 95.10%. Daz-Pernas et al. [11] used MRI images for the classification of brain tumors. They did not perform the pre-processing in their study. Their proposed approach achieved an accuracy of tumor classification of 97.3%. In addition to the MRI scanning, all the imaging techniques produce images in greyscale, except for the color Doppler technique, which produces color images. However, other techniques for tissue segmentation regions such as post-processing do not produce the desired results [12,13].

Many studies focus on the use of deep learning models for brain tumor detection. For example, an intelligent deep learning-based system for brain tumor detection was designed by Khan et al. [7]. They classified brain tumors into three classes: Pituitary Meningioma, and Glioma. The proposed system is HDL2BT (Hierarchical Deep Learning Based Brain tumor) which utilises CNN to classify brain tumours in an exact and precise manner. The proposed model shows a precision of 92.13%. A deep learning-based system DeepTumorNet was designed by Raza et al. [14] for the categorization of the three different kinds of brain tumors, the same used by the [7]. CNN GoogLeNet architecture was utilized as the base of the system. The authors tested the system on the publicly available dataset and achieved good results. They acquired an accuracy score of 98.67%. Ahmad et al. [15] used a number of classical classifiers together with different transfer learning-based deep learning approaches to detect brain tumors. The authors used seven approaches for transfer learning including Xception, ResNet50, InceptionResNetV2, VGG-16 and VGG-19 DenseNet201, and InceptionV3. These transfer learning models were followed by machine learning models. The findings of the study showed an accuracy of 98.39%.

Various researchers have used transfer learning models and achieved robust results for the identification of brain tumors [16,17]. Amran et al. [16] designed a hybrid deep tumor network for brain tumor detection by combining a CNN with GoogleNet. The author achieved 98.91% accuracy using Inceptionresnetv2 in [17]. The study [18] suggested a conditional segmentation strategy based on a residual network, as well as an attention approach based on an extreme gradient boost. The results showed that the CNN-CRF-Resnet system achieved an accuracy of 99.56% across all three classes. Samee et al. designed a hybrid transfer learning system GN-AlexNet for the classification of brain tumors and achieved an accuracy of 99.51% [19].

An ensemble deep learning-based system was designed by Rasool et al. [20] for the categorization of three different kinds of brain tumors. The authors used the ensemble deep learning model with fine-tuned GoogleNet and achieved an accuracy of 93.1%. As opposed to that, when the authors used GoogleNet as a feature extractor they obtained an accuracy of 98.1%. As genetic mutation is the primary reason for brain cancer, classifying and segmenting brain tumors using genomic information can help in diagnosis [21]. Using AI approaches, it is possible to identify disease-related molecular features from radiological medical images by assessing the genomic state of genetic mutations on numerous genes and cell proteins [22,23]. Authors combined AI with radio genomics for brain tumor detection in [24].

Some studies utilized the same dataset used in this study and have shown promising results. The study [25] employs an ensemble learning approach based on machine learning to detect brain cancers. NGBoost classifier was used alongside ETC, RF, GBC, and ADA for comparison. The findings revealed that the use of NGBoost produced a significantly higher accuracy of 98.54%. Aryan Sagar Methil [26] presented a deep learning approach for detecting brain tumors. Several image processing techniques were applied for obtaining better results. The employed CNN model achieves an accuracy of 95%. Shah et al. [27] utilized MR scans to determine the prognosis of brain malignancies. They proposed a refined EfficientNet-B0 for brain tumor prediction and also employed data augmentation techniques to obtain higher-quality photos. The proposed Efficient-B0 system acheived an accuracy of 98.87%. However, the proposed transfer learning model was a complex neural network model that required millions of parameters to train, which was the key drawback of the study.

This paper aims to develop a simple machine learning-based system that uses CNN as the feature engineering technique to classify patients with brain tumors and normal patients using MRI scan data. In summary, the proposed system offers the following advantages

- This study proposes an ensemble model that utilizes convolutional features from a customized CNN model for predicting brain tumors. The proposed ensemble model is based on logistic regression and a stochastic gradient descent classifier with a voting mechanism for making the final output.
- The impact of the original features is analyzed against the performance of models using convolutional features.
- The performance comparison is performed using various machine learning models including random forest (RF), K-nearest neighbor (k-NN), logistic regression (LR), gradient boosting machine (GBM), decision tree (DT), Gaussian Naive Bayes (GNB), extra tree classifier (ETC), support vector machine (SVM), and stochastic gradient descent (SGD). Moreover, the performance of the proposed model is compared with leading-edge methodologies in terms of accuracy, precision, recall, and F1 score.

The remaining sections are arranged as follows. Section 2 discusses the proposed system's components and functions. Section 3 provides the results, whereas Section 4 contains the discussions and conclusion.

2. Materials and Methods

The 'brain tumor' dataset used for the detection of the disease, the proposed approach, and the steps taken for the proposed framework is discussed in this section. The machine learning classifiers utilized in this work are also briefly described in this section.

2.1. Dataset

For the performance comparison, various machine learning models were utilized in this study. The selection of the right dataset is a vital step, this study makes use of the "Brain tumor" dataset which is publicly available on Kaggle [28]. The dataset contained 3762 instances, 13 features, and a target class. Of these 13 features, 5 were first-order features and 8 were texture features. The first-order features were the standard deviation, mean, kurtosis, variance, skewness, and texture features are entropy, contrast, homogeneity, energy, dissimilarity, correlation, coarseness, and ASM (Angular second moment). The target features contained two classes: tumors and non-tumor. Of 3762 instances, 2079 belonged to the non-tumor class and 1683 belonged to the tumor class.

2.2. Machine Learning Models

In this work, nine machine learning algorithms were utilized to identify brain tumors including RF, SVM, k-NN, LR, GBM, DT, GNB, ETC, and SGD. A brief explanation of these machine-learning models is given here.

2.2.1. Random Forest

RF [29,30] is a well-known and widely used tree-based machine learning algorithm. From the previous random vector, RF generates the independent random vector and distributes them among all the trees. It is a step-by-step process in which the root node divides the data into its child nodes, and so on until the leaf nodes are reached. In RF, each node of the tree independently classifies the feature's objective variables, and after that class votes. The classification results from the decision trees depend on the majority voting. Error in RF is calculated using the following formula

$$PE^* = P_{(i,j)}(f(i,j) < 0) \qquad (1)$$

where random vectors are represented by the i and j and these random vectors represent the probability. And f computes the average number of votes across all random vectors for the desired outcome [31], it is calculated as

$$f(i,j) = av_K I(H(i) = j) - max_{y \neq j} av_K I(h_k(i) = y) \qquad (2)$$

2.2.2. Decision Tree

A DT is one of the tree-based methods used for the classification of brain tumors. It handles classification and regression problems efficiently [32,33]. The major issue in DT is the finding of the root node at each level. Attribute selection is the method used to identify the root node. "Gini Index" and "information gain" are the attribute selection techniques. The following formula may be used to compute the Gini value.

$$Gini = 1 - \sum_{i=1}^{classes} p(i|t)^2 \qquad (3)$$

Impurity in the dataset is calculated using Gini. The other method used for attribute selection is information gain. It calculates the purity of the dataset. Information Gain for each attribute can be calculated using the following steps

Step 1: determine the target's entropy.
Step 2: compute each attribute's entropy.

The following formula may be used to get the entropy for a collection of instances D

$$entropy(D) = \sum_{i=1}^{|c|} P_r(C_i) log_2 P_r(C_i), where \sum_{i=1}^{|c|} P_r(C_i) = 1 \qquad (4)$$

For the construction of the trees in all the tree-based classifiers in this work information gain and the Gini index value are used.

2.2.3. K-Nearest Neighbour

k-NN is the first choice for medical data mining. k-NN is a straightforward instance-based classifier [34,35]. A supervised learning model called k-NN compares new data to existing cases to determine how similar they are, then groups the new data with those cases that have the highest similarity. Finding the similarity of the data involves measuring the distance between the new and existing data points. For distance calculation, various methods are available such as Manhattan, Euclidean, Murkowski, etc. Although k-NN is utilized for regression problems it is widely used to solve classification problems. There are multiple parameters in k-NN and these need to be correctly refined for good results.

2.2.4. Logistic Regression

LR is a supervised learning-based machine learning classifier that is statistics-based [36–38]. The input characteristics (X: input) can be categorized by LR into a discrete set of target values (Y: output). A logistic function is employed in LR to determine the likelihood of either class 0 or class 1. A logistic function typically has the shape of an "S" as in the equation below.

$$f(x) = \frac{L}{1 + e^{-m(v-v_0)}} \tag{5}$$

LR uses the sigmoid function for probability prediction. The following formula can be used to determine the sigmoid function.

$$\sigma(x) = e^x(e^x + 1), \sigma(x) = 1(1 + e^{-x}) \tag{6}$$

where $\sigma(x)$ shows output as either 0 or 1 and e is the base of the natural log and x represents the input. For linearly separable data LR is the best choice. It works well to deal with binary classification problems.

2.2.5. Support Vector Machine

A common supervised learning technique used for classification and regression issues is SVM [39]. The dataset is divided using SVM by creating decision paths known as hyperplanes. SVM can effectively handle both linear and nonlinear data. Because the hyperplane separates the dataset into two groups, linear SVM handles the separable data. Data points above the hyperplane are classified as class 1, while those below the hyperplane are classified as class 2. There are support vectors as well. The points that are near the hyperplane are known as support vectors. SVM separates the data on the one-vs-all concept which stops when the dataset separates into several classes. Nonseprable data is handled by the nonlinear SVM. In non-linear SVM the actual coordinate space is converted to separable coordinate space $x = \phi(x)$.

2.2.6. Gradient Boosting Machine

GBM is utilized for both classification and regression issues [40,41]. The main reason for boosting GBM is to enhance the capacity of the model in such a way as to catch the drawbacks of the model and replace them with a strong learner to find the near-to-accurate or perfect solution. This stage is carried out by GBM by gradually, sequentially, and additively training a large number of models. GBM is very sensitive to noisy data. Due to the boosting technique in GBM, it is less susceptible to overfitting problems.

2.2.7. Extra Tree Classifier

ETC is a tree-based learning model that uses the results of multiple correlated DTs for the final prediction [42]. The training samples are used to generate each DT in the forest that will be utilized for further classification. Numerous uncorrelated DTs are constructed using random samples of features. During this process of constructing a tree, the Gini index is used for every feature, and feature selection is performed for data splitting.

2.2.8. Gaussian Naive Bayes

The GNB method is based on the Bayes theorem and assumes that each feature in the model is independent [43,44]. It is used for object classification using uniformly distributed data. It is also known as the GNB classifier because of these features. It can be calculated using the following formula

$$P(c|x) = \frac{P(c|x)P(c)}{p(x)} \quad (7)$$

$$P(c|x) = P(x_1|x) * ...., P(x_1|x) * P(c) \quad (8)$$

2.2.9. Stochastic Gradient Decent

SGD integrates many binary classifiers and has undergone extensive testing on a sizable dataset [45,46]. It is easy to develop and comprehend, and its functioning resembles the regression technique quite a bit. SGD hyperparameter settings need to be correct in order to obtain reliable results. The SGD is sensitive to feature scaling.

2.3. Convolutional Neural Network for Feature Engineering

In this study, a CNN was used for feature engineering [47,48]. The embedding layer, flatten layer, max-pooling layer, and 1D convolutional layer are the four layers that make up CNN. In this study, an embedding layer with an embedding size of 20,000 was used. This layer utilized the features from the brain tumor dataset. The embedding layer had an output dimension of 300. After this layer 1D convolutional layer was used with a filter size of 5000. ReLU was utilized as an activation function and had a kernel size of 2×2. In order to map key features from the output of the 1D convolutional layer, a 2×2 max-pooling layer was utilized. The output was flattened at the end, and the ML models were then converted back to 1D arrays. Let (fs_i, tc_i) be a tuple set of brain tumor data set where the target class columns are represented by the tc, the feature set is represented by the fs and the tuple index is represented by the I. An embedding layer was utilized to get the desired output from the training set.

$$EL = embedding\_layer(Vs, Os, I) \quad (9)$$

$$EOs = EL(fs) \quad (10)$$

where EO_s denotes the embedding layer outputs and is fed to the convolutional layer as input, the embedding layers are denoted by EL. Three parameters are available in EL. V_s as the size of the vocabulary, I as the length of the input, and Os as the dimension of the output.

For brain tumor detection, we set the embedding layer at 20,000. This shows that this layer has the ability to take inputs ranging from 0 to 20,000. The length of the input was set at 13 and the output dimension was set at 300. All the input data in the CNN were processed in the embedding layer which created the output for the models for the next processing. The output dimensions of the embedding layers are

$$1D - Convs = CNN(F, Ks, AF) \leftarrow EOs \quad (11)$$

where the $1D - Convs$ represents the output of 1D convolutional layers.

For brain tumor detection, we used 500 filters for the CNN i.e., $F = 500$ and the Kernel size is $Ks = 2 \times 2$. The activation function not only changes the negative values but also helps to keep other values unchanged.

$$f(x) = max(0, E)s \quad (12)$$

For significant feature mapping the max-pooling layer was utilized in CNN. For brain tumor detection a 2 × 2 pool was used to map the features. Here $Fmap$ represents the features obtained from max-pooling, S-2 shows the stride and $Ps = 2$ is the pooling window size.

$$Cf = Fmap = \lfloor (1 - P_s)/S \rfloor + 1 \qquad (13)$$

A flattened layer was used to transform the 3D data into 1D. The main reason behind this conversion is that the machine learning models work well on the 1D data. For the training of the ML models, the above-mentioned step was implemented and for the training, we obtained the 25,000 features. The architecture of the used CNN along with the predictive model is shown in Figure 1.

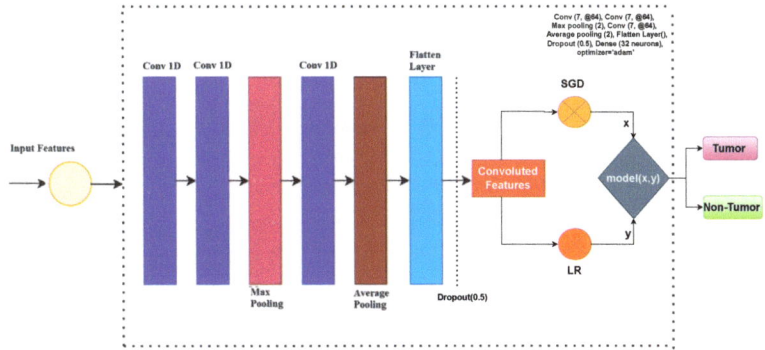

Figure 1. Architecture diagram of the CNN with voting classifier (LR+SGD) model.

2.4. Proposed Voting Classifier

For obtaining better results, several studies preferred ensemble machine learning models. When compared with individual models, the performance of ensemble classifiers is better. Therefore, this study used an ensemble model to detect brain tumors.

Figure 2 displays the pipeline flowchart for detecting brain tumors. Two machine learning models, LR and SGD, were combined to create the proposed model. The brain tumor dataset from the Kaggle was used for experiments. The proposed model was used for the brain tumor dataset for two scenarios. Firstly, all 13 features of the brain tumor dataset were used for brain tumor prediction. In the second experiment, the dataset's characteristics were extracted using CNN, and models were trained on them to distinguish between patient groups with and without tumors. The split of the data is 0.7 to 0.3, with 70% of the data utilized for training and 30% for testing. Accuracy, precision, recall, and F1 score were used to evaluate the model.

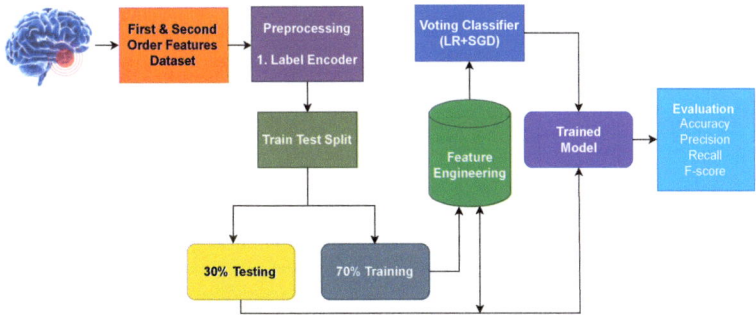

Figure 2. workflow diagram of the proposed voting classifier (LR+SGD) model.

In this work, LR and SGD are combined with soft voting criteria. The architecture of the voting classifier is given in Figure 3. The outcome with high probability is regarded as the final output in soft voting.

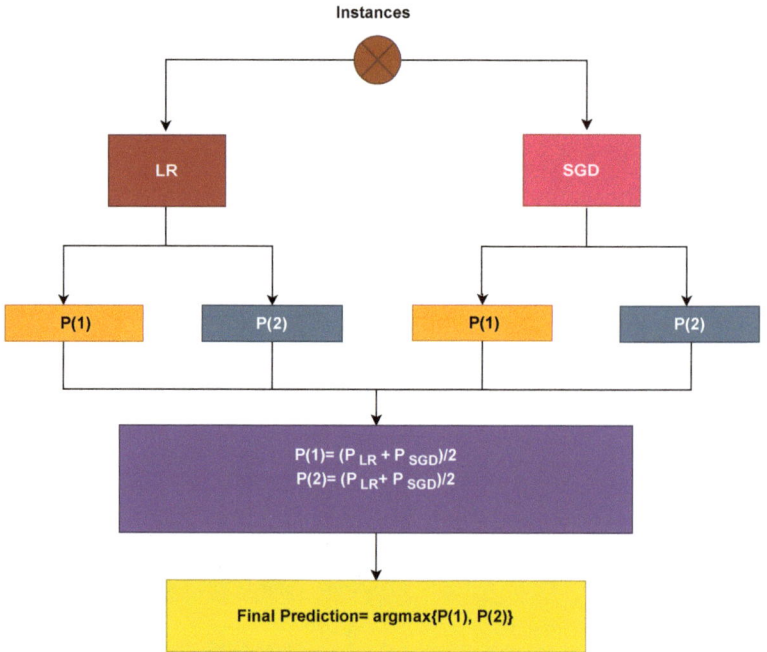

Figure 3. Architecture of the proposed voting classifier (LR+SGD) model.

Mathematically, the soft voting criteria can be represented as

$$\hat{p} = argmax \sum_{i}^{n} LR_i, \sum_{i}^{n} SGD_i \qquad (14)$$

where the probability values against the test sample are denoted by $\sum_{i}^{n} LR_i$ and $\sum_{i}^{n} SGD_i$. The probability values for each instance using LR and SGD are then passed through on the basis of soft voting as shown in Figure 3.

Each sample that has passed through the LR and SGD is given a probability score. For example, if the LR model's probability value is 0.4 and 0.7 for two classes, respectively, and the SGD model's probability value is 0.5 and 0.4 for two classes, respectively, and $P(x)$ represents the probability value of x ranging from 0 to 1, the final probability is determined as

$$P(1) = (0.4 + 0.5)/2 = 0.45$$
$$P(2) = (0.7 + 0.4)/2 = 0.55$$

The final output will be 2 because it has the highest probability. By combining the projected probabilities from both classifiers, VC(LR+SGD) selects the final class based on the maximum average probability for each class. The hyperparameter details of all models used in this research work are listed in Table 1.

Table 1. Hyperparameter values of all models used in this research work.

Classifiers	Parameters
RF	number of trees = 200, maximum depth = 30, random state = 52
DT	number of trees = 200, maximum depth = 30, random state = 52
k-NN	algorithm = 'auto', leaf size = 30, metric = 'minkowski', neighbors = 5, weights = 'uniform'
LR	penalty = 'l2', solver = 'lbfgs'
SVM	C = 2.0, cache size = 200, gamma = 'auto', kernel = 'linear', maximum iteration = −1, probability = False, random state = 52, tol = 0.001
GBM	number of trees = 200, maximum depth = 30, random state = 52, learning rate = 0.1
ETC	number of trees = 200, maximum depth = 30, random state = 52
GNB	alpha = 1.0, binarize = 0.0
SGD	penalty = 'l2', loss = 'log'
CNN	Conv (7, @64), Conv (7, @64), Max pooling (2), Conv (7, @64), Average pooling (2), Flatten Layer(), Dropout (0.5), Dense (32 neurons), optimizer = 'adam'

2.5. Evaluation Metrics

Accuracy, precision, recall, and F1 score are the performance metrics utilized in this study to assess the machine learning models' effectiveness. These measurements are all dependent on the confusion matrix's values.

$$\text{Accuracy} = \frac{TP + TN}{TP + TN + FP + FN} \quad (15)$$

$$\text{Precision} = \frac{TP}{TP + FP} \quad (16)$$

$$\text{Recall} = \frac{TP}{TP + FN} \quad (17)$$

$$\text{F1 score} = 2 \times \frac{\text{Precision} \times \text{Recall}}{\text{Precision} + \text{Recall}} \quad (18)$$

3. Results and Discussion

3.1. Experiment Setup

Several experiments were conducted for the performance analysis, and the performance of the proposed approach was extensively assessed in comparison to the other learning models. All the experiments were performed using a 7th generation Intel Corei7 machine with Windows 10 operating system. Python language was used for the implementation of the proposed approach and the other learning models. Tensor Flow, Sci-kit learn, and Keras libraries were also used. Experiments were carried out in two situations to evaluate the effectiveness of the proposed technique: using original features from the brain tumor dataset and using CNN features.

3.2. Performance of Models Using Original Features

The ML models were applied to the actual dataset in the first set of experiments and the results are shown in Table 2. Results show that the SGD and LR achieved the highest accuracy values of 0.881 and 0.869, respectively among all models. RF received a 0.854 accuracy while the LR+SGD ensemble model attained an accuracy score of 0.845. Tree-based model ETC attained an accuracy score of 0.829 while the GNB showed the worst performance with a 0.769 accuracy score. However, the linear models LR, SGD, and their ensemble outperform when using the original feature set.

Table 2. Results of machine learning models using the original features.

Model	Accuracy	Class	Precision	Recall	F1 Score
Voting Classifier LR+SGD	0.845	Tumour	0.865	0.899	0.878
		Non-Tumour	0.748	0.799	0.776
		Micro Avg.	0.824	0.858	0.856
		Weighted Avg.	0.807	0.843	0.825
GBM	0.805	Tumour	0.795	0.818	0.807
		Non-Tumour	0.818	0.818	0.818
		Micro Avg.	0.805	0.819	0.827
		Weighted Avg.	0.808	0.814	0.826
GNB	0.769	Tumour	0.777	0.788	0.777
		Non-Tumour	0.744	0.766	0.755
		Micro Avg.	0.766	0.777	0.766
		Weighted Avg.	0.766	0.777	0.766
ETC	0.829	Tumour	0.806	0.806	0.806
		Non-Tumour	0.815	0.815	0.815
		Micro Avg.	0.805	0.805	0.805
		Weighted Avg.	0.809	0.820	0.811
LR	0.869	Tumour	0.866	0.899	0.877
		Non-Tumour	0.888	0.899	0.888
		M Avg.	0.855	0.902	0.883
		W Avg.	0.855	0.884	0.876
SGD	0.881	Tumour	0.903	0.892	0.893
		Non-Tumour	0.923	0.924	0.922
		Micro Avg.	0.922	0.922	0.911
		Weighted Avg.	0.919	0.919	0.919
RF	0.854	Tumour	0.827	0.858	0.834
		Non-Tumour	0.844	0.806	0.828
		Micro Avg.	0.844	0.844	0.833
		Weighted Avg.	0.833	0.833	0.833
DT	0.829	Tumour	0.806	0.822	0.811
		Non-Tumour	0.805	0.833	0.814
		Micro Avg.	0.807	0.809	0.818
		Weighted Avg.	0.818	0.804	0.804
SVM	0.788	Tumour	0.788	0.800	0.799
		Non-Tumour	0.777	0.788	0.788
		Micro Avg.	0.788	0.799	0.800
		Weighted Avg.	0.788	0.799	0.800
k-NN	0.828	Tumour	0.788	0.822	0.800
		Non-Tumour	0.777	0.811	0.800
		Micro Avg.	0.777	0.811	0.800
		Weighted Avg.	0.799	0.824	0.824

When compared to other linear models, the performance of the ensemble model was noteworthy. Individually, LR and SGD performed well on the original feature set and their combination further improved the results. Although the proposed voting ensemble model performed well, the obtained accuracy fell short of existing works and lacked the desired accuracy for brain tumor classification. More experiments were conducted for this purpose using CNN as a feature engineering technique and an ensemble learning model.

3.3. Results Using CNN Feature Engineering

In the second set of experiments, the performance of the proposed ensemble model and other models was assessed using CNN as a feature engineering technique to extract features from the dataset. Table 3 presents the results of the models when CNN features were used for model training. Expanding the feature set was the main goal of employing CNN model features, which was anticipated to increase the learning models' accuracy.

The results show that the proposed voting ensemble model LR+SGD leads the performance of all models applied in this study with an accuracy score of 0.995. The proposed ensemble model performs significantly better improving the accuracy by 0.15 over the original feature set. In the same manner, the results of the individual models have also improved using convoluted features. SGD obtained an accuracy score of 0.987 and the regression-based model LR achieves an accuracy score of 0.989. The tree-based models such as ETC and RF obtain accuracy scores of 0.926 and 0.958, respectively. Probability-based model GNB is again the least performer on the CNN features as well and achieved an accuracy score of 0.866. It is noted that GNB also showed some improvement in results as compared to the original features.

3.4. Results of K-Fold Cross-Validation

In order to verify the effectiveness of the proposed model this research work makes use of k-fold cross-validation. Table 4 provides the results of the 10-fold cross-validation. Cross-validation results reveal that the proposed ensemble model provides an average accuracy score of 0.996 while the average scores for precision, recall, and F1 are 0.998, 0.998, and 0.997, respectively.

3.5. Performance Comparison with State-of-the-Art Approaches

The results of the proposed model are compared with existing state-of-the-art studies to show the performance comparison in Table 5. For this purpose, several recently published works are selected so as to report the most recent results. Ref. [25] uses the NGBoost model for brain tumor detection and obtains 0.985 accuracy. Similarly, the study [26] utilizes a CNN deep learning model for the same task and reports a 0.950 accuracy score with the same dataset used in this study. An EfficientNet-B0 is employed in [27] for brain tumor detection that obtains a 0.988 accuracy score. The current study took the benefit of CNN features to train a voting classifier for brain tumor detection and obtained better results than existing state-of-the-art approaches with a classification accuracy of 0.999.

Table 3. Machine Learning Models Performance Using CNN as feature engineering.

Model	Accuracy	Class	Precision	Recall	F1 Score
Voting Classifier LR+SGD	0.995	Tumour	0.999	0.999	0.999
		Non-Tumour	0.999	0.999	0.999
		Micro Avg.	0.999	0.999	0.999
		Weighted Avg.	0.999	0.999	0.999
GBM	0.905	Tumour	0.928	0.944	0.926
		Non-Tumour	0.915	0.923	0.914
		Micro Avg.	0.927	0.931	0.924
		Weighted Avg.	0.915	0.935	0.918
GNB	0.866	Tumour	0.877	0.888	0.877
		Non-Tumour	0.844	0.866	0.855
		Micro Avg.	0.866	0.877	0.877
		Weighted Avg.	0.855	0.877	0.866
ETC	0.926	Tumour	0.907	0.903	0.905
		Non-Tumour	0.914	0.918	0.914
		Micro Avg.	0.913	0.913	0.913
		Weighted Avg.	0.900	0.900	0.900
LR	0.989	Tumour	0.966	0.999	0.977
		Non-Tumour	0.988	0.999	0.988
		M Avg.	0.977	0.999	0.988
		W Avg.	0.977	0.999	0.988
SGD	0.987	Tumour	0.985	0.997	0.986
		Non-Tumour	0.999	0.986	0.988
		Micro Avg.	0.988	0.988	0.988
		Weighted Avg.	0.988	0.988	0.988
RF	0.958	Tumour	0.927	0.954	0.935
		Non-Tumour	0.944	0.960	0.952
		Micro Avg.	0.944	0.960	0.952
		Weighted Avg.	0.934	0.954	0.944
DT	0.936	Tumour	0.900	0.928	0.914
		Non-Tumour	0.900	0.934	0.912
		Micro Avg.	0.900	0.900	0.915
		Weighted Avg.	0.914	0.900	0.900
SVM	0.978	Tumour	0.974	0.922	0.955
		Non-Tumour	0.977	0.944	0.944
		Micro Avg.	0.977	0.933	0.944
		Weighted Avg.	0.988	0.955	0.966
k-NN	0.982	Tumour	0.988	0.988	0.988
		Non-Tumour	0.977	0.977	0.977
		Micro Avg.	0.966	0.966	0.966
		Weighted Avg.	0.977	0.977	0.977

Table 4. Proposed approach k-fold cross-validation result.

Fold Number	Accuracy	Precision	Recall	F-Score
Fold-1	0.992	0.995	0.994	0.995
Fold-2	0.994	0.996	0.995	0.996
Fold-3	0.996	0.997	0.996	0.997
Fold-4	0.998	0.999	1.000	0.998
Fold-5	0.999	0.999	0.998	0.998
Fold-6	1.000	0.999	0.999	0.998
Fold-7	0.995	0.999	0.996	0.997
Fold-8	0.997	0.998	0.997	0.998
Fold-9	0.997	0.997	0.998	0.998
Fold-10	0.999	0.999	0.999	0.999
Average	**0.996**	**0.998**	**0.998**	**0.997**

Table 5. Performance comparison with state-of-the-art studies.

Reference	Year	Approach	Accuracy
[25]	2020	NGBoost	0.985
[26]	2021	CNN	0.950
[27]	2022	EfficientNet-B0	0.988
Proposed	2022	CNN features and voting Classifier	0.999

4. Conclusions and Future Work

The goal of this study was to create a framework that can properly distinguish between brain images with and without tumors and minimize the risks associated with this leading cause of mortality. The proposed method focuses on improving accuracy while reducing prediction errors for brain tumor detection. The experimental finding showed that by employing convolutional features, more accurate results were achieved than by using the original features. Furthermore, the ensemble classifier comprising LR and SGD outperformed individual models. Compared with state-of-the-art methods, the proposed method achieved an accuracy score of 0.999, demonstrating its superiority over existing methods and highlighting the effectiveness of the framework. In the future, we intend to employ deep-learning ensemble models to conduct tumor-type classifications with convolutional features. This study used a single dataset obtained from a single source. In the future, we plan to apply the proposed approach to other datasets to demonstrate its generalizability.

Author Contributions: Conceptualization, N.A. (Nazik Alturki) and M.U.; Data curation, N.A. (Nazik Alturki), A.I. and O.S.; Formal analysis, N.A. (Nazik Alturki), A.I. and A.M.; Funding acquisition, A.M.; Investigation, K.A. and O.S.; Methodology, N.A. (Nihal Abuzinadah); Project administration, K.A.; Resources, N.A. (Nihal Abuzinadah) and A.M.; Software, M.U. and N.A. (Nihal Abuzinadah); Supervision, I.A.; Validation, O.S. and I.A.; Visualization, K.A.; Writing—original draft, M.U. and A.I.; Writing—review & editing, I.A. All authors have read and agreed to the published version of the manuscript.

Funding: Princess Nourah bint Abdulrahman University Researchers Supporting Project number (PNURSP2023R333), Princess Nourah bint Abdulrahman University, Riyadh, Saudi Arabia.

Institutional Review Board Statement: Not applicable.

Informed Consent Statement: Not applicable.

Data Availability Statement: The datasets can be found by the authors at request.

Acknowledgments: Princess Nourah bint Abdulrahman University Researchers Supporting Project number (PNURSP2023R333), Princess Nourah bint Abdulrahman University, Riyadh, Saudi Arabia.

Conflicts of Interest: The authors declare no conflict of interests.

References

1. Umer, M.; Naveed, M.; Alrowais, F.; Ishaq, A.; Hejaili, A.A.; Alsubai, S.; Eshmawi, A.; Mohamed, A.; Ashraf, I. Breast Cancer Detection Using Convoluted Features and Ensemble Machine Learning Algorithm. *Cancers* **2022**, *14*, 6015. [CrossRef]
2. Amin, J.; Sharif, M.; Raza, M.; Saba, T.; Anjum, M.A. Brain tumor detection using statistical and machine learning method. *Comput. Methods Programs Biomed.* **2019**, *177*, 69–79. [CrossRef]
3. McFaline-Figueroa, J.R.; Lee, E.Q. Brain tumors. *Am. J. Med.* **2018**, *131*, 874–882. [CrossRef]
4. Arvold, N.D.; Lee, E.Q.; Mehta, M.P.; Margolin, K.; Alexander, B.M.; Lin, N.U.; Anders, C.K.; Soffietti, R.; Camidge, D.R.; Vogelbaum, M.A.; et al. Updates in the management of brain metastases. *Neuro-oncology* **2016**, *18*, 1043–1065. [CrossRef]
5. Saba, T.; Mohamed, A.S.; El-Affendi, M.; Amin, J.; Sharif, M. Brain tumor detection using fusion of hand crafted and deep learning features. *Cogn. Syst. Res.* **2020**, *59*, 221–230. [CrossRef]
6. Soomro, T.A.; Zheng, L.; Afifi, A.J.; Ali, A.; Soomro, S.; Yin, M.; Gao, J. Image Segmentation for MR Brain Tumor Detection Using Machine Learning: A Review. *IEEE Rev. Biomed. Eng.* **2023**, *16*, 70–90. [CrossRef]
7. Khan, A.H.; Abbas, S.; Khan, M.A.; Farooq, U.; Khan, W.A.; Siddiqui, S.Y.; Ahmad, A. Intelligent model for brain tumor identification using deep learning. *Appl. Comput. Intell. Soft Comput.* **2022**, *2022*, 8104054. [CrossRef]
8. Younis, A.; Qiang, L.; Nyatega, C.O.; Adamu, M.J.; Kawuwa, H.B. Brain Tumor Analysis Using Deep Learning and VGG-16 Ensembling Learning Approaches. *Appl. Sci.* **2022**, *12*, 7282. [CrossRef]
9. Zahoor, M.M.; Qureshi, S.A.; Khan, A.; Rehman, A.u.; Rafique, M. A novel dual-channel brain tumor detection system for MR images using dynamic and static features with conventional machine learning techniques. *Waves Random Complex Media* **2022**, 1–20. [CrossRef]
10. Senan, E.M.; Jadhav, M.E.; Rassem, T.H.; Aljaloud, A.S.; Mohammed, B.A.; Al-Mekhlafi, Z.G. Early Diagnosis of Brain Tumour MRI Images Using Hybrid Techniques between Deep and Machine Learning. *Comput. Math. Methods Med.* **2022**, *2022*, 8330833. [CrossRef]
11. Díaz-Pernas, F.J.; Martínez-Zarzuela, M.; Antón-Rodríguez, M.; González-Ortega, D. A deep learning approach for brain tumor classification and segmentation using a multiscale convolutional neural network. *Healthcare* **2021**, *9*, 153. [CrossRef]
12. Budati, A.; Babu, K. An automated brain tumor detection and classification from MRI images using machine learning techniques with IoT. *Environ. Dev. Sustain.* **2022**, *24*, 1–15. [CrossRef]
13. Akinyelu, A.A.; Zaccagna, F.; Grist, J.T.; Castelli, M.; Rundo, L. Brain Tumor Diagnosis Using Machine Learning, Convolutional Neural Networks, Capsule Neural Networks and Vision Transformers, Applied to MRI: A Survey. *J. Imaging* **2022**, *8*, 205. [CrossRef]
14. Raza, A.; Ayub, H.; Khan, J.A.; Ahmad, I.; Salama, A.S.; Daradkeh, Y.I.; Javeed, D.; Ur Rehman, A.; Hamam, H. A hybrid deep learning-based approach for brain tumor classification. *Electronics* **2022**, *11*, 1146. [CrossRef]
15. Ahmad, S.; Choudhury, P.K. On the Performance of Deep Transfer Learning Networks for Brain Tumor Detection using MR Images. *IEEE Access* **2022**, *10*, 59099–59114. [CrossRef]
16. Amran, G.A.; Alsharam, M.S.; Blajam, A.O.A.; Hasan, A.A.; Alfaifi, M.Y.; Amran, M.H.; Gumaei, A.; Eldin, S.M. Brain Tumor Classification and Detection Using Hybrid Deep Tumor Network. *Electronics* **2022**, *11*, 3457. [CrossRef]
17. Ullah, N.; Khan, J.A.; Khan, M.S.; Khan, W.; Hassan, I.; Obayya, M.; Negm, N.; Salama, A.S. An Effective Approach to Detect and Identify Brain Tumors Using Transfer Learning. *Appl. Sci.* **2022**, *12*, 5645. [CrossRef]
18. Hashmi, A.; Osman, A.H. Brain Tumor Classification Using Conditional Segmentation with Residual Network and Attention Approach by Extreme Gradient Boost. *Appl. Sci.* **2022**, *12*, 10791. [CrossRef]
19. Samee, N.A.; Mahmoud, N.F.; Atteia, G.; Abdallah, H.A.; Alabdulhafith, M.; Al-Gaashani, M.S.; Ahmad, S.; Muthanna, M.S.A. Classification Framework for Medical Diagnosis of Brain Tumor with an Effective Hybrid Transfer Learning Model. *Diagnostics* **2022**, *12*, 2541. [CrossRef]
20. Rasool, M.; Ismail, N.A.; Boulila, W.; Ammar, A.; Samma, H.; Yafooz, W.M.; Emara, A.H.M. A Hybrid Deep Learning Model for Brain Tumour Classification. *Entropy* **2022**, *24*, 799. [CrossRef]
21. DeAngelis, L.M. Brain tumors. *N. Engl. J. Med.* **2001**, *344*, 114–123. [CrossRef]
22. Fathi Kazerooni, A.; Bagley, S.J.; Akbari, H.; Saxena, S.; Bagheri, S.; Guo, J.; Chawla, S.; Nabavizadeh, A.; Mohan, S.; Bakas, S.; et al. Applications of radiomics and radiogenomics in high-grade gliomas in the era of precision medicine. *Cancers* **2021**, *13*, 5921. [CrossRef]
23. Habib, A.; Jovanovich, N.; Hoppe, M.; Ak, M.; Mamindla, P.; Colen, R.R.; Zinn, P.O. MRI-based radiomics and radiogenomics in the management of low-grade gliomas: Evaluating the evidence for a paradigm shift. *J. Clin. Med.* **2021**, *10*, 1411. [CrossRef]
24. Jena, B.; Saxena, S.; Nayak, G.K.; Balestrieri, A.; Gupta, N.; Khanna, N.N.; Laird, J.R.; Kalra, M.K.; Fouda, M.M.; Saba, L.; et al. Brain tumor characterization using radiogenomics in artificial intelligence framework. *Cancers* **2022**, *14*, 4052. [CrossRef]
25. Dutta, S.; Bandyopadhyay, S.K. Revealing brain tumor using cross-validated NGBoost classifier. *Int. J. Mach. Learn. Netw. Collab. Eng.* **2020**, *4*, 12–20. [CrossRef]
26. Methil, A.S. Brain tumor detection using deep learning and image processing. In Proceedings of the 2021 International Conference on Artificial Intelligence and Smart Systems (ICAIS), Tamil Nadu, India, 25–27 March 2021; pp. 100–108.
27. Shah, H.A.; Saeed, F.; Yun, S.; Park, J.H.; Paul, A.; Kang, J.M. A Robust Approach for Brain Tumor Detection in Magnetic Resonance Images Using Finetuned EfficientNet. *IEEE Access* **2022**, *10*, 65426–65438. [CrossRef]

8. Bohaju, J. Brain Tumor Database. July 2020. Available online: https://www.kaggle.com/datasets/jakeshbohaju/brain-tumor (accessed on 10 January 2023).
9. Breiman, L. Bagging predictors. *Mach. Learn.* **1996**, *24*, 123–140. [CrossRef]
10. Breiman, L. Random forests. *Mach. Learn.* **2001**, *45*, 5–32. [CrossRef]
11. Biau, G.; Scornet, E. A random forest guided tour. *Test* **2016**, *25*, 197–227. [CrossRef]
12. Manzoor, M.; Umer, M.; Sadiq, S.; Ishaq, A.; Ullah, S.; Madni, H.A.; Bisogni, C. RFCNN: Traffic accident severity prediction based on decision level fusion of machine and deep learning model. *IEEE Access* **2021**, *9*, 128359–128371. [CrossRef]
13. Kotsiantis, S.B. Decision trees: A recent overview. *Artif. Intell. Rev.* **2013**, *39*, 261–283. [CrossRef]
14. Juna, A.; Umer, M.; Sadiq, S.; Karamti, H.; Eshmawi, A.; Mohamed, A.; Ashraf, I. Water Quality Prediction Using KNN Imputer and Multilayer Perceptron. *Water* **2022**, *14*, 2592. [CrossRef]
15. Keller, J.M.; Gray, M.R.; Givens, J.A. A fuzzy k-nearest neighbor algorithm. *IEEE Trans. Syst. Man Cybern.* **1985**, *SMC-15*, 580–585. [CrossRef]
16. Besharati, E.; Naderan, M.; Namjoo, E. LR-HIDS: Logistic regression host-based intrusion detection system for cloud environments. *J. Ambient Intell. Humaniz. Comput.* **2019**, *10*, 3669–3692. [CrossRef]
17. Khammassi, C.; Krichen, S. A NSGA2-LR wrapper approach for feature selection in network intrusion detection. *Comput. Netw.* **2020**, *172*, 107183. [CrossRef]
18. Kleinbaum, D.G.; Dietz, K.; Gail, M.; Klein, M.; Klein, M. *Logistic Regression*; Springer: Berlin/Heidelberg, Germany, 2002.
19. Noble, W.S. What is a support vector machine? *Nat. Biotechnol.* **2006**, *24*, 1565–1567. [CrossRef]
20. Ashraf, I.; Narra, M.; Umer, M.; Majeed, R.; Sadiq, S.; Javaid, F.; Rasool, N. A Deep Learning-Based Smart Framework for Cyber-Physical and Satellite System Security Threats Detection. *Electronics* **2022**, *11*, 667. [CrossRef]
21. Friedman, J.H. Greedy function approximation: A gradient boosting machine. *Ann. Stat.* **2001**, *29*, 1189–1232. [CrossRef]
22. Umer, M.; Sadiq, S.; Nappi, M.; Sana, M.U.; Ashraf, I.; Karamti, H.; Eshmawi, A.A. ETCNN: Extra Tree and Convolutional Neural Network-based Ensemble Model for COVID-19 Tweets Sentiment Classification. *Pattern Recognit. Lett.* **2022**, *164*, 224–231. [CrossRef]
23. Majeed, R.; Abdullah, N.A.; Faheem Mushtaq, M.; Umer, M.; Nappi, M. Intelligent Cyber-Security System for IoT-Aided Drones Using Voting Classifier. *Electronics* **2021**, *10*, 2926. [CrossRef]
24. Rish, I. An empirical study of the naive Bayes classifier. In Proceedings of the IJCAI 2001 Workshop on Empirical Methods in Artificial Intelligence, Seattle, WA, USA, 4–6 August 2001; Volume 3, pp. 41–46.
25. Umer, M.; Sadiq, S.; Missen, M.M.S.; Hameed, Z.; Aslam, Z.; Siddique, M.A.; Nappi, M. Scientific papers citation analysis using textual features and SMOTE resampling techniques. *Pattern Recognit. Lett.* **2021**, *150*, 250–257. [CrossRef]
26. Bottou, L. Stochastic gradient descent tricks. *Neural Networks: Tricks of the Trade*, 2nd ed.; Springer: Berlin/Heidelberg, Germany, 2012; pp. 421–436.
27. Hameed, A.; Umer, M.; Hafeez, U.; Mustafa, H.; Sohaib, A.; Siddique, M.A.; Madni, H.A. Skin lesion classification in dermoscopic images using stacked Convolutional Neural Network. *J. Ambient. Intell. Humaniz. Comput.* **2021**, *28*, 1–15. [CrossRef]
28. Rustam, F.; Ishaq, A.; Munir, K.; Almutairi, M.; Aslam, N.; Ashraf, I. Incorporating CNN Features for Optimizing Performance of Ensemble Classifier for Cardiovascular Disease Prediction. *Diagnostics* **2022**, *12*, 1474. [CrossRef]

Disclaimer/Publisher's Note: The statements, opinions and data contained in all publications are solely those of the individual author(s) and contributor(s) and not of MDPI and/or the editor(s). MDPI and/or the editor(s) disclaim responsibility for any injury to people or property resulting from any ideas, methods, instructions or products referred to in the content.

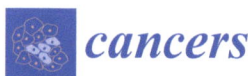

Systematic Review

The Extracellular Matrix in Glioblastomas: A Glance at Its Structural Modifications in Shaping the Tumoral Microenvironment—A Systematic Review

Salvatore Marino [1,†], Grazia Menna [1,*,†], Rina Di Bonaventura [2], Lucia Lisi [3], Pierpaolo Mattogno [2], Federica Figà [1], Lal Bilgin [1], Quintino Giorgio D'Alessandris [1], Alessandro Olivi [1,‡] and Giuseppe Maria Della Pepa [2,‡]

1. Department of Neuroscience, Neurosurgery Section, Università Cattolica del Sacro Cuore, 00168 Rome, Italy
2. Department of Neurosurgery, Fondazione Policlinico Universitario Agostino Gemelli IRCCS, 00168 Rome, Italy
3. Dipartimento di Sicurezza e Bioetica, Università Cattolica del Sacro Cuore, IRCSS-Fondazione Policlinico Universitario Agostino Gemelli, 00168 Rome, Italy
* Correspondence: mennagrazia@gmail.com
† These authors contributed equally to this work.
‡ These authors also contributed equally to this work.

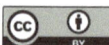

Citation: Marino, S.; Menna, G.; Di Bonaventura, R.; Lisi, L.; Mattogno, P.; Figà, F.; Bilgin, L.; D'Alessandris, Q.G.; Olivi, A.; Della Pepa, G.M. The Extracellular Matrix in Glioblastomas: A Glance at Its Structural Modifications in Shaping the Tumoral Microenvironment—A Systematic Review. *Cancers* **2023**, *15*, 1879. https://doi.org/10.3390/cancers15061879

Academic Editor: Axel H. Schönthal

Received: 23 January 2023
Revised: 5 March 2023
Accepted: 16 March 2023
Published: 21 March 2023

Copyright: © 2023 by the authors. Licensee MDPI, Basel, Switzerland. This article is an open access article distributed under the terms and conditions of the Creative Commons Attribution (CC BY) license (https://creativecommons.org/licenses/by/4.0/).

Simple Summary: The new trends in the research on glioblastomas (GBMs) are focusing on understanding the crosstalk between proper neoplastic tissue and its microenvironment. Against this background, the extracellular matrix (ECM) has been classically linked to a purely structural role. However, it has recently become clear that it actively shapes the functional responses of cells to their environment as well. While many components of the ECM have been isolated and characterized, its modifications in the specific setting of GBMs have only been recently explored in the literature. The aim of this paper is to provide a systematic review on the topic and to assess the ECM's role in shaping tumoral development.

Abstract: Background and aim: While many components of the ECM have been isolated and characterized, its modifications in the specific setting of GBMs have only been recently explored in the literature. The aim of this paper is to provide a systematic review on the topic and to assess the ECM's role in shaping tumoral development. Methods: An online literature search was launched on PubMed/Medline and Scopus using the research string "((Extracellular matrix OR ECM OR matrix receptor OR matrix proteome) AND (glioblastoma OR GBM) AND (tumor invasion OR tumor infiltration))", and a systematic review was conducted in accordance with the PRISMA-P guidelines. Results: The search of the literature yielded a total of 693 results. The duplicate records were then removed (n = 13), and the records were excluded via a title and abstract screening; 137 studies were found to be relevant to our research question and were assessed for eligibility. Upon a full-text review, 59 articles were finally included and were summarized as follows based on their focus: (1) proteoglycans; (2) fibrillary proteins, which were further subdivided into the three subcategories of collagen, fibronectin, and laminins; (3) glycoproteins; (4) degradative enzymes; (5) physical forces (6) and glioma cell and microglia migratory and infiltrative patterns. Conclusions: Our systematic review demonstrates that the ECM should not be regarded anymore as a passive scaffold statically contributing to mechanical support in normal and pathological brain tissue but as an active player in tumor-related activity.

Keywords: glioblastoma; extracellular matrix; cancer; tumor microenvironment

1. Introduction

The new trends in the research on glioblastomas (GBMs) are focusing more and more on the understanding of the crosstalk between proper neoplastic tissue and its microenvironment (TME). The microenvironmental contribution seems to be critical in tumor development, progression, relapse, and resistance to therapies. A definition of the "seed and soil" approach has recently been introduced to describe the glioblastoma landscape: the TME, mainly constituted by inflammatory cells (microglia, monocytes, and macrophages) and stem cells, acts as a fertile "soil" interacting with the "seed", which is represented by proper neoplastic glial cells [1]. Against this background, the extracellular matrix (ECM) has been classically linked to a mere structural role. However, it has recently become clear that it actively shapes the functional responses of cells to their environment as well. Therefore, the ECM should not be regarded anymore as a passive scaffold statically contributing to mechanical support but as an active player in tumor-related activity: it shows dynamic "structural" modifications and interactions under the pressure of the dysregulated TME, it performs active crosstalk with the inflammatory and stem compartment, and it is able to influence cellular migration [2–5]. While many components of the ECM have been isolated and characterized, its modifications in the specific setting of GBMs have only been recently explored in the literature. The aim of this paper is to provide an updated systematic review on the topic and to assess the ECM's role in shaping tumoral development.

2. Materials and Methods

The study presented herein was conducted in accordance with the PRISMA-P (Preferred Reporting Items for Systematic Review and Meta-Analysis Protocols) guidelines [2]. An online literature search was launched on PubMed/Medline and Scopus using the research string "((Extracellular matrix OR ECM OR matrix receptor OR matrix proteome) AND (glioblastoma OR GBM) AND (tumor invasion OR tumor infiltration))"; research was last conducted in September 2022. Two authors, S.M. and F.F., independently conducted the abstract screening for eligibility. Any discordance was solved through consensus with a third senior author, G.M.D.P. No restrictions on date of publication were made. Exclusion criteria were as follows: studies published in languages other than English and meta-analyses. A systematic abstract screening of the references (forward search) was performed to identify additional records.

3. Results

The search of the literature yielded a total of 693 results. The duplicate records were then removed (n = 13), and the records were excluded via a title and abstract screening; 138 studies were found to be relevant to our research question and were assessed for eligibility (Figure 1). Upon a full-text review and forward search, 82 articles were finally included.

The reviewed papers were further divided into six categories based on their focus:
(1) Proteoglycans (Table 1);
(2) Fibrillary proteins, which were further subdivided into three subcategories: collagen (Table 2a), fibronectin (Table 2b), and laminins (Table 2c);
(3) Periostin (Table 3);
(4) Glycoproteins (Table 4);
(5) Degradative Enzymes (Table 5);
(6) Physical forces (Table 6);
(7) Glioma cell and microglia migratory and infiltrative patterns (Table 7).

Table 1. Proteoglycans.

Author	Year	Type of Study	Sample Size	Main Findings
Logun, M.T. [6]	2017	In vitro cell culture	1 human cell line	CS-GAGs directly induce the enhanced cell migration and haptotaxis of glioma cells.
Logun, M.T. [7]	2019	In vitro cell culture	1 murine cell line	GAG promotes GBM cell invasion.
Schrappe, M. [8]	1991	Human GBMs and monoclonal antibodies	5 human GBMs	Human GBMs specifically express a chondroitin sulfate proteoglycan that is recognized by monoclonal antibodies and is localized on the glioma cell surface.
Kim, Y. [9]	2018	Mathematical model		High-molecular-weight CSPGs can regulate the exodus of local reactive astrocytes from the main tumor lesion, leading to an encapsulation of noninvasive tumors and an inhibition of tumor invasion.
Silver, D.J. [10]	2013	In vitro cell culture and xenograft	3 human cell lines	Microenvironmental glycosylated chondroitin sulfate proteoglycans inversely correlate with the invasive character of human gliomas.
Onken, J. [11]	2013	In vitro cell culture and siRNA	2 human cell lines	Versican isoform V1 is a proliferation-enhancing and promigratory molecule in high-grade glioma in vitro.
Tran, V.M. [12]	2018	In vitro cell culture	4 human cell lines and 2 murine cell lines	HPSE has a role in tumor invasion, acting on HSPGs on the cell surface.
Su, G. [13]	2006	In vitro cell culture	5 human cell lines	HSPGs have a great capability to promote FGF-2 signaling. The enhanced HSPG activity correlated with a high level of expression of Gpc-1 and structural HSGAG alterations.
Watanabe, A. [14]	2005	Reverse transcription PCR	10 glioma cell lines, 2 GBM specimens, and 2 normal brain specimens	Syndecan-1 is a key molecule in the motility of cells; it is crucial in coupling the organization of fascin spikes in response to a physiological extracellular ligand, TSP-1, and an overexpression of syndecan-1 in a heterologous cell type is sufficient for causing a dramatic enhancement of cell spreading and formation of fascin spikes in response to TSP-1. It is significantly expressed by GBM cells.
Chen, J.E. [15]	2018	matrix-bound HA and xenograft GBM population	1 patient-derived xenograft GBM population	GBM migration is strongly influenced by HA molecular weight.
Hayen, W. [16]	1999	hyaluronan-containing fibrin gels and GBM cell lines	1 GBM cell line	In complex three-dimensional substrates, the predominant effect of hyaluronan on cell migration might be indirect and requires modulation of fibrin polymerization.
Chen, J.W.E. [17]	2018	In vitro cell culture and hyaluronan synthesis inhibition	2 cell lines	GBM cells under hypoxia show invasive behavior. The lack of matrix-bound HA affects GBM response by inducing compensatory HA secretion of this essential cell adhesive biomolecule, which is associated with increased GBM invasion.
Chen, J.W.E. [18]	2022	culture of patient-derived GBM cells		CD133+ GBM subpopulation increases in response to both hypoxia and matrix-bound hyaluronan.
Akiyama, Y. [19]	2001	Cell culture and surgical specimen	Antibody blockage	HA-receptors contribute to brain tumor adhesion, proliferation, migration, and biological features.
Pibuel, M.A. [20]	2021	In vitro cell culture and hyaluronan synthesis inhibition	2 human cell lines	4MU markedly inhibits cell migration and induces senescence in human GBM cell lines; 4MU modulates the expression and the distribution of CD44, RHAMM, and MMP-2.
Tsatas, D. [21]	2002	In vitro cell culture and antibody blockage	4 glioma cell lines	Hyaluronan induces genes encoding matrix-degrading enzymes (plasminogen cascade).
Zhang, H. [22]	2022	In vitro cell culture and hyaluronan synthesis inhibition	3 cell lines	HA was found to mediate glioma proliferation, progression, and invasion; it potentially promoted macrophage recruitment and M2 polarization through the IL-1/CHI3L1 and TGF-b/CHI3L1 axes.

Table 2. (a) Collagen, (b) fibronectin, and (c) laminins.

(a)

Author	Year	Type of Study	Sample Size	Main Findings
Calori, I.R. [23]	2022	GBM cell lines and type I collagen	4 cell lines	The enzymatic cleavage of collagen affects spheroid morphology and increases cell migration while maintaining cell viability.
Wang, Y. [24]	2022	GBM cell lines and COL1A2 siRNA	3 cell lines	COL1A2 plays an important role in driving GBM progression. COL1A2 inhibition attenuates GBM proliferation by promoting cell cycle arrest.
Chintala, et al. [25]	1996	In vitro cell culture	4 cell lines	Collagen type II is involved in migration and invasion of glioblastoma cells.
Mammoto, T. et al. [26]	2013	In vitro cell culture and antibody blockage	3 cell lines	D-penicillamine decreases collagen expression, disrupts collagen structure in tumors, and inhibits brain tumor growth.
Senner, V. [27]	2008	In vitro cell culture and siRNA	5 cell lines	Glioma cell lines can utilize collagen type XVI as a substrate for adhesion.
Huijbers, I.J., et al. [28]	2010	Human cell culture and antibody blockage	79 gliomas	Fibrillar collagens are extensively deposited in GBMs; the collagen type I internalization receptor Endo180 is both highly expressed in these tumors and serves to mediate the invasion of tumor cells through collagen-containing matrices.
Lin, J. [29]	2021	In vitro cell culture and xenograft	58 gliomas	P4HA2 is a prognostic marker and exerts oncogenic functions to promote the malignancy of gliomas (grade II to grade IV). The underlying mechanism may be regulating the collagen-dependent PI3K/AKT signaling pathway.
Jiang, X. [30]	2017	In vitro cell culture and xenograft	2 cell lines	HSP47 promotes GBM stem-like cell survival by modulating tumor microenvironment ECM through TGF-β pathway.

(b)

Author	Year	Type of Study	Sample Size	Main Findings
Ohnishi, T. [31]	1998	In vitro human cell culture and antibody blockage	9 GBM samples	Fibronectin concentration seems to be higher in tumor cells and promotes migration of glioma cells.
Chintala, S.K. [32]	1996	In vitro human cell culture and antibody blockage	13 GBM samples	Glioblastoma cells produce collagen type IV, laminins, and fibronectin.
Caffo, M. [33]	2004	In vitro human cell culture and antibody blockage	6 GBM samples	Integrins appear to be of great interest in GBM treatment either as targeted therapies, drug-delivering vectors, or diagnostic tools for tumor imaging.
Serres, E. [34]	2013	In vitro human cell culture and antibody blockage	3 GBM lines	FN produced by tumor cells has a role in GBM pathophysiology.
Sengupta, S. [35]	2010	Xenograft and siRNA	Murine glioma cell line	Fibronectin silencing aborts integrin signaling in GL261 cells and fails to initiate Src kinase and STAT3 activity, thus aggressively reducing survivin expression.
Huang, J.M. [36]	2006	In vitro cell culture and GBM cell line	1 GBM cell line	The interaction between beta1-integrin and FN may stimulate U251MG cell migration, changing the structure of the microfilament skeleton and the number of pseudopodia. Beta1-integrin may play a role in the LN-mediated in vitro invasion of U251MG cells.
Yu, S. [37]	2020	Xenograft and siRNA	3 cell lines	GBP2 dramatically promotes GBM tumor growth and invasion in mice and significantly reduces the survival time of the mice with a tumor.
Kabir, F. [38]	2022	Mathematical model—bioinformatics model	7 data sets	FN1 has prognostic value in GBMs.

(c)

Author	Year	Model Used	Sample Size	Main Findings
Tysnes, B.B. [39]	1999	Xenograft	5 GBM samples	Laminins can be produced by GFAP positive cells during glioma cell invasion in humans.

Table 2. Cont.

Author	Year	Type of Study	Sample Size	Main Findings
Caffo, M. [33]	2004	In vitro human cells and antibody blockage	6 GBM samples	Integrins appear to be of great interest in GB treatment either as targeted therapies, drug-delivering vectors, or diagnostic tools for tumor imaging.
Sun, T. [40]	2022	Xenograft culture	107 GBMS samples	Inhibition of the vascular BM component laminin-411, which is produced by tumor cells like many other tumor ECM components, disrupts the perivascular CSC niche, negatively affects CSCs, and may enhance the efficacy of glioma therapy.
Khazenzon, N.M. [41]	2003	In vitro human cell culture and antibody blockage	2 cell lines	Laminin-8 may play an important role in glioma invasion.
Gamble, J.T. [42]	2018	Xenograft culture	1 cell line	Laminin alpha 5 significantly lowers the invasion of mobile U251MG cells.

Table 3. Periostin.

Author	Year	Model Used	Sample Size	Main Findings
Wang, H. [43]	2013	Frozen glioma tissue and microarray	220 frozen glioma tissues	The expression levels of POSTN are relative to glioma grade progression and are inversely correlated with overall survival in high-grade glioma patients.
Landré, V. [44]	2016	In vitro human cell culture, plasmids, and antibodies	2 cell lines	TAp73 controls glioblastoma cell invasion by regulating the expression of the matricellular protein POSTN.
Ouanouki, A. [45]	2018	In vitro human cell culture	1 cell line	Periostin acts as a central element in TGF-β-induced EMT.

Table 4. Glycoprotein—tenascin.

Author	Year	Model Used	Sample Size	Main Findings
Xia, S. [46]	2016	Xenograft culture	2 human cell lines	TNC expression levels or gene copy numbers do not significantly affect patient survival, and TNC knockdown cells are more sensitive to antiproliferative strategies.
Hirata, E. [47]	2009	Xenograft culture	1 human cell line	Endogenous tenascin facilitates GBM cell invasion by regulating focal adhesion, and, therefore, GBMs with higher Tenascin C expression have a more aggressive behavior.
Zhang, J.F. [48]	2019	In vitro human cell culture and siRNA	2 cell lines	IL-33/NF-κB/TNC supports cancer progression.
Sarkar, S. [49]	2015	Xenograft culture	7 human cell lines	TNC is a promoter of the invasiveness of BTICs through a mechanism involving ADAM-9 proteolysis via the c-Jun NH2-terminal kinase pathway.
Sarkar, S. [50]	2006	In vitro human cell culture	2 cell lines	Tenascin-C is a favorable substrate for glioma invasiveness; its effect is mediated through MMP-12.
Mai, J. [51]	2002	In vitro human cell culture		Cathepsin B and Tenascin-C are highly expressed in malignant anaplastic astrocytomas and glioblastomas when compared to normal brain tissues and are associated with tumor neovessels.

Table 5. Degradative enzymes.

Author	Year	Model Used	Sample Size	Main Findings
Li, Q. [52]	2016 Mar	Data set and genome mRNA	23 types of MMPs and 305 gliomas	Patients expressing MMP9 may have a longer survival and may benefit from temozolomide chemotherapy.
Lakka, S.S. [53]	2004	In vitro human cell culture and siRNA	1 cell line	Simultaneous RNAi-mediated targeting of MMP-9 and cathepsin B has potential application in the treatment of human gliomas.
Kargiotis, O. [54]	2008	In vitro human cell culture and xenograft	4 cell lines	MMP-2 inhibition induces apoptotic cell death and suppresses tumor growth.
Schuler, P.J. [55]	2012	Xenograft	1 cell line	uPA, uPAR, MMP-2, and MMP-9 play an important role in GBM growth.
Sun, J. [56]	2019	In vitro human cell culture	12 GBMs	TRAF6 and MMP9 have higher expression in GBMs compared to adjacent tissues. High expression of TRAF6 and MMP9 is significantly associated with unfavorable prognoses.
Zhao, Y. [57]	2008	In vitro human cell culture and recombinant protein	1 cell line	uPA directly cleaves the latent form of MMP-9 both at the N- and C-terminus, and this novel activation pathway promotes U1242 GBM cell invasion.
Chang, L. [58]	2015	In vitro human cell culture	1 cell line	The hedgehog signaling pathway promotes the invasion and migration of GBM cells by enhancing MMP-2 and MMP-9 expression via the PI3K/AKT pathway.
Zheng, Q. [59]	2019	In vitro human cell culture	2 cell lines	IL-17A promotes GBM cell migration and invasion via PI3K/AKT signaling pathway.
Das, G. [60]	2011	Human cell culture and antibodies	2 cell lines	Rictor bridges two major pathways—Akt (PKB)/mTOR and Raf-1-MEK-ERK—for regulation of MMP-9 activity and invasion of glioma tumor cells.
Djediai, S. [61]	2021	Human cell culture and RNA isolation	1 cell line	MT1-MMP and TGF-β mediate EMT-like induction in glioblastoma cells.
Zhai, Y. [62]	2022	Immunostaining with rabbit monoclonal antibodies	214 gliomas	MT1-MMP, β1-integrin, and YAP1 are prognostic biomarkers.
Held-Feindt, J. [63]	2005	Human GBM samples, GBM cell lines, and RT-PCR	4 GBM cell lines	In human glioblastomas, secretory proteases, such as ADAMTS4 and ADAMTS5, are expressed at the mRNA and protein levels in considerable amounts.
Siney, E.J. [64]	2017	Excised high-grade glioma and antibody inhibition	12 excised GBMs	ADAM10 and ADAM17 inhibition selectively increases GSC migration, and the migrated GSCs exhibit a differentiated phenotype.

Table 6. Physical forces.

Author	Year	Model Used	Sample Size	Main Findings
Herrera-Perez, M. [65]	2015	In vitro human cell culture in 3D matrix		Migration of glioblastoma stem cells is reduced by the presence of hyaluronan.
Ulrich, T.A. [66]	2009	In vitro human cell culture	2 cell lines	Increasing ECM rigidity can induce a cascade of phenotypic changes in human glioma cells, which includes increased cell spreading, faster motility, and enhanced proliferation.
Kaufman, L.J. [67]	2005	Human cells encapsulated in 3D hydrogel	1 cell line	GBM tumors are affected significantly by the total collagen concentration in the gel, and there are distinct growth patterns in low- and high-concentration collagen type I gels. Specifically, increasing concentrations of collagen type I correlate positively with invasion but negatively with MTS growth.
Wang, C. [68]	2014	In vitro human cell culture	15 primer sequences	Matrix stiffness modulates GBM progression.
Lim, E.J. [69]	2018	In vitro cell culture and siRNA	1 cell line	tMSLCs, as stromal cells, provide force-mediated proinvasive ECM remodeling in the GBM microenvironment.
Pu, W. [70]	2020	In vitro human cell culture	2 cell lines	MPs play pivotal roles in the invasiveness of GBMs by degrading the surrounding tissue, activating signal transduction, and releasing ECM-bound growth factors.

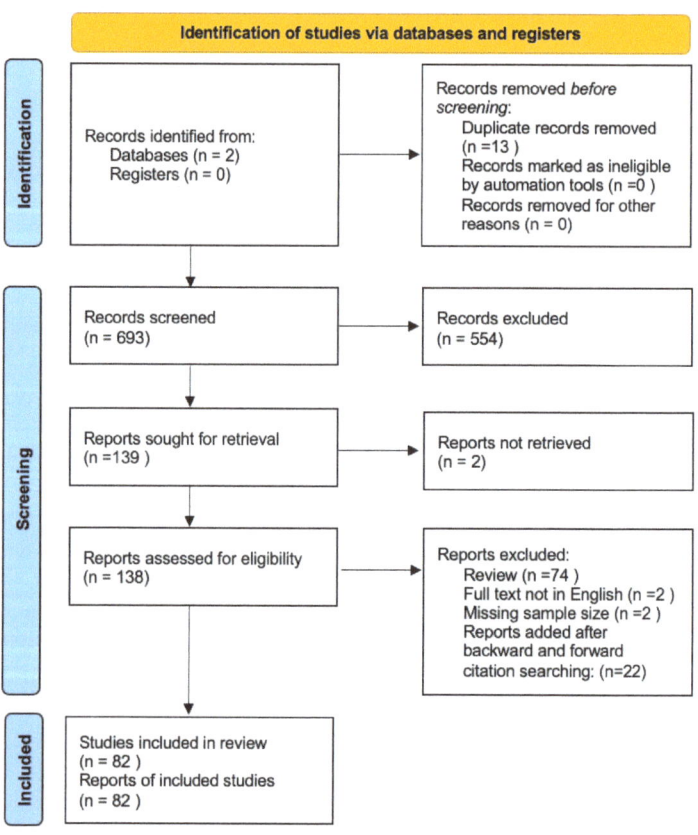

Figure 1. Prisma flowchart summarizing the results of our research.

Table 7. Glioma cell and microglia migratory and infiltrative patterns.

Author	Year	Model Used	Sample Size	Main Findings
Koh, I. [71]	2018	In vitro human cell culture	1 cell line	MMP9 and HAS2 are highly upregulated in pdGCs cultured within the pdECM. In fact, both MMPs and HASs have been implicated in playing crucial roles in GBM invasiveness.
Herrera-Perez, M. [65]	2015	In vitro human cell culture		GSC migration is not limited to a unique migration mode that is usually observed in in vitro studies but is able to concomitantly exhibit multiple migration modes (collective and single) as a response to the heterogeneity of the environment.
Rao, S.S. [72]	2013	In vitro human cell culture and 3D matrix	1 cell line	GBM migration is an inverse function of HA concentration, with HA impeding and eventually stopping cell movement.
Cui, Y. [73]	2020	In vitro human cell culture and 3D matrix	1 cell line	HA addition to the collagen culture environment induces many changes consistent with the amoeboid migratory phenotype, including rounded morphology, squeezing or gliding motility, cortical actin expression, reduced cell–fiber interactions, and reduced integrin expression.
Hirata, E. [74]	2012	Xenograft and shRNA	3 cell lines	Zizimin1 appears to play an important role in the formation of multiple pseudopodia and invasion of the brain parenchyma.
Lively, S. [75]	2013	Cultured rat microglial cells	1 cell line	Microglial cells migrate during CNS development and after CNS damage or disease.
de Vrij, J. [76]	2015	Human cell culture	2 cell lines	EVs are mechanisms for GBMs to use to induce MT1-MMP expression in GBM associated microglia, supporting tumor growth.
Gabrusiewicz, K. [77]	2011	Murine glioma cells and xenograft	1 cell line	Resident microglia and blood-derived macrophages contribute to a pool of glioma-infiltrating immune cells and regulate tumor angiogenesis and invasion, which are essential for glioma progression.
Bettinger, I. [78]	2002	Murine glioma cell and mouse microglial cell cultures	1 cell line	Microglial cells promote the invasive phenotype of diffuse astrocytoma cells.
Markovic, D.S. [79]	2005	Murine glioma cell and microglial cell cultures		The presence of microglia in a GBM has a protumorigenic effect.
Markovic, D.S. [80]	2009	Murine glioma cells and shRNA	1 cell line	Protumorigenic role of microglial cells is substantial and may put microglial cells into focus as a target for new brain tumor therapies. Therapeutic TLR blockade, which may be achieved with TLR subtype-specific antagonists, could serve as a future tool to attenuate microglia-promoted tumor invasion.
Wu, C.Y.J. [81]	2020	Human cell culture and poli- and monoclonal antibodies	3 cell lines	Chemokine axis in the glioma microenvironment is subject to CCL5-mediated invasion, and such regulation is facilitated by GAM activation. Restriction of calcium-dependent pathways may be pivotal in eliminating CCL5/GAM-regulated glioma invasion.
Kulla, A. [82]	2000	Human cell culture	90 gliomas	Higher numbers of tumor-infiltrating macrophagic/microglial cells are present in TN-positive areas of human gliomas; TN serves as a permissive substrate for macrophage migration and may have a certain role in modulating and possibly promoting the trafficking of cells of monocyte lineage in malignant human gliomas.
Xia, S. [46]	2016	Xenograft culture and shRNA	2 cell lines	TNC knockdown cells are more sensitive to antiproliferative strategies, which could ultimately lead to novel combinatory antitumor strategies that can target both tumor invasion and proliferation.
Hu, F. [83]	2015	Murine and human cells and animal xenograft	5 cell lines	Versican, released from gliomas, promotes tumor expansion through glioma-associated microglial/macrophage TLR2 signaling and subsequent expression of MT1-MMP.
Juliano, J. [84]	2018	Animal model and retrovirus injection		Increased density of glioma cells is correlated with increased activation of microglia.

3.1. Proteoglycans

Proteoglycans are a heterogeneous group of complex extracellular and cell surface macromolecules composed of a central core protein with covalently linked glycosaminoglycan (GAG) chains. Through interactions with chemokines, neurotrophins, growth factors and the other components of the ECM, proteoglycans (PGs) play a critical role in many basic processes of the CNS, including cellular proliferation, migration, specification, synaptogenesis, plasticity, and regeneration [6]. For these reasons, it has been proposed that PGs could be involved in several aspects of tumor biology, including cell proliferation, tumor cell adhesion and migration, inflammation, and angiogenesis. Indeed, recent studies have proven that heparan sulfate proteoglycans (HSPGs) and chondroitin sulfate proteoglycans (CSPGs) are largely upregulated in GBM samples relative to normal brain tissue [7].

Chondroitin sulfate proteoglycans (CSPGs) consist of a protein core and covalently attached chondroitin sulfate side chains. It has been noticed that CSPGs and related enzymes are upregulated in the GBM microenvironment relative to normal tissue [8]. Similarly, in vitro studies have shown an upregulation of focal adhesion proteins, such as FAK and Vinculin, and a faster migration of glioma cells in oversulfated hydrogel matrices when compared to nonsulfated hydrogels. Moreover, these data suggest that CSPGs can modulate glioma invasiveness in a GAG-sulfation-dependent manner. Indeed, CSPGs show a different affinity to chemokines and chemokine receptors according to the sulfatation rate of CS-GAG [7]. Beyond the sulfatation rate, even the pure concentration of CSPGs in the microenvironment has been identified as a major parameter in the regulation of glioma cell invasiveness. In fact, low-CSPG levels in the microenvironment are associated with the downregulation of the LAR (leukocyte common antigen-related)-CSGAG complex while high-CSPG levels induce its upregulation. LAR is a CS-GAG receptor that regulates cell adhesion to the ECM components. When LAR-CSGAG is downregulated, adhesion between the tumor cells and the ECM components is weak, therefore allowing the tumor cells to spread. On the other hand, high levels of CSPGs and, consequently, an upregulation of LAR-CSGAG induces strong adhesion, preventing the dispersion of the glioma cells. Moreover, LAR-CSGAG seems to influence the activation and migration of the microglia toward the tumor periphery [9,10].

Versican is one of the most represented proteins among the CSPGs in the ECM. An in vitro cell culture study revealed an important role of Versican in the regulation of glioma cell migration and adhesion. Indeed, the downregulation of Versican in the isoform V1 by siRNAs is associated with a significant reduction in proliferation and migration in glioblastoma cell lines, and TGF-beta 2, a well-known modulator of glioma cell invasion, was identified as the primary inductor of Versican 1 [11].

HSPGs consist of a core protein and covalently attached heparan sulfate (HS) glycosaminoglycan chains. Extensive co- and posttranslational enzymatic modifications particularly involving the 6-O-sulfate (6OS) of glucosamine, generate great structural heterogeneity. An analysis conducted on human GBM cell lines and murine GBM cell lines demonstrated great heterogeneity in the content and in the structure of HS glycosaminoglycans between different glioma cell lines, suggesting a role in tumorigenesis and subtype differentiation. Heparanase is an enzyme involved in the biological regulation of HSPGs since it cleaves HS chains to reduce the HS chain length and to release smaller biologically active oligosaccharides. Heparanase induces the modification of the HS content and structure in the microenvironment and, therefore, is thought to be involved in GBM genesis. Indeed, a study on cell invasion into a three-dimensional matrix showed that clones with heterozygous deletions in HPSE and reduced HPSE expression exhibit a marked decrease in tumor cell invasion and cell adhesion to laminins [12].

Glypicans and Syndecans represent the most expressed families of heparan sulfate proteoglycans in the brain. Glypicans are overexpressed in the glioma microenvironment when compared to normal brain tissue and, according to the literature, can stimulate glioma growth by inducing the upregulation of the FGF-2 signal [13,14]. Similarly, the Syndecan family is overexpressed in the glioma microenvironment. Particularly, Syndecan-1 is overexpressed in almost all glioma cell lines studied and is poorly expressed in normal specimens. It has been suggested that the overexpression of Syndecan-1 in the glioma microenvironment induces tumor invasion through the upregulation of thrombospondin-1 [14].

Hyaluronan is a linear and nonsulfated GAG which can bind ECM proteins and proteoglycans, building a three-dimensional network. HA serves as a ligand for the membrane receptor CD-44 and the RHAMM and MEK/ERK signaling pathways, participating in cellular growth, cellular proliferation, and cellular differentiation. In vitro studies have demonstrated that glioma cell behavior differs on the base of the HA structure in the tumor microenvironment since hydrogel matrices containing high-molecular-weight HA (500K) showed significantly reduced invasion when compared to all other hydrogel groups (-HA, 10, and 60K) [15]. Moreover, gels resulting from fibrin polymerization in the presence of HA stimulate glioma cell migration, suggesting that HA could regulate glioma cell invasiveness by modulating the fibrin fiber architecture [16]. The recent data show that hypoxia could enhance endogenous HA production by glioblastoma cells [17] and that HA could stimulate glioblastoma growth by upregulating CD133+ GBM cell fractions [18]. Concerning HA downstream signaling inducing glioma cell migration, receptor CD-44 and RHAMM appear to be involved [19]. CD44-HA mediated cell invasion can be modulated by EGFR, a well-known receptor overexpressed in gliomas. In fact, CD-44 binds to EGFR, leading to an upregulation of urokinase-type plasminogen activator (uPA), urokinase-type plasminogen activator receptor (uPAR), and plasminogen activator inhibitor-1 (PAI-1) in response to HA [20,21]. Moreover, recent studies have suggested that HA potentially promotes macrophage recruitment and M2 polarization through the IL-1/CHI3L1 and TGF-b/CHI3L1 axes and that it also regulates the expression of PD-L1 [22].

3.2. Fibrillar Proteins

3.2.1. Collagen

Normal brain tissue ECMs are poor in collagen, whereas its content in the glioma microenvironment and especially around vessels presents a large increase. Actually, different subtypes of collagen have been investigated over the years and are related to GBM invasiveness. Recent findings have shown that GBM cell lines form tight spheroids in the presence of type I collagen and that the enzymatic cleavage of collagen affects spheroid morphology and increases cell migration [23]. In particular, the collagen alpha-2(I) chain (COL1A2) was found to be upregulated in GBMs compared with normal brain tissue, and it is related to poor progression-free survival and overall survival [24]. Similarly, collagen type III was found to play a role in the modulation of migration and the invasion of glioblastoma cell lines in a dose-related manner; moreover, migration and invasion were inhibited in the presence of monoclonal type III collagen antibodies [25]. In vitro studies revealed that, under the specific conditions of physical compaction, human glioblastoma cell lines induce the expression of collagen type IV and type VI. Moreover, collagen disruptors such as β-aminopropionitrile induced the inhibition of glioblastoma growth in the mouse orthotopic brain tumor model [26]. Collagen type XVI mRNA was also found to be upregulated in glioblastoma cell lines. It seems to play a role in glioma cell adhesion to the ECM since a SiRNA knockdown resulted in decreased cell adhesion, although migration remained unchanged [27].

Different families of receptors and different pathways have been supposed to be involved in collagen-related GBM invasion. Functionally, Endo180 (CD280), a collagen-binding receptor overexpressed in GBMs, serves as the major collagen internalization receptor in GBMs and is critical in glioma cell invasion into the ECM [28]. Prolyl-4-hydroxylase subunit 2 (P4HA2) is a member of the collagen modification enzymes involved in the remodeling of the extracellular matrix (ECM). The main transcriptional P4HA2 level was found to be higher in glioma samples compared to normal brain tissue, and this correlates with glioma grading and patient survival; moreover, a P4HA2 knockdown significantly decreased cellular invasion and migration in Matrigel. An in vivo subcutaneous xenograft assay in a nude mouse model led to the same conclusions. Since P4HA2 overexpression correlates with higher levels of collagen types I, IV, and VI, a pathway was hypothesized in which P4HA4 promotes an overexpression of the collagen content, which serves as a major ligand for the activation of PI3K/AKT signaling [29]. HSP47 serves as a human chaperone protein for collagen. Recent findings suggest that HSP47 is significantly overexpressed in GBMs and that it promotes GBM stem-like cell survival by modulating the tumor microenvironment through the TGF-β pathway [30].

3.2.2. Fibronectin

Fibronectin (FN) is a high-molecular-weight glycoprotein poorly represented in normal brain tissue ECMs that binds cellular receptors such as integrins and the other components of the ECM, playing an important role in cellular growth, cellular differentiation, migration and embryonic development. In vitro and in vivo immunohistochemical studies revealed that fibronectin, especially the isoform containing the ED-A and ED-B sequences, and fibronectin cellular receptors are present in almost all glioblastoma microenvironments especially around the vessels [31–33]. In cell cultures, glioblastoma cells showed chemotactic migration towards fibronectin in a dose-dependent manner; moreover, cell adhesion to fibronectin appeared to be dose-related and dependent on glioma invasiveness [34]. In 3D matrix cultures, the depletion of FN by targeted short hairpin RNA expression compromised collective invasion. Similarly, in orthotopic grafts, FN depletion significantly reduced tumor growth and angiogenesis [35,36].

It has been hypothesized that FN-related GBM invasion downstream involves the Integrin B1 fibronectin receptor and the Src kinase/STAT3 signaling pathways [36]. Moreover, recent findings suggest that GBP2, an interferon-inducible large GTPase, is essential in inducing FN expression via the Stat3-pathway [37]. These data suggest the role of fibronectin in regulating in vivo and in vitro glioblastoma cell invasion; moreover, it has been recently proposed as a prognostic biomarker since high FN1 expression appears to be related to poor prognoses [38].

3.2.3. Laminins

Laminins are a large group of glycoproteins consisting of three long polypeptides (the alpha, beta, and gamma chains present in different isoforms) that are not abundant in normal brain tissue and that are mainly present in the basal lamina. The proteins are multifunctional and play roles in development, differentiation, and cell migration, as they can interact with many cell surface proteins. Laminins are abundant in the glioma microenvironment and are mostly associated with the basal lamina of blood vessels, especially in the brain/tumor confrontation zone. In vitro studies revealed that, in the presence of laminins, glioma cell lines form F-actins, form strong and dense stress fibers, and increase the number of pseudopodia on the cell surface, stimulating cell adhesion and invasion. Moreover during the progression of glial tumors, laminin-9 (alpha4beta2gamma1) is switched to laminin-8 (alpha4beta1gamma1), which is, therefore, considered to be primarily involved in glioblastoma invasion [39]. According to these findings, the overexpression of Laminin isoform-411 (Laminin 8) has been identified to be correlated with higher recurrence rates and the shorter survival of GBM patients. As expected, the depletion of laminin-411 with CRISPR/Cas9 in human GBM cells led to the reduced growth of the resultant intracranial tumors in mice and significantly increased the survival of the host animals by suppressing the Notch pathways compared to mice with untreated cells [40]. Similar in vitro studies have shown that antisense oligonucleotides against both the alpha4 and beta1 chains of laminin-8 are able to significantly block the invasion of cocultures in Matrigel [41]. The debate is on the role of Laminin alpha-5. Recent zebrafish xenograft models with knocked down Laminin alpha-5 indicate that lama5 discourages glioblastoma cell dispersal and decreases invasion despite previous evidence indicating laminin alpha-5 to be promigratory in in vitro settings [42].

3.2.4. Periostin

The implication of PRO in GBM growth has been enquired in the last decade. Indeed, it was found that the expression of PRO is related to glioma grading and is inversely related to OS. Moreover, in cases of the overexpression of PRO, the genes related to cell migration and proliferation, such as MMP-9, were significantly enriched [43]. Recent evidence suggests p73 to be a main inductor of glioblastoma cell invasion through the direct activation of PRO [44]. It is thought that PRO could stimulate the transforming growth factor β (TGF-β)-induced epithelial–mesenchymal transition via the Akt and Fak signaling pathways [45].

3.3. Glycoproteins
Tenascin

Tenascins are large hetero- or homohexameric glycoproteins in which the subunits are held together with disulfide bonds. Four members are known in this family: Tenascin-C, -R, -X, and -W. Tenascins are involved in the modulation of cell adhesion, migration, and growth. Tenascin–C is found to be overexpressed in the glioblastoma microenvironment. In vitro, TNC knockdown glioblastoma cell lines were characterized by increased adhesion to the ECM components mediated through the upregulation of the FAK-pathway [46]. Moreover, in the presence of endogenous or exogenous TNC, glioblastoma cell lines expressed an increase in cell migration in a dose-related manner, while no differences in cellular growth were detected. Similarly, mouse xenograft models showed that tumors derived from TNC knockdown cells were less invasive, with tumor cells confined to better-defined tumor borders compared to the control tumors, while tumor size was approximately equal [47]. These data suggest the role of tenascin-C in modulating glioma cell invasion and migration through the ECM without interfering with cell proliferation.

Recently, it has been proposed that TNC expression in glioma tissue may be promoted by the IL-33-ST2-NFkB pathway [48]. Although the details of the role of downstream Tenascin-C in GBM invasion are not clear up to date, proteases, Cathepsin-B, MMP-12, and the ADAM-9-MAPK8 pathway were found to play a pivotal role in TNC-mediated GBM invasion [49–51].

3.4. Degradative Enzymes

MMPs are a group of zinc-dependent endopeptidases that degrade several components of the ECM via integrin mediation, participating in tissue structural changes, cell proliferation, and cell migration. At least 23 members of the human MMP family have been identified. GBM cells are known to secrete various MMPs through which they degrade various ECM proteins, including fibronectin, laminins, collagen, and gelatin, promoting cell migration and releasing activated proteins through cleavage [85]. Specifically, a specific subgroup of MMPs (including MMP-1, -2, -7, -9, -11, -12, -14, -15, and -25) was shown to be strictly related to glioma grading and glioblastoma development. In particular, high levels of MMP-9 and MMP-2 were found to be associated with a higher tumor grade, a lesser response to chemotherapy, and a worse survival outcome [52–54].

Different pathways of MMP activation have been investigated. The role of the uPA-uPAR pathway in the activation of MMP-9 and MMP-2 in GBMs is well established [55]. uPA is a protease, which is overexpressed in high-grade gliomas, that converts plasminogen to plasmin with a better efficacy when anchored to its receptor, uPAR. Both uPA and plasmin are responsible for MMP activation [56,57]. Moreover, uPA/uPAR, through an interaction with the integrin receptor, has been proven to activate downstream signaling through the activation of FAK, ERK, and Src, which lead to F-Actin assembly, membrane protrusion, and cell migration. Recently, other signaling pathways have been identified. The activation of Sonic Hedgehog signaling is related to an increase in the migration and invasion of GBM cells, which is mediated through the overexpression of MMP-9/-2 via the PI3K/AKT pathway [58]. In a similar way, it has been suggested that even IL-17A might control glioma cell invasiveness by inducing the overexpression of MMP-9/-2 via PI3K/AKT [59].

However, Rictor, a component of the mTOR complex, induces glioma cell migration increasing MMP-9 expression through the Raf-1-MEK-ERK signaling pathway [60].

Membrane-type MMPs are a subgroup of metalloproteinases that are membrane associated and have cytoplasmic domains, which may be important in cellular signaling. It has been proven that MT-MMP plays a role in the cleavage of pro-MMP to the active form of MMP-2 [86]. MT1-MMP was found to be involved in the epithelial-to-mesenchymal-transition of glioblastoma cells through pathway signaling, which involves transforming growth factor beta and SNAIL [61]. Similarly, other studies found a correlation between the expression of the MT1-MMP, Beta1-integrin, YAP1 pathways and the grading of gliomas [62].

The subfamily of adamalysins (ADAM proteases) was shown to be overexpressed in glioblastoma cell lines in vitro and in glioblastoma patients and may contribute to cell invasion. ADAM-10 and ADAM-17 are overexpressed in the glioblastoma microenvironment. In vitro studies reported that ADAM10 and ADAM17 inhibition selectively increases glioma sphere-forming cells but not neural stem cell migration and that the migrated GSCs exhibit a differentiated phenotype, suggesting a role in retaining the cells in the tumorigenic environment in an undifferentiated state [63,64].

3.5. Physical Forces

Many studies have proven that ECM mechanical changes influence glioma cell invasion, migration, and morphology [65]. Particularly, in vitro studies revealed that, in highly rigid ECMs, tumor cells spread extensively and migrate rapidly, whereas, in lower rigidity ECMs, comparable to normal brain tissue, tumor cells appear rounded and fail to migrate productively [66,67]. Moreover, a variation in matrix stiffness induced the differential expression of enzymes in which HA-synthases and MMP-1 were upregulated in the stiff condition [68]. It has been proposed that tumor-associated mesenchymal stem-like cells could play an important role in glioblastoma ECM remodeling through CCL2/JAK1/MLC2 signaling [69].

Other in vitro studies reported that, in response to hyperosmolarity and hydrostatic pressure, GBM cell lines upregulated the expression of urokinase-type plasminogen activator (uPA) and matrix metalloproteinases (MMPs), promoting cell invasion [70].

3.6. Glioma Cell and Microglia Migration and Invasion Patterns

Carcinoma cell invasion is a complex reciprocal process in which cells induce the reorganization of the structure and composition of the ECM, and, in turn, the microenvironment influences cancer cell function, migration pathways, and cell morphology [71].

GBM cells are regulated through several environmental mechanisms that facilitate the spread of these tumors. For example, the invasion pattern of malignant GBMs is associated with the distinct anatomic pathways following the myelinated fiber tracts and blood vessels. In addition to the anatomical and physical aspects, there is accumulating evidence that specific ECM components (such as hyaluronan, vitronectin, and tenascin C) are unregulated at the border of the spreading GBMs, and this may alter cellular invasiveness. Molecular guidance during cell invasion is often dependent on the ECM and the underlying mechanism of glioblastoma invasion and the GBM-specific ECM microenvironment represent interesting and potentially meaningful fields of research [65].

In vitro studies, using patient-tissue-derived decellularized ECMs and glioblastoma cell lines, revealed that cancer cells that move through the ECM can be distinguished by their invasion mode. The mesenchymal mode is based on the MMP proteolytic degradation of the matrix, and, in this mode, cells have an elongated morphology and show a polarized extension of the leading edge; additionally, in the ameboid mode, rounded cells tend to migrate in the absence of proteolytic ECM degradation and squeeze through the ECM space [71]. Different ECM compositions have been proven to play a pivotal role in regulating the cell morphology and the migration pathway. For example, in 3D collagen matrices, glioma cells typically show mesenchymal-like migration, whereas, in the presence of HA cells they assume an ameboid-like pattern [72]. Moreover, GBM cells treated with MMP2/9 inhibitors have a rounded-ameboid mode of invasion, whereas the inhibition of HA synthases (HASs) promotes the morphological transition from a rounded-amoeboid to an elongated-mesenchymal morphology [73]. These findings, together, suggest that the ECM-cell interaction could lead to a switch between these two patterns of migration, enhancing glioma cells' ability for invasion and representing a mechanism of target therapy escaping.

According to the literature, glioma cell invasion develops preferentially along preexisting tracks such as myelinated axons and blood vessels. Indeed, in vivo studies have shown that the glioma cells that spread along blood vessels and those directly invading the brain parenchyma exhibit different morphological features, the former being spindle-shaped with a single pseudopodium towards the direction of movement and the latter exhibiting multiple pseudopodia with random invasion directions. Moreover, the former exhibits an overexpression of Rho family GTPase activity in contrast with the latter, which exhibits an overexpression of Rac1 and Cdc42 activity [74]. In support of these findings, recent in vitro studies showed that the glioma neurospheres located close to the rods tend to assume a collective strand and to perform fast migration along this physical support, maintaining cell–cell contact, whereas the cells facing the matrix directly exhibit single-cell and random migration in 3D matrices with pseudo vessels recreated using sterile microrods coated with Matrigel [75].

According to recent findings, the nontumoral cells in the glioma microenvironment may reciprocally interact with the ECM components and with glioma cells themselves, representing a further cell migration and invasiveness modulation system. Macrophages/microglia account for up to 30% of the cells in the glioma microenvironment. It is known that macrophages can assume two different forms in tissue repair and, most of all, in ECM remodeling: classical M1-activation, in which the macrophages present an ameboid or round shape and which has been supposed to sustain a proinflammatory role, and alternative M2-activation, in which unipolar macrophages are present and which has a role in antagonizing proinflammatory mediators [76]. In vitro studies showed that microglia can degrade and migrate through the ECM by using a wide range of degradative enzymes. Interestingly, M2-activated macrophages present a higher rate of migration compared to M1-activated macrophages, which is sustained, most of all, by the overexpression of MMP2, Cat-k, and Cat-s [77]. Glioma cells may directly influence the activity of surrounding nontumoral cells with extracellular vesicles, leading, in this instance, to a differentiation of macrophages toward the M2-activated form [78], which, indeed, is the most represented in the glioma microenvironment among the macrophage phenotypes, suggesting a role of activated macrophages/microglia in tumor growth.

Previous in vitro studies have shown that, in presence of microglia, glioma cells show a higher rate of migration and invasiveness. Moreover, such a phenomenon seems to be microglial-specific since replacing microglial with nonmicroglial cells, such as oligodendrocytes or endothelial cells, did not show any significant impact on glioma cell migration. It has been proposed that macrophages/microglia directly affect glioma cell migration through the ECM by secreting MMPs and that they indirectly affect it by promoting the activation of pro-MMP secreted in the microenvironment by glioma cells by means of membrane-type metalloproteases (MT-MMP), which has been proven to be overexpressed in tumor-associated microglia. Among all the different forms of degradative enzymes, MMP-2 seems to play a pivotal role. In fact, in organotypical brain slice models, MMP-2 activity was found to be much higher when glioma cells were cultured in the presence of microglia. Altogether, these data suggest that microglia could play an important role in tumor cell invasion by cooperating with glioma cells themselves in the remodeling of the extracellular matrix, providing a favorable substrate for migration [79]. In support of the data, in vitro studies revealed that glioma cells tend to migrate, in a heterogeneous shape, toward activated microglia-conditioned media and that such migration is sustained through an overexpression of MMP-2 [80,81].

Moreover, not only may the microglia modify the structure of the ECM, but the latter can also have an effect on the former: it has been proven that different components of the ECM could influence microglial activity. Indeed, tumor specimen studies revealed a close relation between the number of macrophages and the Tenascin-C content in the glioma extracellular matrix, suggesting that Tenascin-C may represent a permissive substrate for macrophagic migration in gliomas [82]. Moreover, microglia expressed different morphologies in the Tenascin knockdown glioma xenograft when compared to the control group, exhibiting the first ameboid-like morphology, resembling activated microglia, and the latter resembling inactivated microglia with long and thin processes, pointing out once again the reciprocal interaction between microglial cells and the extracellular matrix. Similarly, mouse xenograft studies revealed that Versican acts as a major ligand for the Toll-like receptors expressed on the macrophage surface, inducing the activation of the latter through an overexpression of MT-MMP [46,83].

In a recent study, the migratory behavior of the microglia and tumor glioma cells at the tumor infiltrative edge was studied and compared to better understand the dynamics of tumor infiltration and, eventually, the reciprocal interactions between the microglia and glioma cells. As reported, in a mouse brain slice model, microglial cells exhibited a migration pattern termed "simple diffusive" characterized by a random walk in a nonrestricted environment, whereas glioma cells exhibited a migration pattern termed "super diffusive" characterized by a persistent directionality of cell migration. At the infiltrative edge, microglial cells present a higher migration speed and a lower directionality compared to the microglial cells located in the peritumoral area, whereas glioma cells present, on average, a higher speed and directionality compared to microglial cells. Moreover, both the microglial and glioma cells exhibit little motility when located further away from the tumor infiltrative edge. Considering these findings, it has been proposed that glioma cells stimulate the activity and motility of microglial cells towards the infiltrative edge and that, in turn, activated microglial cells condition the infiltrative edge microenvironment by modifying the extracellular matrix to reduce the impedance to migration, allowing efficacious glioma cell invasion [84].

4. Discussion

The ECM forms a critical and dynamic scaffold that supports the normal brain architecture. It is a complex nonhomogenous structure which physiologically displays a vast and complex interaction with neural and supporting cells. Normal brain tissue has unique components that are not expressed in other tissues. In fact, the brain ECM presents small amounts of fibrous proteins, such as collagen, fibronectin, and laminins, and high amounts of glycosaminoglycans (either bound to proteins, chondroitin sulfate, dermatan sulfate, heparan sulfate, and keratan sulfate, or unbounded in the form of hyaluronan) proteoglycans, called lecticans (versican, aggrecan, neurocan, brevican, and decorin); and glycoproteins, such as tenascin-C.

A large number of studies have proven that the ECM does not only have a mechanical supporting role in the regulation of neural stem cell behavior, neuronal migration, the formation of axonal processes and their myelin sheaths, synapse formation, etc. [4]. Indeed, cells interact with the components of the ECM through membrane receptors (integrins, CD44, BEHAB/brevican, and N-CAM), producing molecular responses and establishing mutual interactions in which cells can modify the microenvironment and vice versa.

Functional studies in vitro and genetic studies in mice have provided evidence that the ECM affects virtually all the aspects of nervous system development and function and that it ultimately plays a significant role in all the phases of GBM development and progression. The ECM in GBMs shows significant remodeling compared to the ECM in a healthy brain. Recent evidence highlights that the three-dimensional ECM architecture and its mechanical properties affect the cell behavior in the TME both at the tumoral core and in its periphery. The ECM elements have been shown to display either an attractant or repellant action respective to the glioma cells, microglia, monocytes, macrophages, and stem cells that constitute the TME. We will herein examine the different ECM structural component modifications in GBMs (Figure 2).

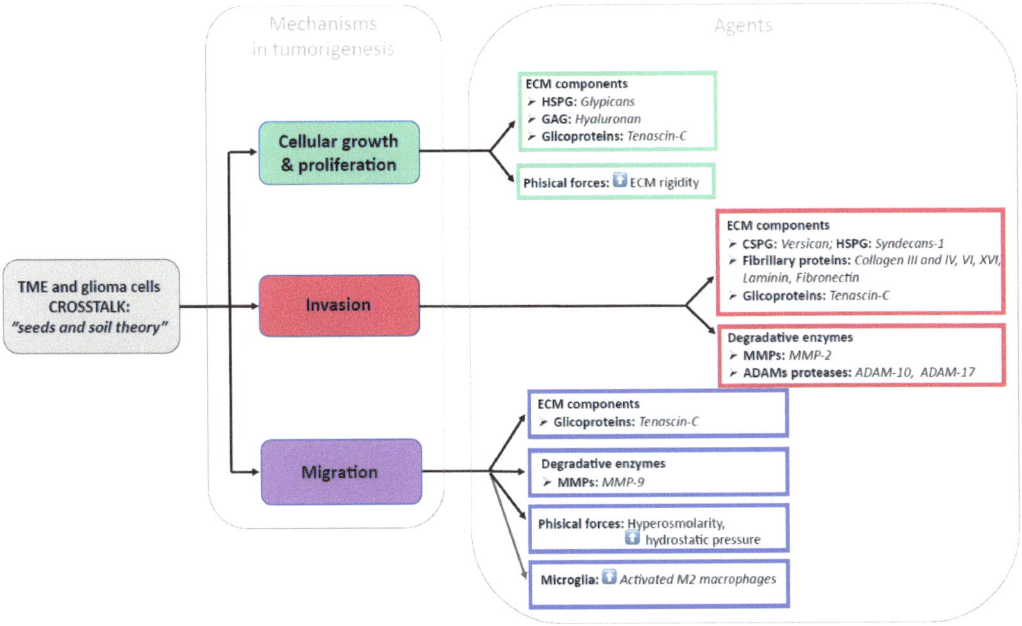

Figure 2. Pictorial summary of our findings.

5. Conclusions

Our systematic review demonstrates that the ECM should not be regarded anymore as a passive scaffold statically contributing to mechanical support in normal and pathological brain tissue but as an active player in tumor-related activity. Further research is necessary to fully understand the clinical implications of these preliminary findings.

Author Contributions: Conceptualization, G.M.D.P. and S.M.; methodology, G.M. and G.M.D.P.; investigation, F.F. and S.M.; writing—original draft preparation, S.M.; writing—review and editing, G.M., L.B., Q.G.D.A., P.M., L.L. and R.D.B.; supervision, A.O. All authors have read and agreed to the published version of the manuscript.

Funding: This research received no external funding.

Conflicts of Interest: The authors declare no conflict of interest.

Abbreviations

BEHAB	Brain-enriched hyaluronan-binding protein
CD44	Cluster of differentiation 44
CD280	Endo180
CHI3L1	Chitinase-3-like protein 1
CNS	Central nervous system
COL1A2	Collagen alpha-2(I) chain
CSPG	Chondroitin sulfate proteoglycan
ECM	Extracellular matrix
ED-A	Extra domain A
ED-B	Extra domain B

EGFR	Epidermal growth factor receptor
FAK	Focal adhesion kinase
GAG	Glycosaminoglycan
GBM	Glioblastoma
HSPG	Heparan sulfate proteoglycan
IL-1	Interleukin-1
LAR	Leukocyte common antigen-related
MEK/ERK	Mitogen-activated protein kinase/extracellular signal-regulated kinase
MMP	Matrix metalloproteinase
NFkB	Nuclear factor kappa-light-chain enhancer of activated B cells
N-CAM	Neural cell adhesion molecule
PAI-1	Plasminogen activator inhibitor-1
P4HA2	Prolyl-4-hydroxylase subunit 2
PRISMA-P	Preferred Reporting Items for Systematic Review and Meta-Analysis Protocols
PRO	Periostin
RHAMM	Receptor for hyaluronan-mediated motility
siRNA	Small interfering RNA
TGF-β	Transforming growth factor beta
TME	Tumor microenvironment
uPA	Urokinase-type plasminogen activator
uPAR	Urokinase-type plasminogen activator receptor

References

1. Menna, G.; Manini, I.; Cesselli, D.; Skrap, M.; Olivi, A.; Ius, T.; Della Pepa, G.M. Immunoregulatory effects of glioma-associated stem cells on the glioblastoma peritumoral microenvironment: A differential PD-L1 expression from core to periphery? *Neurosurg. Focus* **2022**, *52*, E4. [CrossRef] [PubMed]
2. Ruoslahti, E. Brain extracellular matrix. *Glycobiology* **1996**, *6*, 489–492. [CrossRef] [PubMed]
3. Novak, U.; Kaye, A.H. Extracellular matrix and the brain: Components and function. *J. Clin. Neurosci.* **2000**, *7*, 280–290. [CrossRef] [PubMed]
4. Barros, C.S.; Franco, S.J.; Müller, U. Extracellular matrix: Functions in the nervous system. *Cold Spring Harb. Perspect. Biol.* **2011**, *3*, a005108. [CrossRef] [PubMed]
5. Moher, D.; Liberati, A.; Tetzlaff, J.; Altman, D.G.; the PRISMA Group. Preferred reporting items for systematic reviews and meta-analyses: The PRISMA statement. *BMJ* **2009**, *339*, b2535. [CrossRef]
6. Logun, M.T.; Bisel, N.S.; Tanasse, E.A.; Zhao, W.; Gunasekera, B.; Mao, L.; Karumbaiah, L. Glioma cell invasion is significantly enhanced in composite hydrogel matrices composed of chondroitin 4- and 4,6-sulfated glycosaminoglycans. *J. Mater. Chem.* **2016**, *4*, 6052–6064. [CrossRef]
7. Logun, M.T.; Wynens, K.E.; Simchick, G.; Zhao, W.; Mao, L.; Zhao, Q.; Mukherjee, S.; Brat, D.J.; Karumbaiah, L. Surfen-mediated blockade of extratumoral chondroitin sulfate glycosaminoglycans inhibits glioblastoma invasion. *FASEB J.* **2019**, *33*, 11973–11992. [CrossRef]
8. Schrappe, M.; Klier, F.G.; Spiro, R.C.; Waltz, T.A.; Reisfeld, R.A.; Gladson, C.L. Correlation of chondroitin sulfate proteoglycan expression on proliferating brain capillary endothelial cells with the malignant phenotype of astroglial cells. *Cancer Res.* **1991**, *51*, 4986–4993.
9. Kim, Y.; Kang, H.; Powathil, G.; Kim, H.; Trucu, D.; Lee, W.; Lawler, S.; Chaplain, M. Role of extracellular matrix and microenvironment in regulation of tumor growth and LAR-mediated invasion in glioblastoma. *PLoS ONE* **2018**, *13*, e0204865. [CrossRef]
10. Silver, D.J.; Siebzehnrubl, F.A.; Schildts, M.J.; Yachnis, A.T.; Smith, G.M.; Smith, A.A.; Scheffler, B.; Reynolds, B.A.; Silver, J.; Steindler, D.A. Chondroitin sulfate proteoglycans potently inhibit invasion and serve as a central organizer of the brain tumor microenvironment. *J. Neurosci.* **2013**, *33*, 15603–15617. [CrossRef]
11. Onken, J.; Moeckel, S.; Leukel, P.; Leidgens, V.; Baumann, F.; Bogdahn, U.; Vollmann-Zwerenz, A.; Hau, P. Versican isoform V1 regulates proliferation and migration in high-grade gliomas. *J. Neuro-Oncol.* **2014**, *120*, 73–83. [CrossRef]
12. Tran, V.M.; Wade, A.; McKinney, A.; Chen, K.; Lindberg, O.R.; Engler, J.R.; Persson, A.I.; Phillips, J.J. Heparan sulfate glycosaminoglycans in glioblastoma promote tumor invasion. *Mol. Cancer Res.* **2017**, *15*, 1623–1633. [CrossRef]
13. Su, G.; Meyer, K.; Nandini, C.D.; Qiao, D.; Salamat, S.; Friedl, A. Glypican-1 is frequently overexpressed in human gliomas and enhances FGF-2 signaling in glioma cells. *Am. J. Pathol.* **2006**, *168*, 2014–2026. [CrossRef]
14. Watanabe, A.; Mabuchi, T.; Satoh, E.; Furuya, K.; Zhang, L.; Maeda, S.; Naganuma, H. Expression of syndecans, a heparan sulfate proteoglycan, in malignant gliomas: Participation of nuclear factor-κB in upregulation of syndecan-1 expression. *J. Neuro-Oncol.* **2006**, *77*, 25–32. [CrossRef]
15. Chen, J.-W.E.; Pedron, S.; Shyu, P.; Hu, Y.; Sarkaria, J.N.; Harley, B.A.C. Influence of hyaluronic acid transitions in tumor microenvironment on glioblastoma malignancy and invasive behavior. *Front. Mater.* **2018**, *5*, 39. [CrossRef]

16. Hayen, W.; Goebeler, M.; Kumar, S.; Riessen, R.; Nehls, V. Hyaluronan stimulates tumor cell migration by modulating the fibrin fiber architecture. *J. Cell Sci.* **1999**, *112*, 2241–2251. [CrossRef]
17. Chen, J.-W.E.; Lumibao, J.; Blazek, A.; Gaskins, H.R.; Harley, B. Hypoxia activates enhanced invasive potential and endogenous hyaluronic acid production by glioblastoma cells. *Biomater. Sci.* **2018**, *6*, 854–862. [CrossRef]
18. Chen, J.-W.E.; Leary, S.; Barnhouse, V.; Sarkaria, J.N.; Harley, B.A. Matrix hyaluronic acid and hypoxia influence a CD133$^+$ subset of patient-derived glioblastoma cells. *Tissue Eng.* **2022**, *28*, 330–340. [CrossRef]
19. Akiyama, Y.; Jung, S.; Salhia, B.; Lee, S.; Hubbard, S.; Taylor, M.; Mainprize, T.; Akaishi, K.; van Furth, W.; Rutka, J.T. Hyaluronate receptors mediating glioma cell migration and proliferation. *J. Neuro-Oncol.* **2001**, *53*, 115–127. [CrossRef]
20. Pibuel, M.A.; Poodts, D.; Díaz, M.; Molinari, Y.A.; Franco, P.G.; Hajos, S.E.; Lompardía, S.L. Antitumor effect of 4MU on glioblastoma cells is mediated by senescence induction and CD44, RHAMM and p-ERK modulation. *Cell Death Discov.* **2021**, *7*, 280. [CrossRef]
21. Tsatas, D.; Kanagasundaram, V.; Kaye, A.H.; Novak, U. EGF receptor modifies cellular responses to hyaluronan in glioblastoma cell lines. *J. Clin. Neurosci.* **2002**, *9*, 282–288. [CrossRef] [PubMed]
22. Zhang, H.; Zhang, N.; Dai, Z.; Wang, Z.; Zhang, X.; Liang, X.; Zhang, L.; Feng, S.; Wu, W.; Ye, W.; et al. Hyaluronic acids mediate the infiltration, migration, and M2 polarization of macrophages: Evaluating metabolic molecular phenotypes in gliomas. *Mol. Oncol.* **2022**, *16*, 3927–3948. [CrossRef] [PubMed]
23. Calori, I.R.; Alves, S.R.; Bi, H.; Tedesco, A.C. Type-I collagen/collagenase modulates the 3D structure and behavior of glioblastoma spheroid models. *ACS Appl. Bio Mater.* **2022**, *5*, 723–733. [CrossRef]
24. Wang, Y.; Sakaguchi, M.; Sabit, H.; Tamai, S.; Ichinose, T.; Tanaka, S.; Kinoshita, M.; Uchida, Y.; Ohtsuki, S.; Nakada, M. COL1A2 inhibition suppresses glioblastoma cell proliferation and invasion. *J. Neurosurg.* **2022**, *138*, 639–648. [CrossRef] [PubMed]
25. Chintala, S.K.; Sawaya, R.; Gokaslan, Z.L.; Rao, J.S. The effect of type III collagen on migration and invasion of human glioblastoma cell lines in vitro. *Cancer Lett.* **1996**, *102*, 57–63. [CrossRef]
26. Mammoto, T.; Jiang, A.; Jiang, E.; Panigrahy, D.; Kieran, M.W.; Mammoto, A. Role of collagen matrix in tumor angiogenesis and glioblastoma multiforme progression. *Am. J. Pathol.* **2013**, *183*, 1293–1305. [CrossRef]
27. Senner, V.; Ratzinger, S.; Mertsch, S.; Grässel, S.; Paulus, W. Collagen XVI expression is upregulated in glioblastomas and promotes tumor cell adhesion. *FEBS Lett.* **2008**, *582*, 3293–3300. [CrossRef]
28. Huijbers, I.J.; Iravani, M.; Popov, S.; Robertson, D.; Al-Sarraj, S.; Jones, C.; Isacke, C.M. A role for fibrillar collagen deposition and the collagen internalization receptor Endo180 in glioma invasion. *PLoS ONE* **2010**, *5*, e9808. [CrossRef]
29. Lin, J.; Jiang, L.; Wang, X.; Wei, W.; Song, C.; Cui, Y.; Wu, X.; Qiu, G. P4HA2 promotes epithelial-to-mesenchymal transition and glioma malignancy through the collagen-dependent PI3K/AKT pathway. *J. Oncol.* **2021**, *2021*, 1406853. [CrossRef]
30. Jiang, X.; Zhou, T.; Wang, Z.; Qi, B.; Xia, H. HSP47 promotes glioblastoma stemlike cell survival by modulating tumor microenvironment extracellular matrix through TGF-β pathway. *ACS Chem. Neurosci.* **2017**, *8*, 128–134. [CrossRef]
31. Ohnishi, T.; Hiraga, S.; Izumoto, S.; Matsumura, H.; Kanemura, Y.; Arita, N.; Hayakawa, T. Role of fibronectin-stimulated tumor cell migration in glioma invasion in vivo: Clinical significance of fibronectin and fibronectin receptor expressed in human glioma tissues. *Clin. Exp. Metastasis* **1998**, *16*, 729–741. [CrossRef]
32. Chintala, S.K.; Sawaya, R.; Gokaslan, Z.L.; Fuller, G.; Rao, J.S. Immunohistochemical localization of extracellular matrix proteins in human glioma, both in vivo and in vitro. *Cancer Lett.* **1996**, *101*, 107–114. [CrossRef]
33. Caffo, M.; Caruso, G.; Meli, F.; Galatioto, S.; Sciacca, M.P.; Tomasello, F.; Germano, A. An immunohistochemical study of extracellular matrix proteins laminin, fibronectin and type IV collagen in paediatric glioblastoma multiforme. *Acta Neurochir.* **2004**, *146*, 1113–1118. [CrossRef]
34. Serres, E.; Debarbieux, F.; Stanchi, F.; Maggiorella, L.; Grall, D.; Turchi, L.; Burel-Vandenbos, F.; Figarella-Branger, D.; Virolle, T.; Rougon, G.; et al. Fibronectin expression in glioblastomas promotes cell cohesion, collective invasion of basement membrane in vitro and orthotopic tumor growth in mice. *Oncogene* **2013**, *33*, 3451–3462. [CrossRef]
35. Sengupta, S.; Nandi, S.; Hindi, E.S.; Wainwright, D.A.; Han, Y.; Lesniak, M.S. Short hairpin RNA-mediated fibronectin knockdown delays tumor growth in a mouse glioma model. *Neoplasia* **2010**, *12*, 837–847. [CrossRef]
36. Huang, J.M.; Tian, X.X.; Zhong, Y.F.; Ma, D.L.; Ma, Y.; You, J.F.; Zhang, Y. Effects of beta1-integrin, fibronectin and laminin on invasive behavior of human gliomas. *Zhonghua Bing Li Xue Za Zhi* **2006**, *35*, 478–482. (In Chinese)
37. Yu, S.; Yu, X.; Sun, L.; Zheng, Y.; Chen, L.; Xu, H.; Jin, J.; Lan, Q.; Chen, C.C.; Li, M. GBP2 enhances glioblastoma invasion through Stat3/fibronectin pathway. *Oncogene* **2020**, *39*, 5042–5055. [CrossRef]
38. Kabir, F.; Apu, M.N.H. Multi-omics analysis predicts fibronectin 1 as a prognostic biomarker in glioblastoma multiforme. *Genomics* **2022**, *114*, 110378. [CrossRef]
39. Tysnes, B.B.; Mahesparan, R.; Thorsen, F.; Haugland, H.K.; Porwol, T.; Enger, P.Ø.; Lund-Johansen, M.; Bjerkvig, R. Laminin expression by glial fibrillary acidic protein positive cells in human gliomas. *Int. J. Dev. Neurosci.* **1999**, *17*, 531–539. [CrossRef]
40. Sun, T.; Patil, R.; Galstyan, A.; Klymyshyn, D.; Ding, H.; Chesnokova, A.; Cavenee, W.K.; Furnari, F.B.; Ljubimov, V.A.; Shatalova, E.S.; et al. Blockade of a Laminin-411-notch axis with CRISPR/Cas9 or a nanobioconjugate inhibits glioblastoma growth through tumor-microenvironment cross-talk targeting tumor microenvironment to treat glioblastoma. *Cancer Res.* **2019**, *79*, 1239–1251. [CrossRef]
41. Khazenzon, N.M.; Ljubimov, A.V.; Lakhter, A.J.; Fujita, M.; Fujiwara, H.; Sekiguchi, K.; Sorokin, L.M.; Petäjäniemi, N.; Virtanen, I.; Black, K.L.; et al. Antisense inhibition of laminin-8 expression reduces invasion of human gliomas in vitro. *Mol. Cancer Ther.* **2003**, *2*, 985–994. [PubMed]

42. Gamble, J.T.; Reed-Harris, Y.; Barton, C.L.; La Du, J.; Tanguay, R.; Greenwood, J.A. Quantification of glioblastoma progression in zebrafish xenografts: Adhesion to laminin alpha 5 promotes glioblastoma microtumor formation and inhibits cell invasion. *Biochem. Biophys. Res. Commun.* **2018**, *506*, 833–839. [CrossRef] [PubMed]
43. Wang, H.; Wang, Y.; Jiang, C. Stromal protein periostin identified as a progression associated and prognostic biomarker in glioma via inducing an invasive and proliferative phenotype. *Int. J. Oncol.* **2013**, *42*, 1716–1724. [CrossRef] [PubMed]
44. Landré, V.; Antonov, A.; Knight, R.; Melino, G. p73 promotes glioblastoma cell invasion by directly activating POSTN (periostin) expression. *Oncotarget* **2016**, *7*, 11785–11802. [CrossRef]
45. Ouanouki, A.; Lamy, S.; Annabi, B. Periostin, a signal transduction intermediate in TGF-β-induced EMT in U-87MG human glioblastoma cells, and its inhibition by anthocyanidins. *Oncotarget* **2018**, *9*, 22023–22037. [CrossRef]
46. Xia, S.; Lal, B.; Tung, B.; Wang, S.; Goodwin, C.R.; Laterra, J. Tumor microenvironment tenascin-C promotes glioblastoma invasion and negatively regulates tumor proliferation. *Neuro Oncol.* **2016**, *18*, 507–517. [CrossRef]
47. Hirata, E.; Arakawa, Y.; Shirahata, M.; Yamaguchi, M.; Kishi, Y.; Okada, T.; Takahashi, J.A.; Matsuda, M.; Hashimoto, N. Endogenous tenascin-C enhances glioblastoma invasion with reactive change of surrounding brain tissue. *Cancer Sci.* **2009**, *100*, 1451–1459. [CrossRef]
48. Zhang, J.-F.; Tao, T.; Wang, K.; Zhang, G.-X.; Yan, Y.; Lin, H.-R.; Li, Y.; Guan, M.-W.; Yu, J.-J.; Wang, X.-D. IL-33/ST2 axis promotes glioblastoma cell invasion by accumulating tenascin-C. *Sci. Rep.* **2019**, *9*, 20276. [CrossRef]
49. Sarkar, S.; Zemp, F.J.; Senger, D.; Robbins, S.M.; Yong, V.W. ADAM-9 is a novel mediator of tenascin-C-stimulated invasiveness of brain tumor—Initiating cells. *Neuro-Oncol.* **2015**, *17*, 1095–1105. [CrossRef]
50. Sarkar, S.; Nuttall, R.K.; Liu, S.; Edwards, D.R.; Yong, V.W. Tenascin-C stimulates glioma cell invasion through matrix metalloproteinase-12. *Cancer Res.* **2006**, *66*, 11771–11780. [CrossRef]
51. Mai, J.; Sameni, M.; Mikkelsen, T.; Sloane, B. Degradation of extracellular matrix protein tenascin-C by cathepsin B: An interaction involved in the progression of gliomas. *Biol. Chem.* **2002**, *383*, 1407–1413. [CrossRef]
52. Li, Q.; Chen, B.; Cai, J.; Sun, Y.; Wang, G.; Li, Y.; Li, R.; Feng, Y.; Han, B.; Li, J.; et al. Comparative analysis of matrix metalloproteinase family members reveals that MMP9 predicts survival and response to temozolomide in patients with primary glioblastoma. *PLoS ONE* **2016**, *11*, e0151815. [CrossRef]
53. Lakka, S.S.; Gondi, C.S.; Yanamandra, N.; Olivero, W.C.; Dinh, D.H.; Gujrati, M.; Rao, J.S. Inhibition of cathepsin B and MMP-9 gene expression in glioblastoma cell line via RNA interference reduces tumor cell invasion, tumor growth and angiogenesis. *Oncogene* **2004**, *23*, 4681–4689. [CrossRef]
54. Kargiotis, O.; Chetty, C.; Gondi, C.S.; Tsung, A.J.; Dinh, D.H.; Gujrati, M.; Lakka, S.S.; Kyritsis, A.P.; Rao, J.S. Adenovirus-mediated transfer of siRNA against MMP-2 mRNA results in impaired invasion and tumor-induced angiogenesis, induces apoptosis in vitro and inhibits tumor growth in vivo in glioblastoma. *Oncogene* **2008**, *27*, 4830–4840. [CrossRef]
55. Schuler, P.J.; Bendszus, M.; Kuehnel, S.; Wagner, S.; Hoffmann, T.K.; Goldbrunner, R.; Vince, G.H. Urokinase plasminogen activator, uPAR, MMP-2, and MMP-9 in the C6-glioblastoma rat model. *Vivo* **2012**, *26*, 571–576.
56. Sun, J.; Zhao, B.; Du, K.; Liu, P. TRAF6 correlated to invasion and poor prognosis of glioblastoma via elevating MMP9 expression. *Neuroreport* **2019**, *30*, 127–133. [CrossRef]
57. Zhao, Y.; Lyons, C.E.; Xiao, A.; Templeton, D.J.; Sang, Q.A.; Brew, K.; Hussaini, I.M. Urokinase directly activates matrix metalloproteinases-9: A potential role in glioblastoma invasion. *Biochem. Biophys. Res. Commun.* **2008**, *369*, 1215–1220. [CrossRef]
58. Chang, L.; Zhao, D.; Liu, H.-B.; Wang, Q.-S.; Zhang, P.; Li, C.-L.; DU, W.-Z.; Wang, H.-J.; Liu, X.; Zhang, Z.-R.; et al. Activation of sonic hedgehog signaling enhances cell migration and invasion by induction of matrix metalloproteinase-2 and -9 via the phosphoinositide-3 kinase/AKT signaling pathway in glioblastoma. *Mol. Med. Rep.* **2015**, *12*, 6702–6710. [CrossRef]
59. Zheng, Q.; Diao, S.; Wang, Q.; Zhu, C.; Sun, X.; Yin, B.; Zhang, X.; Meng, X.; Wang, B. IL-17A promotes cell migration and invasion of glioblastoma cells via activation of PI3K/AKT signalling pathway. *J. Cell Mol. Med.* **2019**, *23*, 357–369. [CrossRef]
60. Das, G.; Shiras, A.; Shanmuganandam, K.; Shastry, P. Rictor regulates MMP-9 activity and invasion through Raf-1-MEK-ERK signaling pathway in glioma cells. *Mol. Carcinog.* **2011**, *50*, 412–423. [CrossRef]
61. Djediai, S.; Suarez, N.G.; El Cheikh-Hussein, L.; Torres, S.R.; Gresseau, L.; Dhayne, S.; Joly-Lopez, Z.; Annabi, B. MT1-MMP cooperates with TGF-β receptor-mediated signaling to trigger snail and induce epithelial-to-mesenchymal-like transition in U87 glioblastoma cells. *Int. J. Mol. Sci.* **2021**, *22*, 13006. [CrossRef] [PubMed]
62. Zhai, Y.; Sang, W.; Su, L.; Shen, Y.; Hu, Y.; Zhang, W. Analysis of the expression and prognostic value of MT1-MMP, β1-integrin and YAP1 in glioma. *Open Med.* **2022**, *17*, 492–507. [CrossRef] [PubMed]
63. Held-Feindt, J.; Paredes, E.B.; Blömer, U.; Seidenbecher, C.; Stark, A.M.; Mehdorn, H.M.; Mentlein, R. Matrix-degrading proteases ADAMTS4 and ADAMTS5 (disintegrins and metalloproteinases with thrombospondin motifs 4 and 5) are expressed in human glioblastomas. *Int. J. Cancer* **2006**, *118*, 55–61. [CrossRef] [PubMed]
64. Siney, E.J.; Holden, A.; Casselden, E.; Bulstrode, H.; Thomas, G.J.; Willaime-Morawek, S. Metalloproteinases ADAM10 and ADAM17 mediate migration and differentiation in glioblastoma sphere-forming cells. *Mol. Neurobiol.* **2017**, *54*, 3893–3905. [CrossRef]
65. Herrera-Perez, M.; Voytik-Harbin, S.L.; Rickus, J.L. Extracellular matrix properties regulate the migratory response of glioblastoma stem cells in three-dimensional culture. *Tissue Eng.* **2015**, *21*, 2572–2582. [CrossRef]
66. Ulrich, T.A.; de Juan Pardo, E.M.; Kumar, S. The mechanical rigidity of the extracellular matrix regulates the structure, motility, and proliferation of glioma cells. *Cancer Res.* **2009**, *69*, 4167–4174. [CrossRef]

67. Kaufman, L.; Brangwynne, C.; Kasza, K.; Filippidi, E.; Gordon, V.; Deisboeck, T.; Weitz, D. Glioma expansion in collagen I matrices: Analyzing collagen concentration-dependent growth and motility patterns. *Biophys. J.* **2005**, *89*, 635–650. [CrossRef]
68. Wang, C.; Tong, X.; Yang, F. Bioengineered 3D brain tumor model to elucidate the effects of matrix stiffness on glioblastoma cell behavior using peg-based hydrogels. *Mol. Pharm.* **2014**, *11*, 2115–2125. [CrossRef]
69. Lim, E.-J.; Suh, Y.; Kim, S.; Kang, S.-G.; Lee, S.-J. Force-mediated proinvasive matrix remodeling driven by tumor-associated mesenchymal stem-like cells in glioblastoma. *BMB Rep.* **2018**, *51*, 182–187. [CrossRef]
70. Pu, W.; Qiu, J.; Riggins, G.J.; Parat, M.-O. Matrix protease production, epithelial-to-mesenchymal transition marker expression and invasion of glioblastoma cells in response to osmotic or hydrostatic pressure. *Sci. Rep.* **2020**, *10*, 2634. [CrossRef]
71. Koh, I.; Cha, J.; Park, J.; Choi, J.; Kang, S.-G.; Kim, P. The mode and dynamics of glioblastoma cell invasion into a decellularized tissue-derived extracellular matrix-based three-dimensional tumor model. *Sci. Rep.* **2018**, *8*, 4608. [CrossRef]
72. Rao, S.; DeJesus, J.; Short, A.R.; Otero, J.J.; Sarkar, A.; Winter, J.O. Glioblastoma behaviors in three-dimensional collagen-hyaluronan composite hydrogels. *ACS Appl. Mater. Interfaces* **2013**, *5*, 9276–9284. [CrossRef]
73. Cui, Y.; Cole, S.; Pepper, J.; Otero, J.J.; Winter, J.O. Hyaluronic acid induces ROCK-dependent amoeboid migration in glioblastoma cells. *Biomater. Sci.* **2020**, *8*, 4821–4831. [CrossRef]
74. Hirata, E.; Yukinaga, H.; Kamioka, Y.; Arakawa, Y.; Miyamoto, S.; Okada, T.; Sahai, E.; Matsuda, M. In vivo fluorescence resonance energy transfer imaging reveals differential activation of Rho-family GTPases in glioblastoma cell invasion. *J. Cell Sci.* **2012**, *125*, 858–868. [CrossRef]
75. Lively, S.; Schlichter, L.C. The microglial activation state regulates migration and roles of matrix-dissolving enzymes for invasion. *J. Neuroinflamm.* **2013**, *10*, 843. [CrossRef]
76. de Vrij, J.; Maas, S.N.; Kwappenberg, K.M.; Schnoor, R.; Kleijn, A.; Dekker, L.; Luider, T.M.; de Witte, L.D.; Litjens, M.; van Strien, M.E.; et al. Glioblastoma-derived extracellular vesicles modify the phenotype of monocytic cells. *Int. J. Cancer* **2015**, *137*, 1630–1642. [CrossRef]
77. Gabrusiewicz, K.; Ellert-Miklaszewska, A.; Lipko, M.; Sielska, M.; Frankowska, M.; Kaminska, B. Characteristics of the alternative phenotype of microglia/macrophages and its modulation in experimental gliomas. *PLoS ONE* **2011**, *6*, e23902. [CrossRef]
78. Bettinger, I.; Thanos, S.; Paulus, W. Microglia promote glioma migration. *Acta Neuropathol.* **2002**, *103*, 351–355. [CrossRef]
79. Markovic, D.S.; Glass, R.; Synowitz, M.; van Rooijen, N.; Kettenmann, H. Microglia stimulate the invasiveness of glioma cells by increasing the activity of metalloprotease-2. *J. Neuropathol. Exp. Neurol.* **2005**, *64*, 754–762. [CrossRef]
80. Markovic, D.S.; Vinnakota, K.; Chirasani, S.; Synowitz, M.; Raguet, H.; Stock, K.; Sliwa, M.; Lehmann, S.; Kälin, R.; van Rooijen, N.; et al. Gliomas induce and exploit microglial MT1-MMP expression for tumor expansion. *Proc. Natl. Acad. Sci. USA* **2009**, *106*, 12530–12535. [CrossRef]
81. Wu, C.Y.-J.; Chen, C.-H.; Lin, C.-Y.; Feng, L.-Y.; Lin, Y.-C.; Wei, K.-C.; Huang, C.-Y.; Fang, J.-Y.; Chen, P.-Y. CCL5 of glioma-associated microglia/macrophages regulates glioma migration and invasion via calcium-dependent matrix metalloproteinase 2. *Neuro-Oncol.* **2020**, *22*, 253–266. [CrossRef]
82. Kulla, A.; Liigant, A.; Piirsoo, A.; Rippin, G.; Asser, T. Tenascin expression patterns and cells of monocyte lineage: Relationship in human gliomas. *Mod. Pathol.* **2000**, *13*, 56–67. [CrossRef] [PubMed]
83. Hu, F.; Dzaye, O.D.; Hahn, A.; Yu, Y.; Scavetta, R.J.; Dittmar, G.; Kaczmarek, A.K.; Dunning, K.R.; Ricciardelli, C.; Rinnenthal, J.L.; et al. Glioma-derived versican promotes tumor expansion via glioma-associated microglial/macrophages toll-like receptor 2 signaling. *Neuro-Oncol.* **2015**, *17*, 200–210. [CrossRef] [PubMed]
84. Juliano, J.; Gil, O.; Hawkins-Daarud, A.; Noticewala, S.; Rockne, R.C.; Gallaher, J.; Massey, S.C.; Sims, P.A.; Anderson, A.R.A.; Swanson, K.R.; et al. Comparative dynamics of microglial and glioma cell motility at the infiltrative margin of brain tumours. *J. R. Soc. Interface* **2018**, *15*, 20170582. [CrossRef]
85. Sternlicht, M.D.; Werb, Z. How matrix metalloproteinases regulate cell behavior. *Annu. Rev. Cell Dev. Biol.* **2001**, *17*, 463–516. [CrossRef]
86. Fillmore, H.L.; VanMeter, T.E.; Broaddus, W.C. Membrane-type matrix metalloproteinases (MT-MMP)s: Expression and function during glioma invasion. *J. Neuro-Oncol.* **2001**, *53*, 187–202. [CrossRef]

Disclaimer/Publisher's Note: The statements, opinions and data contained in all publications are solely those of the individual author(s) and contributor(s) and not of MDPI and/or the editor(s). MDPI and/or the editor(s) disclaim responsibility for any injury to people or property resulting from any ideas, methods, instructions or products referred to in the content.

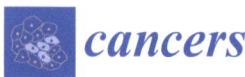

Article

Extracellular Vesicles Potentiate Medulloblastoma Metastasis in an EMMPRIN and MMP-2 Dependent Manner

Hannah K. Jackson [1,2], Christine Mitoko [1], Franziska Linke [1,3], Donald Macarthur [4], Ian D. Kerr [5] and Beth Coyle [1,*]

1. Children's Brain Tumour Research Centre, School of Medicine, Biodiscovery Institute, University Park, University of Nottingham, Nottingham NG7 2RD, UK; hj363@cam.ac.uk (H.K.J.); f.linke@erasmusmc.nl (F.L.
2. Department of Pathology, University of Cambridge, Cambridge CB2 1QP, UK
3. Department of Experimental Urology, Erasmus MC Cancer Institute, University Medical Center Rotterdam, 3015 GD Rotterdam, The Netherlands
4. Department of Neurosurgery, Nottingham University Hospital, Nottingham NG7 2UH, UK
5. School of Life Sciences, University of Nottingham, Queen's Medical Centre, Nottingham NG7 2UH, UK; ian.kerr@nottingham.ac.uk
* Correspondence: beth.coyle@nottingham.ac.uk

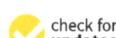

Citation: Jackson, H.K.; Mitoko, C.; Linke, F.; Macarthur, D.; Kerr, I.D.; Coyle, B. Extracellular Vesicles Potentiate Medulloblastoma Metastasis in an EMMPRIN and MMP-2 Dependent Manner. *Cancers* 2023, *15*, 2601. https://doi.org/10.3390/cancers15092601

Academic Editors: David Wong, Annunziato Mangiola and Gianluca Trevisi

Received: 27 March 2023
Revised: 19 April 2023
Accepted: 23 April 2023
Published: 4 May 2023

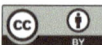

Copyright: © 2023 by the authors. Licensee MDPI, Basel, Switzerland. This article is an open access article distributed under the terms and conditions of the Creative Commons Attribution (CC BY) license (https://creativecommons.org/licenses/by/4.0/).

Simple Summary: Medulloblastoma is the most prevalent malignant paediatric brain tumour, where metastasis and recurrence account for 95% of medulloblastoma-associated deaths. Secretion of extracellular vesicles (EVs) has emerged as a pivotal mediator for communication in the tumour microenvironment during metastasis. We investigated whether sEVs and exosomes mediate communication between medulloblastoma cells and their surroundings to drive metastasis. Metastatic exosomes were shown to potentiate medulloblastoma migration via the active protease, matrix metalloproteinase-2 (MMP-2), on their surface, resulting in degradation of the extracellular matrix (ECM) and creating routes for medulloblastoma cells to invade into the surrounding environment. Knockdown of MMP-2 and its activator extracellular matrix metalloproteinase inducer (EMMPRIN) reduced this invasive potential. Our observations also highlight the potential of MMP-2 as a biomarker for metastatic medulloblastoma. Together, our findings reveal unique insights into the pathogenesis of medulloblastoma and highlight the need to explore alternative therapeutic approaches to impair MMP-driven mechanisms of tumour invasion and migration.

Abstract: Extracellular vesicles (EVs) have emerged as pivotal mediators of communication in the tumour microenvironment. More specifically, nanosized extracellular vesicles termed exosomes have been shown to contribute to the establishment of a premetastatic niche. Here, we sought to determine what role exosomes play in medulloblastoma (MB) progression and elucidate the underlying mechanisms. Metastatic MB cells (D458 and CHLA-01R) were found to secrete markedly more exosomes compared to their nonmetastatic, primary counterparts (D425 and CHLA-01). In addition, metastatic cell-derived exosomes significantly enhanced the migration and invasiveness of primary MB cells in transwell migration assays. Protease microarray analysis identified that matrix metalloproteinase-2 (MMP-2) was enriched in metastatic cells, and zymography and flow cytometry assays of metastatic exosomes demonstrated higher levels of functionally active MMP-2 on their external surface. Stable genetic knockdown of MMP-2 or extracellular matrix metalloproteinase inducer (EMMPRIN) in metastatic MB cells resulted in the loss of this promigratory effect. Analysis of serial patient cerebrospinal fluid (CSF) samples showed an increase in MMP-2 activity in three out of four patients as the tumour progressed. This study demonstrates the importance of EMMPRIN and MMP-2-associated exosomes in creating a favourable environment to drive medulloblastoma metastasis via extracellular matrix signalling.

Keywords: medulloblastoma; extracellular vesicles; exosomes; MMP-2; EMMPRIN; metastasis

1. Introduction

Metastatic medulloblastoma is a devastating disease with a poor prognosis of less than 10% five-year survival in affected paediatric patients [1,2]. Whilst primary medulloblastoma tumours have been well characterised on the basis of their epigenetic and transcriptomic features, there is very little information regarding the molecular signatures of metastatic tumours due to the rarity of reoperation. The resulting scarcity of metastatic tumour samples from these patients limits data available on the metastatic tumour microenvironment, which has been increasingly postulated to exert a role in the dissemination of solid tumours.

The secretion of extracellular vesicles (EVs) as vehicles for cell-to-cell communication has gained prominence in recent years. The most common nomenclature divides EVs into three subclasses based on their biogenesis; exosomes, approximately 30–150 nm in diameter, originating in multivesicular endosomes (MVEs) which fuse with the plasma membrane; microvesicles, which range from 100–1000 nm and form via direct budding of the plasma membrane; and apoptotic bodies, vesicles ranging around 1–4 μm and are formed from of dying cells [3]. The most investigated are small EVs (sEVs or exosomes), which are nanometer-sized vesicles secreted by all cell types and able to cross the blood–brain barrier (BBB) [4]. The role of exosomes as vehicles for cell-to-cell communication between a tumour and its microenvironment is a relatively new concept, with only limited study of their role in medulloblastoma [5–9]. Exosomes represent a unique form of information delivery operating at short and long distances [10]. Tumour-derived exosomes can transfer signals and convey information from tumours to distant tissues and organs. They are also present in circulation and can therefore disseminate their cargo throughout the body. Exosomes have been shown to carry surface components that enable direct contact with recipient cells to activate intracellular signalling [11–13]. In addition, exosomes interact with target cells by fusion with the cell membrane followed by the transfer of exosomal cargoes (protein, mRNA, miRNA) into the cell cytoplasm [14]. Cancer cell-derived exosomes have been shown to participate in the crucial steps of the metastatic spread of a primary tumour, ranging from oncogenic reprogramming of malignant cells to the formation of premetastatic niches [15]. These effects are achieved through the mediation of intercellular cross talk and subsequent modification of both local and distant microenvironments. In the context of brain tumours, sEVs originating from primary tumour cells have been demonstrated to enhance the growth of brain metastases, modulate immune responses to support tumour cell proliferation, regulate tumour cell stability, and have been identified as potential diagnostic or prognostic biomarkers [10,16,17]. This study focussed on how medulloblastoma exosomes interact with the recipient cells utilizing direct extracellular matrix signalling, via surface-associated proteins, to activate intracellular signalling pathways.

In this context, we assessed the expression of tumour-supporting proteins EMMPRIN and MMP-2. Increased levels of MMP-2 and EMMPRIN have been associated with more aggressive metastatic disease in other solid tumours [18,19]. Therefore, we sought to investigate whether the secretion of exosomes containing MMPs and EMMPRIN might be necessary for tumour progression and thereby a potential mechanism of dissemination in medulloblastoma. We demonstrated that metastatic exosomes significantly enhanced the migration and invasiveness of primary and nonmalignant cells. Moreover, the promigratory function of metastatic exosomes was, in part, due to EMMPRIN and MMP-2 enriched on their external surface. Furthermore, metastatic exosomes were shown to potentiate medulloblastoma migration resulting in the degradation of the extracellular matrix components, via the active protease, MMP-2, on their surface. In support of this, stable genetic knockdown of the genes encoding MMP-2 and EMMPRIN (namely *MMP-2* or *BSG*) antagonised the promigratory function of exosomes, confirming that MMP-2 and EMMPRIN are promigratory factors on medulloblastoma exosomes. Finally, we observed increased levels of functionally-active MMP-2 in medulloblastoma patients' CSFs, which correlated with disease progression and appeared to correlate with prognosis, highlighting the biomarker potential of functional MMP-2.

2. Materials and Methods

2.1. Cell Culture

CHLA-01 and CHLA-01R brain tumour cell lines (primary-tumour-derived cell line and recurrent metastatic line derived from pleural fluid, respectively) were obtained from Geoff Pilkington (University of Portsmouth, Portsmouth, UK). DAOY (nonmetastatic primary-tumour derived) and D283 (derived from peritoneal metastases) brain tumour cell lines were obtained from ATCC (Manassas, VA, USA), UW228-3 (nonmetastatic primary tumour derived), D458 (derived from metastatic cells in the CSF) brain tumour cell lines were a gift from John R. Silber (University of Washington, Seattle, DA, USA), HD-MB03 (metastatic primary-tumour derived) brain tumour cell lines were a gift from Till Milde, D425 (derived from the primary-tumour counterpart of D458) from Marcel Kool (both at DKFZ, Heidelberg, Germany), and ONS76 (metastatic primary-tumour derived) brain tumour cell lines were a gift from Annette Künkele (Charité Universitätsmedizin Berlin, Germany). FB83 was derived inhouse from human foetal brain tissue as previously described [20]. CHLA-01 and CHLA-01R were cultured in Dulbecco's Modified Eagle Medium (DMEM) supplemented with 2% B-27, 20 ng/mL Epidermal growth factor (EGF, Gibco, PHG0315), and 20 ng/mL basic fibroblast growth factor (bFGF, Gibco, PHG0266). DAOY, D283, D425 and D458 cells were cultured in DMEM with 10% foetal bovine serum (FBS). FB83 cells were cultured in DMEM with 15% FBS. UW-228-3 cells in DMEM/F-12 with 15% FBS and 1% sodium pyruvate. ONS76 and HD-MB03 cells were cultured in RPMI 1640 with 10% FBS. In all cases, FBS used was (HyClone SH30541.03 (Logan, UT, USA)).

All cell lines were grown under antibiotic-free culture conditions at 37 °C in a humidified atmosphere with 5% CO_2. Prior to EV isolation, CHLA-01 and CHLA-01R cell lines were grown without EGF and bFGF, and D425 and D458 cell lines were grown in DMEM with 2% exosome-depleted FBS for 48 h. Exosome-depleted FBS was generated by the pelleting of extracellular vesicles by overnight ultracentrifugation at $100,000 \times g$ at 4 °C. Mycoplasma testing was performed monthly using a PlasmoTest™ mycoplasma detection kit (InvivoGen (San Diego, CA, USA); rep-pt1) as per the manufacturer's instructions.

2.2. PrestoBlue® Assay

To measure changes in cell viability and the proliferation of cells, a PrestoBlue® (ThermoFisher (Waltham, MA, USA), A13262) assay was used. Cells were assayed at a final dilution of 1:10 for 60 min at 37 °C and 5% CO_2 and fluorescence was measured at 560/590 nm using a FLUOstar Omega (BMG Labtech, (Ortenberg, Germany)) microplate reader.

2.3. Isolation of Exosomes

To isolate exosome cell populations, cells were cultured in 10 T-75 flasks up to 30% confluence, washed twice with Hanks' Balanced Salt Solution (HBSS, Gibco (Loughborough, UK)) and incubated in media supplemented with exosome-depleted FBS for 48 h. Cell culture supernatants were collected and cells were removed by centrifugation for 5 min at $750 \times g$ at 4 °C. The pellet was discarded and the supernatant was centrifuged for 15 min at $1500 \times g$ at 4 °C to remove smaller cell debris. To remove larger EVs, the supernatant was then centrifuged for 35 min at $14,000 \times g$ at 4 °C. The remaining supernatant was filtered through a 0.22 µm filter (Millipore, Burlington, MA, USA) and then centrifuged for 2 h at $100,000 \times g$ at 4 °C. The pellet was washed by resuspension in phosphate-buffered saline (PBS, Gibco (Loughborough, UK)) and centrifuged again for 2 h at $100,000 \times g$ at 4 °C.

2.4. Migration and Invasion Assays

Cell migration and invasion were quantified in a modified Boyden chamber assay. In both, the lower wells of the chamber were filled with DMEM + 10% FBS (D425 and D458 cells) or EGF, FGF (20 ng/mL) and 2% B-27 (CHLA-01 and CHLA-01R cells) and sealed with a polycarbonate transwell insert with a pore diameter of 8 µm (Greiner Bio One Greiner (Kremsmünster, Austria 662638)). For the invasion experiments, transwell inserts were coated with Collagen IV (Bio-Techne (Abingdon, UK) 3410-010-02)) diluted to 200 µg/mL in H$_2$O and laminin I (Cultrex, 3400-010-02) and diluted to 100 µg/µL in serum-free media. This setting is thought to resemble the in vivo situation of tumour migration through the basement membrane. The 1×10^5 cells were seeded in the upper wells in a medium devoid of FBS. The chamber was incubated for 24 h at 37 °C, 5% CO$_2$ and subsequently, the number of invasive cells in the lower chamber was quantified relative to the standard curve. For the exosome treatments, cells were pretreated with the indicated concentrations of exosomes 24 h prior to the seeding of tumour cells in the upper wells.

2.5. Generation of Stable Knockdown Cell Lines

Cell lines with stable knockdown of *BSG* and *MMP-2* expression were generated through shRNA-mediated gene silencing using commercialised virus particles. GIPZ™ Lentiviral particle starter kits (Horizon Discovery, (Waterbeach, UK) *BSG*; VGH5526-EG4313, *MMP-2*; VGH5526-EG682) were used for subsequent transduction of the CHLA-01R and D458 cell lines, following the GIPZ™ lentiviral shRNA manual.

2.6. Preparation of Cerebrospinal Fluid Samples

Cerebrospinal fluid (CSF) samples were obtained from paediatric patients who had lumbar punctures within a fortnight of the surgical resection of their primary or recurrent/relapsed medulloblastoma at our institution. The samples were twice centrifuged at approximately $100 \times g$ for 10 min and the resulting supernatant was further centrifuged at $300 \times g$ for 10 min before storing them at -80 °C. The CSF samples were then defrosted over ice and equal volumes were assayed in gelatin zymography experiments.

2.7. Detection of Metalloproteinase Activity by Zymography

The activity of gelatinases MMP-2 and MMP-9 was determined using gelatin zymography. Cell supernatants (15 µL), CSF (15 µL) or exosomes (20 µg) were mixed 1:4 with 4X NuPage LDS sample buffer (11836170001, Roche (Basel, Switzerland)) (without β-mercaptoethanol) and loaded onto 10% SDS-PAGE gels that had been supplemented with 3 mg/mL gelatin (Sigma Aldrich (St. Louis, MO, USA). Recombinant MMP-2 (Sigma Aldrich (St. Louis, MO, USA), 86607) was also added as a reference marker. Electrophoresis was used to separate proteins according to their molecular weight. Subsequently, to restore MMP activity, gels were incubated in zymogram renaturing buffer (Thermo Fisher Scientific (Waltham, MA, USA) at room temperature for 30 min. Renaturing buffer was removed and replaced with a zymogram developing buffer (Thermo Fisher Scientific (Waltham, MA, USA) and incubated overnight at 37 °C, during which time gelatinases degrade the gel. This degradation was visualised by the staining of the gels with 0.5% w/v Coomassie blue R-250 in 40% v/v methanol, 10% v/v glacial acetic acid (Bio-Rad (Hercules, CA, USA) at room temperature for 15 min. To reduce background staining, gels were washed in a destaining solution (40% v/v methanol, 10% v/v glacial acetic acid) for two hours to reveal the gelatinase bands. Gels were fixed in a fixative solution (2% paraformaldehyde, 0.075 M lysine, and 0.01 M sodium periodate, pH 7.4) for 15 min before being dried and photographed.

2.8. Western Blot

Cells and exosomes were lysed in a lysis buffer (1% Triton-x100, 1 mM EDTA, 150 mM NaCl, 20 mM Tris pH 7.5) supplemented with $1 \times$ cOmplete™ EDTA-free Protease Inhibitor Cocktail (11836170001, Roche (Basel, Switzerland)) and protein concentrations were determined using a Bradford assay (Bio-Rad) in relation to a BSA standard curve. Proteins were separated according to molecular weight by SDS-PAGE and transferred onto a PVDF membrane (Scientific Lab Supplies 10600023). For protein detection, membranes were blocked with 5% nonfat milk and 1% Tween/PBS, and subsequently incubated with primary antibodies against MMP-2 (Abcam, 86607, 1:500), EMMPRIN (Santa Cruz, 46700, 1:500), CD9 (Cell signalling, 13174, 1:1000), Alix (Cell signalling, 2171, 1:1000), Annexin V (Cell signalling, 8555, 1:1000) and Histone 4 (Cell signalling, 41328, 1:1000). Appropriate horseradish peroxidase-conjugated secondary antibodies were applied. GAPDH (Sigma-Aldrich, 406609, 1:2000) was used as the loading control. Protein signals were detected using an enhanced chemiluminescence (ECL) solution (Thermo Fisher Scientific (Waltham, MA, USA); 32106). Chemiluminescence was then measured in the LAS-3000 mini biomolecular imager.

2.9. Quantitative Real-Time Polymerase Chain Reaction

RNA isolation was performed using the miRNeasy micro kit (Qiagen (Hilden, Germany)). RNA samples were transcribed into cDNA using reverse transcriptase (Invitrogen (Waltham, MA, USA); 1080-044). Gene expression of the resultant cDNA template was assessed by quantitative reverse transcription PCR (CFX96 real-time PCR machine; BIORAD (Hercules, CA, USA)) and iQ SYBR SuperMix (BIORAD, (Hercules, CA, USA)). Primer sequences: *MMP-2* forward: 5' GCCTTTAACTGGAGCAAAAACAA 3', reverse: 5' TCCATTTTCTTCTTCACCTCATTG 3', *BSG* forward: 5' GTTCTTGCCTTTGTCATTCTG 3' reverse: 5' TCACCATCATCTTCATCTACGA 3'. The house-keeping gene *GAPDH* forward 5' ATGTTCGTCATGGGTGTAA 3', reverse: 5' GTCTTCTGGGTGGCAGTGAT 3' was used as a control to normalize the data and the relative mRNA expression level was calculated using the ΔCt method.

2.10. Transmission Electron Microscopy

To visualize exosomes, vesicle pellets were resuspended in 2% paraformaldehyde and applied to Cu-Rh formvar-coated 200 mesh grids (Agar 53 Scientific, (Los Angeles, CA, USA)) for 3 min. Absorbent paper was used to gently remove any excess suspension. Negative contrast was achieved by incubating the grid for 30 s in 1% uranyl acetate, and excess liquid was blotted off. Subsequent analyses of vesicles were carried out using a JEOL 2100+ transmission electron microscope and iTEM software (Olympus, (Tokyo, Japan)).

2.11. NanoFCM

Exosome samples were diluted in PBS (phosphate buffered saline) 1:10–1:100 and analysed using the Flow Nano Analyzer (NanoFCM Inc. (Nottingham, UK)), according to the manufacturer's protocol [21]. Briefly, lasers were calibrated using 200 nm control beads (NanoFCM Ltd.), which were analysed as a reference for particle concentration. A mixture of various-sized beads (NanoFCM Inc.) was analysed to set a reference for size distribution. PBS was analysed as a background signal. Particle concentrations and size distributions were calculated using NanoFCM software (NanoFCM profession V1.0) and normalised to the cell number and dilution necessary for adequate NanoFCM reading.

2.12. Nanoparticle Tracking Analysis

Particle counts and size distributions were determined for each extracellular vesicle preparation using a nanoparticle tracking analysis (NTA) (NanoSight Ltd. (Malvern, UK). The instrument was configured with a 488 nm LM14 laser module and a high-sensitivity digital camera system (OrcaFlash2.8, Hamamatsu C11440, NanoSight Ltd., Amesbury, UK). Prior to the analysis of extracellular vesicle samples, 100 nm standard latex beads were tested as a control to confirm that the NTA measurements were accurate. Samples were diluted in PBS, to a concentration of between 2×10^6 and 5×10^7 particles/mL within the linear range of the instrument. Five replicate videos of 20 s were taken at 25 °C, with samples under controlled flow, and analysed using NTA software (version 2.5), with the minimal expected particle size set to automatic, and camera sensitivity set at 12–16. The detection thresholds were set at 1–3 to reveal small particles.

2.13. Statistical Analysis

Results are shown as mean ± SEM of the indicated number of independent experiments. The statistical significance of differences in the group results was compared using a one- or two-way analysis of variance (ANOVA) with multiple comparison testing as indicated. All statistical analyses and plots were carried out using GraphPad Prism 8 (GraphPad Software Inc., La Jolla, CA, USA).

2.14. Bioinformatic Analysis of Published Datasets

Published medulloblastoma patient datasets were accessed and analysed using the R2: Genomics Analysis and Visualization Platform (http://r2.amc.nl, (accessed on 3 October 2022)).

3. Results

3.1. Metastatic Cell Lines Release More Exosomes Than Their Primary Counterparts

The current international consensus recognises four distinct molecular subgroups of medulloblastoma each associated with different patterns of metastasis and overall prognosis—wingless (WNT), sonic hedgehog; (SHH), group three and group four—these can now be further categorised into second-generation subgroups [22,23]. WNT patients classically have a favourable prognosis (>90% 5-year survival); SHH patients display heterogeneous outcomes associated with the age of diagnosis and specific genetics (TP53 mutation status). The underlying biology of group three and group four patients remains less clear, and a substantial number of these patients relapse and are associated with high levels of metastasis [22,23].

Exosomes were isolated from cultured cell lines that represent pairs of metastatic and primary-tumour origins. Since group three and group four medulloblastoma molecular subgroups have the highest occurrence of metastasis at diagnosis [23–25] cell lines were used from these subgroups. The two group three cell lines were the primary cell line D425 and the metastatic D458 cell line. The two group four cell lines were the primary CHLA-01 cell line and the metastatic CHLA-01R cell line. These cell lines were valuable in gaining insight into the molecular, genetic, and proteomic signature changes that occurred between the primary-tumour stage and the dissemination to a secondary site.

Exosomes were isolated by ultracentrifugation and characterised according to MISEV criteria [26]. We observed enrichment for the exosome-associated markers CD9, Annexin V, and Alix, and an absence of histone four, a nuclear marker that would indicate contamination with cellular debris (Figure 1Ai,Aii; full-length blots in Supplementary Figure S1). Exosomes were visualised by transmission electron microscopy (TEM), revealing that medulloblastoma cell lines release a heterogeneous population of "cup-shaped" spherical vesicles (Figure 1B), characteristic of exosomes under TEM [27,28]. There was some heterogeneity in size (diameters varying between 30–150 nm) and appearance of the structures visualized, though little evidence of nonvesicular contamination [29]. Similarly, particle size distribution and particle concentrations, as measured by NTA and NanoFCM (Figure 1C,D), further supported that the isolated particles were indeed exosomes.

A notable feature of cancer cells is that they produce exosomes in greater amounts than normal cells. Several studies have shown that exosome numbers are elevated in the plasma of cancer patients compared to healthy controls; an increase in the levels of extracellular vesicles released correlates with poor prognosis and survival outcomes [30,31]. Exosomes were therefore isolated from a series of medulloblastoma cell lines representing different subgroups and metastatic capacities. Using both particle concentrations and total protein measurements, metastatic cells produce more exosomes relative to primary cells (Figure 1E,F), indicating that they may play a vital role in increasing medulloblastoma metastasis.

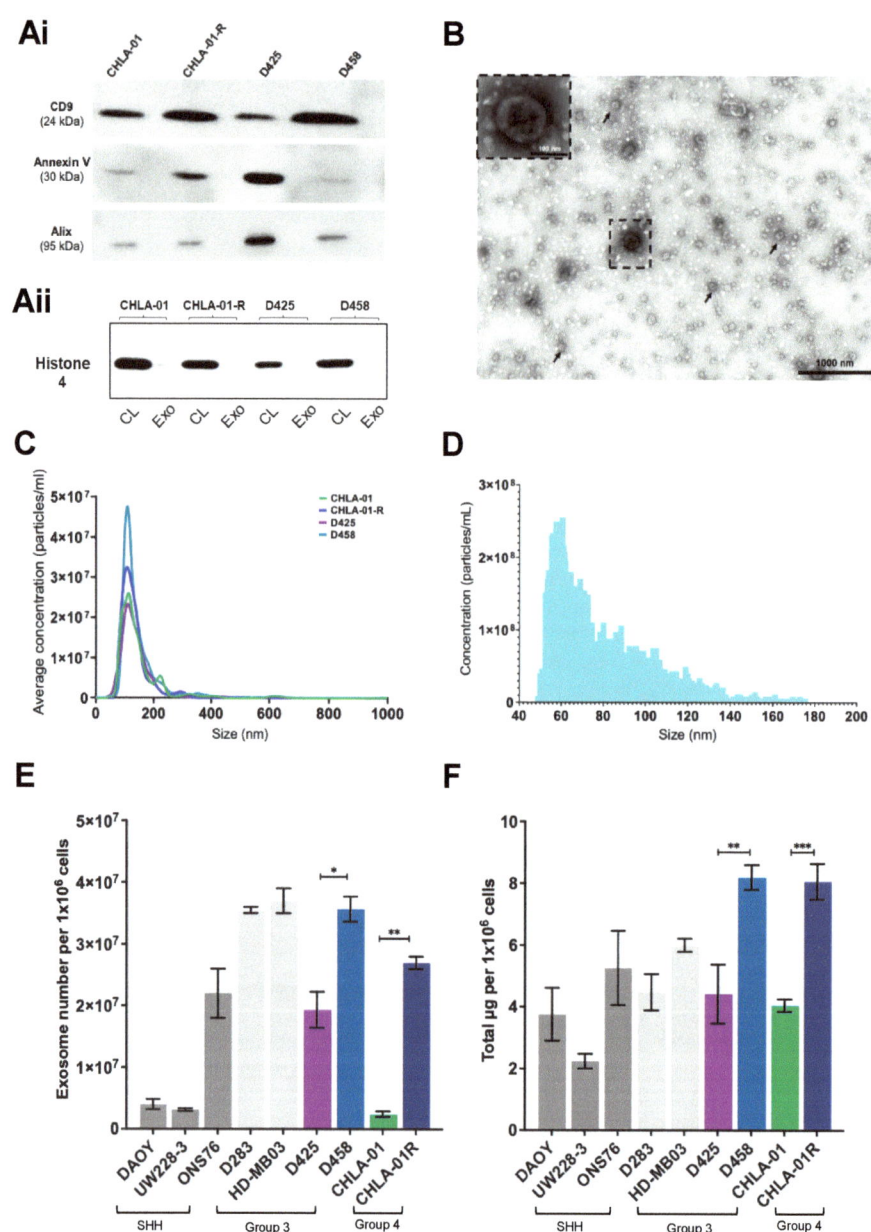

Figure 1. Isolation and characterisation of exosomes from medulloblastoma cell lines. Western blot confirmation that exosomes (**Ai**) express the marker proteins CD9, Annexin V, and Alix, and show no cross contamination with the nuclear protein histone 4 which is only detected in cell lysate (CL) rather than exosome (Exo) fractions (**Aii**). The uncropped blots are shown in Figure S1. (**B**) Exosomes from CHLA-01 cells were imaged by transmission electron microscopy (TEM) and identified as multiple cup-shaped structures ranging from 30–150 nm in size (arrowheads). Scale bar 1000 nm. (**C,D**) Exosomal particle concentrations were measured by NTA (**C**) and NanoFCM (**D**). NTA data represent the average

of at least three independent repeats. Representative NanoFCM data is shown for CHLA-01-derived exosomes. (**E,F**) Metastatic cell lines (D283, HD-MB03, D458, and CHLA-01-R) typically secrete more exosomes than the primary cell lines as determined by exosomal number (**E**) and exosomal protein content (**F**), both corrected for cell density. SHH (sonic hedgehog). Significant differences were calculated using one-way ANOVA analyses with Sidak's multiple-comparisons test, (* $p \leq 0.05$, ** $p \leq 0.01$, *** $p \leq 0.005$). Data represent the average of three independent experiments with error bars indicating the standard error of the mean (SEM).

3.2. Treatment of Medulloblastoma Cells with Migratory-Derived Exosomes Enhances Cell Invasion and Migration

To determine whether metastatic cell-derived exosomes conferred a phenotype upon the recipient cell lines, primary cell lines were cocultured with exosomes isolated from their matched metastatic cell line pair. Migration and invasion of cell lines were measured using a modified Boyden chamber transwell model, recapitulating invasion through the blood–brain barrier (schematic representation Figure 2A). Initially, the migration of cell lines in the absence of added exosomes was measured. When comparing matched cell line pairs, there was a higher level of cell migration in the metastatic cells compared to the primary cells (Supplementary Figure S2A,B). The effects of exosomes on cell invasion and migration were then assessed by adding exosomes derived from metastatic cells to primary cells in the insert. Interestingly, CHLA-01 cells showed significantly enhanced tumour migration and invasion in response to metastatic exosome addition, compared to the vesicle-free supernatant (Figure 2B). Similarly, D425 cells showed a significant increase in invasion in response to metastatic exosome addition (Figure 2C). Moreover, exosome-free supernatant or PBS had no effect on cell migration rates (Supplementary Figure S2C), confirming that metastatic exosome-induced tumour cell migration and invasion is a specific and not an artefactual effect. In both cell lines tested, there was only a small increase in proliferation after metastatic exosome stimulation (Figure 2D,E), suggesting that the direct impacts on recipient cell migration and invasion are conveyed by exosome stimulation.

Since exosomes have been described as transferring malignant characteristics to surrounding cells, the influence of exosomes on a nonmalignant cell line (FB83) derived from foetal neuronal stem cells was also explored. As shown in Figure 2F, stimulation with metastatic exosomes (derived from CHLA-01R cells) alone was able to induce an invasive phenotype in the FB83 cells ($p \leq 0.01$), suggesting that recipient cells did not need to be predisposed to an invasive phenotype, or even a cancerous one, prior to exosome stimulation. A significant increase in proliferation was not observed until 72 h (Figure 2G), again indicative of migratory effects only in this cell line.

3.3. MMP-2 and EMMPRIN Are Abundant in Proinvasive Exosomes

Having established that metastatic cells were able to release exosomes that endowed an invasive capability on the recipient cells, we then investigated the protease content of our matched lines. In each pair, we were able to identify higher relative expression of MMP-2 in the metastatic line (Supplementary Figure S3, Supplementary Method). Matrix metalloproteinases (MMPs) are proteases that have been heavily implicated in the modulation of the TME and demonstrated to be upregulated in the metastasis of several solid tumours [32,33]. Their tight regulation is, in part, mediated by an extracellular matrix metalloproteinase inducer (EMMPRIN), a glycoprotein commonly enriched on the surface of tumour cells and associated with tumour progression and poor patient outcomes [34,35]. EMMPRIN has been shown to mediate MMP release [36] and, more recently, it has been found in tumour-derived extracellular vesicles [37] where it also mediated an MMP-inducing effect [38].

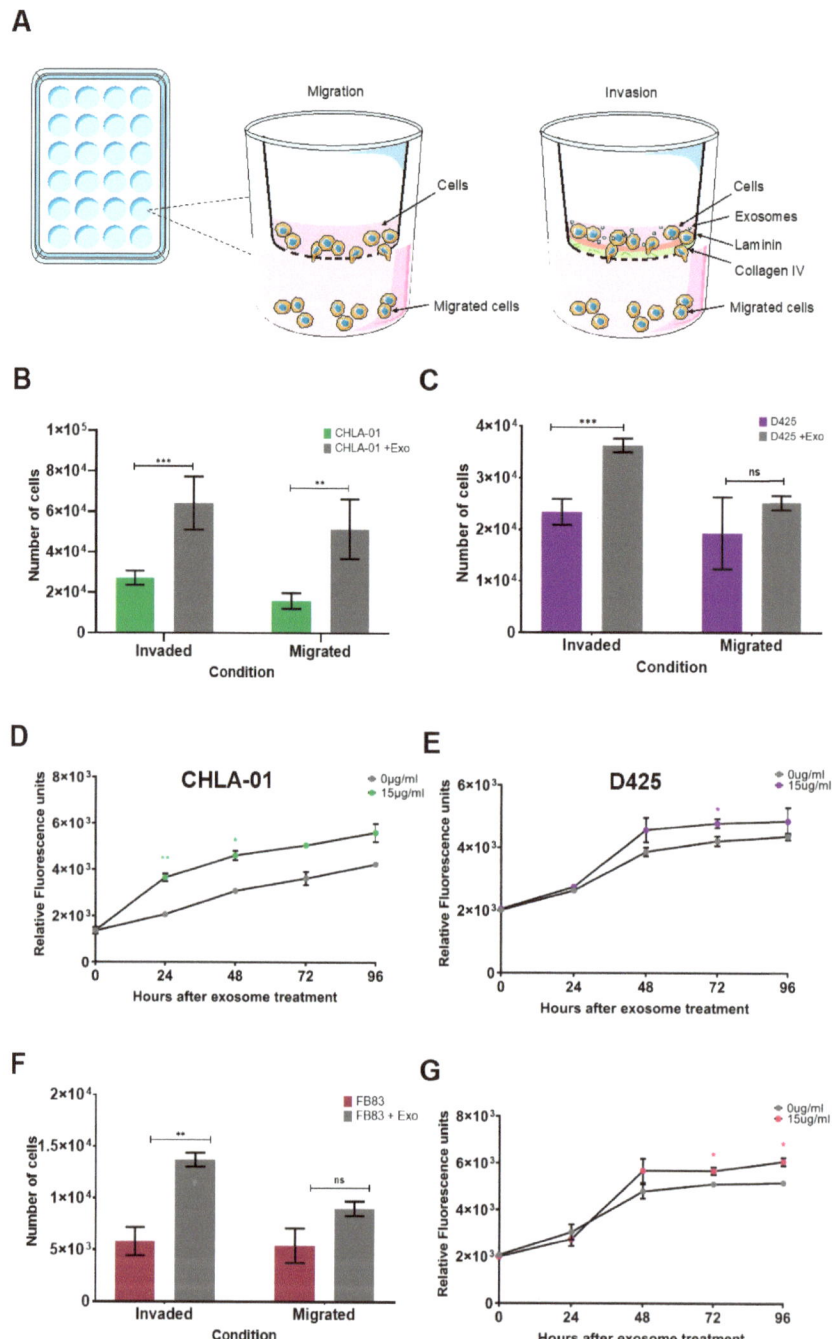

Figure 2. Exosomes from metastatic cell lines can confer a proinvasive phenotype on recipient cells (**A**) Experimental setup for migration through an uncoated chamber insert, or invasion and migration through a collagen IV- and laminin I-coated insert. (**B,C**) Exosomes derived from the metastatic cell lines CHLA-01R and D458 were applied (+Exo) to matched primary cell lines CHLA-01 (**B**) and D425

(C), respectively, and led to an increase in cell invasion behaviour (grey bars) compared to exosome-free supernatant control cells (coloured bars). (D,E) Exosomes from metastatic cell lines conferred only a modest effect on cell proliferation determined by Presto Blue viability assays. (F,G) Exosomes from the metastatic CHLA-01R cell line were able to confer an invasive phenotype on the noncancerous FB83 cell line (F), independent of an effect on cell proliferation (G). Significant differences in migration were calculated using one-way ANOVA analyses with Dunnett's multiple-comparisons post hoc test, (* $p \leq 0.05$, ** $p \leq 0.01$, *** $p \leq 0.005$) (ns = not significant). Data represent the average of three independent experiments with error bars indicating the standard error of the mean (SEM).

Elevated EMMPRIN expression levels have been correlated with a higher metastatic stage in medulloblastoma [19,39]. Further analysis of large-scale publicly-available datasets shows that when medulloblastoma patients were stratified according to the mRNA levels at diagnosis. Those with higher *BSG* expression had significantly worse five- and ten-year overall survival than patients with lower *BSG* expression (Supplementary Figure S4A), suggesting that the expression level of *BSG* may represent a negative prognostic factor for overall survival in medulloblastoma patients. Moreover, *BSG* gene expression was assessed across a panel of subgrouped medulloblastoma cell lines with known metastatic status. Interestingly, expression was observed to be higher in group three and group four cell lines, the two subgroups commonly associated with poor prognosis and a higher potential for metastatic dissemination (Supplementary Figure S4B). A significant biochemical property of EMMPRIN is that it can appear in diverse glycosylated forms, with large variation in molecular weights. Previous research has suggested that differential glycosylation of EMMPRIN exhibits functional relevance in tumour cells, with the highly glycosylated form being associated with enhanced cell adhesion, cell migration, and MMP-1 and MMP-2 production [36]. We, therefore, aimed to identify the expression patterns and glycosylation forms of EMMPRIN in matched medulloblastoma cell lines. Metastatic cell lines were significantly enriched with highly glycosylated EMMPRIN, compared to the primary cell lines which were distinguished by the low glycosylation variant of EMMPRIN (Supplementary Figure S4C–E).

Having been shown to correlate with poor patient outcomes and a higher grade in multiple cancers [40], it was postulated that the expression of MMP-2 would represent a poor prognosis factor in medulloblastoma. However, when medulloblastoma patients were stratified according to mRNA levels at diagnosis, those with elevated MMP-2 expression displayed a better five- and ten-year overall survival than patients with low MMP-2 expression (Supplementary Figure S5A). Additionally, when comparing MMP-2 gene expression in matched-primary and metastatic medulloblastoma cell lines there was not a consistent pattern of high MMP-2 in metastatic cells and low MMP-2 expression in the primary cells. However, this "high is worse" pattern was observed at the protein level, indicative that MMP-2 protein levels may be a more physiologically relevant marker of medulloblastoma metastasis (Supplementary Figure S5B–D).

Since medulloblastoma cell lines exhibit high EMMPRIN and MMP-2 levels and their expression was differentially enriched in metastatic cell lines compared to the primary cell lines, we hypothesised that MMP-2, and its inducer EMMPRIN, could be packaged into exosomes for extracellular release, thus contributing to medulloblastoma invasion and migration. A Western blot analysis of exosomes was therefore performed to assess whether the proinvasive phenotype correlated with increased MMP-2 and EMMPRIN levels. An analysis revealed an enrichment of EMMPRIN and MMP-2 in metastatic-derived exosomes compared to primary-derived exosomes (Figure 3Ai–Aiii, full-length blot in Supplementary Figure S6). Of note, the analysis of EMMPRIN protein size revealed that only metastatic CHLA-01R exosomes were enriched with highly glycosylated EMMPRIN compared to the low glycosylation variant of EMMPRIN. In contrast, the CHLA-01, D458, and D425 exosomes were distinguished by the low glycosylation variant of EMMPRIN.

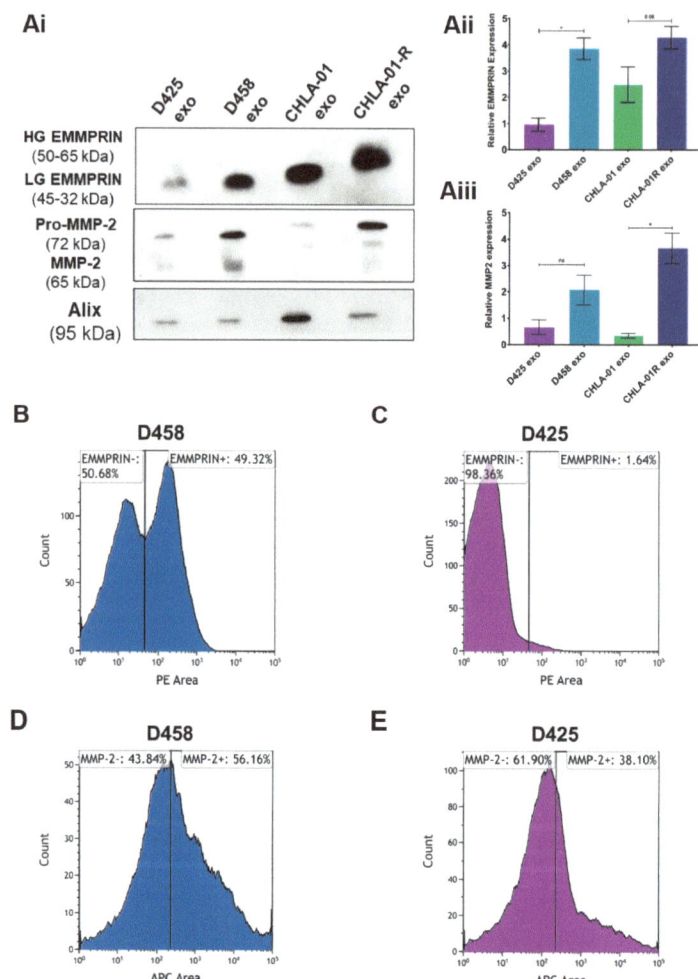

Figure 3. MMP-2 and EMMPRIN are expressed on exosomes released by medulloblastoma cell lines. Exosomal EMMPRIN and MMP2 protein expression was determined by Western blotting (representative image in panel (**Ai**) and was quantified relative to Alix protein expression (**Aii**,**Aiii**) (**B**). Flow-cytometry analysis of EMMPRIN (**B**,**C**) and MMP-2 (**D**,**E**) in medulloblastoma-derived exosomes. Exosomes from the metastatic and primary matched pair of cell lines (D458 and D425) were labelled with anti-EMMPRIN or anti-MMP-2 antibodies and secondary antibodies conjugated to either PE (EMMPRIN) or APC (MMP-2). Gating was identical across cell lines and the percentage of cells in populations representing high and low expression is shown. One representative experiment out of two performed with similar results is shown. Data in (**Ai**–**Aiii**) represent the average of three independent experiments with error bars indicating SEM. Significant differences in protein expression between exosomes derived from the matched cell lines were calculated using the Kruskal–Wallis test with Dunn's multiple-comparisons post hoc test (* $p \leq 0.05$, ns = not significant). The uncropped blots are shown in Supplementary Figure S6.

Since proinvasive exosomes promote cell migration and invasion, we predicted that this effect is mediated by MMP-2 and/or EMMPRIN on the exosomal surface. To investigate this hypothesis, flow cytometry of the exosomes was carried out. The exosomes isolated from the metastatic D458 cell line clearly resolved into two populations based upon

EMMPRIN expression (49.2% EMMPRIN positive compared to 50.7% EMMPRIN negative) whereas only a single, lower expressing, population was observed in the D425-derived exosomes (1.6% EMMPRIN positive compared to 98.3% EMMPRIN negative) (Figure 3B,C). For MMP-2 expression, the difference was more subtle, with exosomes isolated from the metastatic D458 cell lines clearly resolved into two populations based upon MMP-2 expression (56.2% MMP-2 positive compared to 43.8% MMP-2 negative) and a lower population of MMP-2-expressing exosomes was observed in the D425 exosomes (38.1% MMP-2 positive compared to 61.9% MMP-2 negative) (Figure 3D,E). These findings reinforced our hypothesis that EMMPRIN and MMP-2 are enriched on metastatic exosomes and are involved in conveying a proinvasive phenotype.

3.4. Stimulation of Medulloblastoma Cells with Migratory-Derived Exosomes Enhances Cell Invasion and Migration

MMPs can either be bound to the cell's membrane or secreted from the cytosol into the extracellular matrix, where they function as modulators of the extracellular space [40]. MMPs are synthesised as inactive proenzymes, termed zymogens, which require activation prior to being functionally active. Importantly, several MMPs in exosomes have been shown to exhibit proteolytic activities and can directly contribute to the degradation of ECM proteins in the extracellular space [41]. We hypothesised that surface-bound MMPs may degrade the extracellular matrix more effectively, creating a path for tumour cells or exosomes to migrate in the extracellular space. To determine whether the exosomal MMP-2 was catalytically active, gelatin zymography of exosomes suspended in PBS was performed and the functional activity of MMP-2 was determined. In accordance with the Western blot results, the metastatic-derived exosomes demonstrated the highest levels of functional MMP-2 activity compared to the primary exosomes (Figure 4A). The inherent differences in the basal levels of exosome-associated MMP-2 present in metastatic-derived exosomes compared to primary exosomes, further suggests that the MMP-2-associated exosomes promote tumour progression.

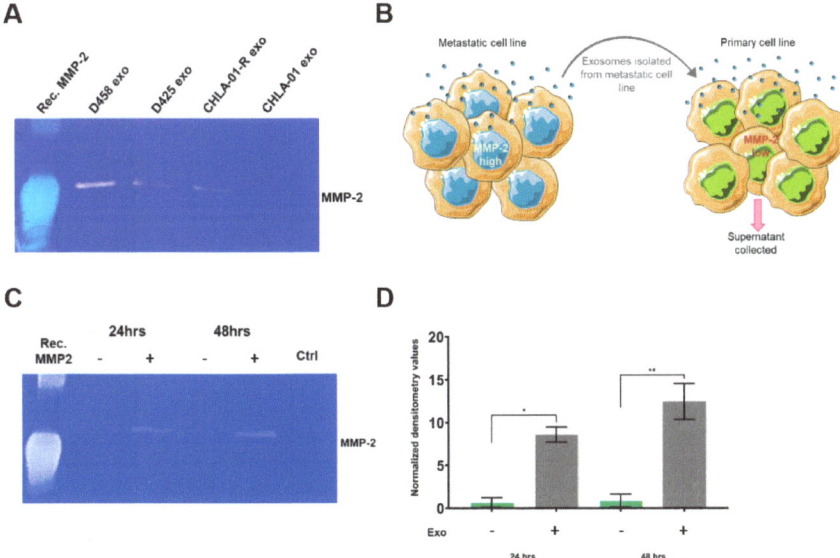

Figure 4. Exosomes contain functionally active MMP-2 and can transfer gelatinase activity onto recipient cell lines. (**A**) Gelatin zymography was used for the detection of MMP-2 activity in medulloblastoma-derived exosomes. The 5 µg of exosomes suspended in PBS were loaded onto gelatin-incorporated zymography gels and the functional activity of the gelatinase and MMP-2 was

determined. Data are representative of three independent experiments. (**B**) Schematic representation of the stimulation of a low MMP-2 expressing cell line (CHLA-01) with 10 µg of exosomes from a high MMP-2 expressing cell lines (CHLA-01R). After 24 and 48 h, supernatant from the recipient cell line was collected and loaded onto the gelatin-containing gel. Proteolysis was detected as a white band. MMP-2 levels shown in (**C**) were quantified and displayed graphically in (**D**). Data represent the average of two independent experiments with error bars indicating the standard error of the mean (SEM). Significant differences were calculated using one-way ANOVA analyses with Dunnett's multiple-comparisons post hoc test, (* $p \leq 0.05$, ** $p \leq 0.01$). The uncropped blots are shown in File S1.

Since proinvasive exosomes were found to express EMMPRIN and MMP-2 at high levels, and the role of exosome-bound EMMPRIN for the induction of MMPs is well established [42,43], MMP-2 secretion by medulloblastoma cells after exosome stimulation was explored (schematic representation shown in Figure 4B). After preconditioning with proinvasive exosomes, a time-dependent increase in the levels of functionally active MMP-2 secreted into the media compared to buffer-treated cells was observed (Figure 4C,D).

3.5. Knockdown of MMP-2 and EMMPRIN Reduces Exosome-Mediated Migration and Invasion

Given that exosomes from metastatic medulloblastoma cells, carrying higher levels of MMP-2 and EMMPRIN could confer an invasive phenotype on recipient cells, we decided to test the direct contribution of MMP-2 and EMMPRIN by genetic knockdown (Supplementary Figure S7A,B). In group four, medulloblastoma cells' knockdown of *BSG* or *MMP-2* at the genetic level resulted in a reduction of the ability of cells to invade a collagen-IV–laminin matrix (Figure 5A). Knockdown of *BSG* or *MMP-2* had little effect on either the distribution or the amounts of exosomes secreted by the corresponding cells (Figure 5B). Exosomes isolated from these cell lines did, however, result in a significant decrease in MMP-2 and EMMPRIN exosomal levels (Figure 5Ci–Ciii).

Primary cell lines were cocultured with exosomes isolated from knockdown metastatic cell lines or exosomes isolated from nontargeting controls. The addition of exosomes does not affect *MMP-2* mRNA levels in recipient cells (Figure 5D). However, a significant reduction in the migration of primary group four cell lines was observed when cells were pretreated with exosomes isolated from knockdown EMMPRIN and MMP-2 cell lines (Figure 5E). In addition, the preconditioning with exosomes isolated from MMP-2 knockdown cell lines also reduced the secretion of MMP-2 in primary medulloblastoma cell lines compared to controls (Figure 5Fi). Since EMMPRIN is known to induce MMP-2 production and secretion, it was slightly surprising that an increase in MMP-2 function was observed when primary medulloblastoma cell lines were preconditioned with exosomes isolated from *BSG* knockdown cell lines, (Figure 5Fii). The incomplete knockdown of EMMPRIN in exosomes may account for this observation (Figure 5Ci–Ciii), thus MMP-2 activation persists to some extent. Together, these results indicate that exosomal EMMPRIN has the ability to initiate MMP-2 secretion in the recipient medulloblastoma cells, while exosomal MMP-2 can further stimulate MMP-2 secretion in a positive feedback loop. Increased levels of secreted MMP-2 would support extracellular-matrix degradation, in turn facilitating tumour cell invasion and metastasis.

Group three primary MB cells showed a similar pattern in reduction when using knock down exosomes; however, the results were not statistically significant (Supplementary Figure S7). In accordance with the findings that depletion of MMP-2 or EMMPRIN slightly reduced migration of medulloblastoma cells, these results strongly indicate that exosomal MMP-2 and EMMPRIN facilitate the progression of medulloblastoma. This is particularly apparent for group four medulloblastoma.

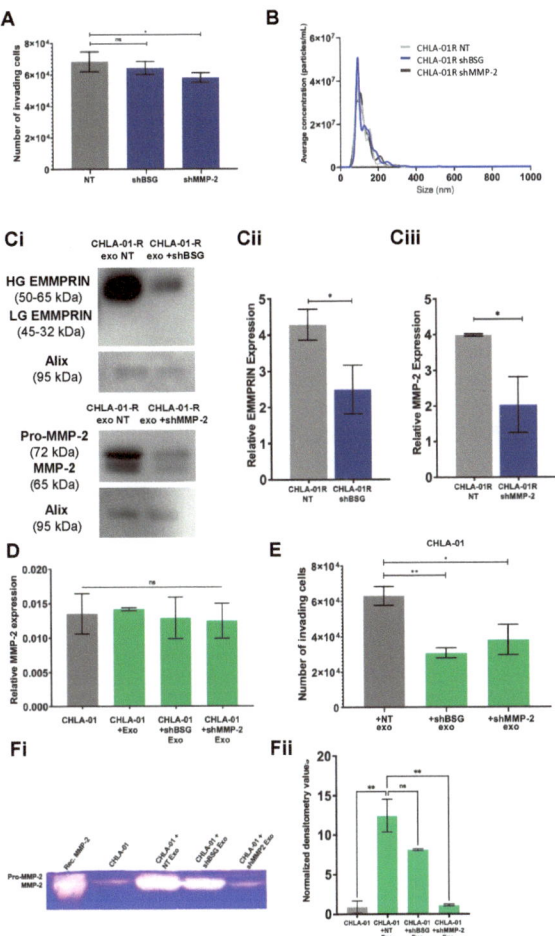

Figure 5. Knockdown of MMP-2 and EMMPRIN appears to reduce exosome-mediated migration and invasion in group four medulloblastoma cell lines. (**A**) Group four cell invasion through a collagen and laminin IV coated transwell chamber insert was quantified by PrestoBlue metabolic staining and compared to cell lines transduced with nontargeting (NT). (**B**) Exosomes from the CHLA-01R knockdown cell lines and nontransduced cells were isolated and their size and concentration were measured by NanoFCM. (**Ci**) Western blot analysis and concurrent densitometry revealed both EMMPRIN (**Cii**) and MMP-2 (**Ciii**) protein levels to be significantly depleted in exosomes isolated from the knockdown cell lines. Densitometry data are presented relative to the Alix loading control and compared to the appropriate nonsilencing control cell line. (**D**) Exosomes from the CHLA-01R knockdown cell lines were applied to the matched parental cell line CHLA-01 (+NT exo: nontargetting, +shBSG exo, knockdown *BSG*, or shMMP-2 exo knockdown MMP-2) following which MMP-2 mRNA expression levels in recipient cells was determined by qRT-PCR. (**E**) The ability of these recipient cell lines to invade through a laminin and collage IV matrix was determined by metabolic assay. MMP-2 activity in the medium of CHLA-01 cells receiving exosomes was determined by gelatin zymography. Proteolysis was detected as a white band. MMP-2 levels shown in (**Fi**) were quantified and displayed graphically in (**Fii**). Significance was assessed by ordinary one-way ANOVA analysis with Sidak's multiple-comparison tests (* $p \leq 0.05$, ** $p \leq 0.01$) (ns = not significant). Data represent the average of at least two independent experiments with error bars indicating the standard error of the mean (SEM). The uncropped blots are shown in File S1.

3.6. CSF Levels of Functionally Active MMP2 Increase at Disease Progression

Having consistently demonstrated higher levels of functionally active MMP-2 are secreted from the group four metastatic MB cell line CHLA-01R in comparison to its primary counterpart, we sought to determine whether this finding would be replicated in an ex-vivo pilot study of cerebrospinal fluid (CSF) derived from paediatric medulloblastoma patients. Their key features are tabulated in Figure 6A. Disease progression was defined as patients presenting with the growth of their residuum (Figure 6B), recurrence or relapse of their medulloblastoma. We explored whether the levels of functional active MMP-2 secreted into CSF could be employed as surrogate markers of disease progression, irrespective of their starting point. The examined CSF samples were derived from four patients, all of whom were male and between the ages of 5 and 20 years old. Molecular subgrouping was unfortunately only available for two of the four patients both of whom were determined to be group four MB. While the size of our pilot study was limited by the availability of the matched CSF samples, we observed increased levels of functionally active MMP-2 in three of four patients, which correlated with disease progression in patients one, three, and four (Figure 6C). Furthermore, the observation of a strong MMP-2 signal in the CSF derived from patients one and four at the point of disease progression, appeared to correlate with prognosis, in contrast to CSF cytology, which was negative in both cases (Figure 6A).

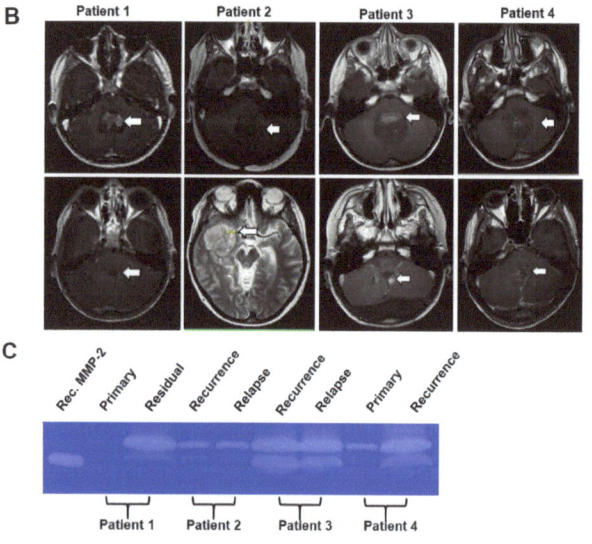

Figure 6. Determination of MMP-2 activity in clinical CSF samples from medulloblastoma patients indicates MMP-2 activity as a possible marker of disease progression. (**A**) Clinical characteristics of 4 medulloblastoma patients. (**B**) Axial MRI with gadolinium T1 and T2 images taken at presentation (top row) and at disease progression (bottom row) with tumours highlighted with white arrows (**C**) Paired CSF sampled from the patients was examined and the levels of functional activity of MMP 2 determined and normalised to recombinant MMP-2, at their presentation and disease progression. The uncropped blots are shown in File S1.

4. Discussion

Metastatic dissemination is the predominant cause of the mortality of patients with medulloblastoma [44]. Increasing evidence suggests that exosomes serve as key mediators in tumour metastasis [45]. It has been reported that exosomes from highly metastatic tumour cell lines could significantly enhance the migration capacity of less migratory recipient cells [35]. Similarly, the present study revealed that exosomes isolated from migratory medulloblastoma cell lines directly enhanced the invasive potential of less-migratory matched primary-tumour cells in a heterologous stimulation loop. The effect was specific to exosomes since the exosome-free supernatant had no influence on tumour invasion.

Several studies have demonstrated that exosomes are able to transfer malignant characteristics from highly invasive tumour cells to surrounding nonmalignant cells [46,47]. In line with this, the invasive capacity of nonmalignant foetal neuronal stem cells was enhanced when stimulated with heterologous exosomes derived from highly migratory medulloblastoma cell lines, indicating that recipient cells did not need to be predisposed to an invasive phenotype prior to exosome stimulation.

Although some studies have already demonstrated the tumour-supporting functions of EMMPRIN or MMP-2 in medulloblastoma metastasis [39,48–50], the presence of these proteins on medulloblastoma exosomes has not yet been investigated. In this current study, we have advanced the understanding of the mechanism of action of MMP-2 and its inducer EMMPRIN in medulloblastoma progression by demonstrating that MMP-2 and EMMPRIN are associated with secreted exosomes. Importantly, Western blot and flow cytometry analysis revealed that proinvasive metastatic exosomes were significantly enriched with membrane-associated EMMPRIN and MMP-2 compared to the primary exosomes. It is therefore reasonable to propose that exosomal MMP-2 and EMMPRIN are surface-associated in invasive exosomes, as this location is required for a protease to exert its proteolytic activity on extracellular proteins. Recently, it has been suggested that EVs possess a protein corona [51,52], which includes extracellular matrix components such as fibronectin. It would be interesting to see if this protein corona is present in medulloblastoma-derived exosomes and if MMP-2 or EMMPRIN might either be interacting with it or constituting it.

The role of exosomes in ECM degradation has been described recently [50,53]. Activated MMP-2 has a wide range of substrates and can degrade basement-membrane collagen IV, elastin, and several other ECM molecules, including interstitial-collagen types I, II, and III [54], and is therefore associated with ECM remodelling as a prerequisite for cellular invasion and migration [55]. Our finding, that functional activated MMP-2 is carried by exosomes and released by metastatic cell lines into the extracellular space, reveals a possible mechanism by which MMP-2 may facilitate the breakdown of the ECM. Degradation of the ECM would create routes for medulloblastoma cells to directionally invade the surrounding environment, and functional MMP-2 on the external surface of exosomes could allow exosomes to reach long-distance target locations. Moreover, shRNA-mediated knockdown of EMMPRIN or MMP-2 in exosomes decreased the promigratory effect of exosomes on recipient cells.

The association between exosomal EMMPRIN/MMP-2 and ECM degradation was reinforced by zymography assays, demonstrating that secretion of active MMP-2 was activated in primary medulloblastoma cell lines upon coculture with metastatic exosomes enriched with high glycosylated EMMPRIN and MMP-2. Validation of this was provided by a significant reduction in this heterologous stimulation when exosomes were isolated from the metastatic cell lines stably transfected with EMMPRIN or MMP-2 shRNAs. Future research is needed to determine how MMP-2 and EMMPRIN are recruited into and out of the exosomes, as modulation of these mechanisms could potentially prevent or limit the establishment of a premetastatic niche that is conducive to MB dissemination throughout the neuroaxis. Achieving absolute purification or complete isolation of EVs from other entities poses significant challenges. Future proteomic and transcriptomic analyses of the sEVs could serve as a valuable approach to elucidate the molecular mechanisms underlying the metastatic effects of these extracellular vesicles.

Additionally, the positive correlation between the increased secretion of functionally active MMP-2, as detected in the CSF zymography, and their disease progression, may improve our accuracy of disease surveillance and potentially provide a surrogate biomarker of prognosis and response to treatment. However, given our modest sample size, this work would need to be replicated with a larger patient cohort, to gain further insight into the generalisability of our findings.

5. Conclusions

Taken together, this work demonstrated that medulloblastoma cells release exosomes into the local tumour microenvironment. This creates a favourable milieu within the neuroaxis, driving medulloblastoma metastasis, through extracellular matrix signalling, via surface-associated proteins. Our findings provide important and unique insights into the pathogenesis of medulloblastoma and highlight the need to explore alternative therapeutic approaches to impair MMP-driven mechanisms of tumour invasion and migration.

Supplementary Materials: The following supporting information can be downloaded at https://www.mdpi.com/article/10.3390/cancers15092601/s1, Supplementary Figures: Figure S1 Characterisation of exosomes from medulloblastoma cell lines; Figure S2: Comparisons of cell line migration and invasion in transwell assays; Figure S3: Densitometry of protease microarrays of the matched Group 3/4 medulloblastoma cell lines; Figure S4: EMMPRIN gene and protein expression in medulloblastoma; Figure S5: MMP-2 gene and protein expression in medulloblastoma; Figure S6 Representative full-length western blot images from Figure 3A confirming exosomal EMMPRIN and MMP2 protein expression; and Figure S7: *BSG* and *MMP-2* were significantly depleted using shRNA in D458 and CHLA-01-R cell lines. Supplementary Method: Protease arrays. File S1: Full length western blots.

Author Contributions: Conceptualization, H.K.J., I.D.K. and B.C.; Data curation, H.K.J., I.D.K. and B.C.; Formal analysis, H.K.J., C.M. and F.L.; Funding acquisition, H.K.J., I.D.K. and B.C.; Investigation H.K.J. and C.M.; Methodology, H.K.J., C.M. and F.L.; Supervision, D.M., I.D.K. and B.C.; Validation H.K.J. and C.M.; Visualization, H.K.J., I.D.K. and B.C.; Writing—original draft, H.K.J., I.D.K. and B.C Writing—review & editing, H.K.J., C.M., F.L., D.M., I.D.K. and B.C. All authors have read and agreed to the published version of the manuscript.

Funding: James Tudor Fund (awarded to H.K.J., I.D.K., and B.C.), Haydn Green Institute for Innovation and Entrepreneurship (awarded C.M.), and Stoneygate Trust (awarded to B.C.).

Institutional Review Board Statement: The study was conducted in accordance with the Declaration of Helsinki, and approved by the National Research Ethics Service Committee East Midlands—Nottingham 2 of the National Health Service (REC reference: 11/EM/0076 approved 5 May 2011; amendment approved 20 February 2019).

Informed Consent Statement: For all patients, informed consent was obtained from the patient, or a parent and/or legal guardian where the patient was under 18 years of age, prior to their inclusion in the study.

Data Availability Statement: Data is contained within the article or Supplementary Material.

Acknowledgments: Transmission Electron Microscope sample processing and image acquisition were kindly performed by Zubair Nizamudeen. NanoFCM readings and instrument calibration were conducted by Ben Peacock (NanoFCM application scientist).

Conflicts of Interest: The authors declare no conflict of interest. The funders had no role in the design of the study; in the collection, analyses, or interpretation of data; in the writing of the manuscript; or in the decision to publish the results.

References

1. Hill, R.M.; Richardson, S.; Schwalbe, E.C.; Hicks, D.; Lindsey, J.C.; Crosier, S.; Rafiee, G.; Grabovska, Y.; Wharton, S.B.; Jacques, T.S.; et al. Time, Pattern, and Outcome of Medulloblastoma Relapse and Their Association with Tumour Biology at Diagnosis and Therapy: A Multicentre Cohort Study. *Lancet Child Adolesc. Health* **2020**, *4*, 865–874. [CrossRef] [PubMed]
2. Ramaswamy, V.; Remke, M.; Bouffet, E.; Bailey, S.; Clifford, S.C.; Doz, F.; Kool, M.; Dufour, C.; Vassal, G.; Milde, T.; et al. Risk Stratification of Childhood Medulloblastoma in the Molecular Era: The Current Consensus. *Acta Neuropathol.* **2016**, *131*, 821–831. [CrossRef]
3. Van Niel, G.; D'Angelo, G.; Raposo, G. Shedding Light on the Cell Biology of Extracellular Vesicles. *Nat. Rev. Mol. Cell Biol.* **2018**, *19*, 213–228. [CrossRef]
4. Banks, W.A.; Sharma, P.; Bullock, K.M.; Hansen, K.M.; Ludwig, N.; Whiteside, T.L. Transport of Extracellular Vesicles across the Blood-Brain Barrier: Brain Pharmacokinetics and Effects of Inflammation. *Int. J. Mol. Sci.* **2020**, *21*, 4407. [CrossRef] [PubMed]
5. Magaña, S.M.; Peterson, T.E.; Evans, J.E.; Decker, P.A.; Simon, V.; Eckel-Passow, J.E.; Daniels, D.J.; Parney, I.F. Pediatric Brain Tumor Cell Lines Exhibit MiRNA-Depleted, Y RNA-Enriched Extracellular Vesicles. *J. Neurooncol.* **2022**, *156*, 269–279. [CrossRef]
6. Epple, L.M.; Griffiths, S.G.; Dechkovskaia, A.M.; Dusto, N.L.; White, J.; Ouellette, R.J.; Anchordoquy, T.J.; Bemis, L.T.; Graner, M.W. Medulloblastoma Exosome Proteomics Yield Functional Roles for Extracellular Vesicles. *PLoS ONE* **2012**, *7*, e42064. [CrossRef] [PubMed]
7. Bisaro, B.; Mandili, G.; Poli, A.; Piolatto, A.; Papa, V.; Novelli, F.; Cenacchi, G.; Forni, M.; Zanini, C. Proteomic Analysis of Extracellular Vesicles from Medullospheres Reveals a Role for Iron in the Cancer Progression of Medulloblastoma. *Mol. Cell. Ther.* **2015**, *3*, 1–12. [CrossRef]
8. Huang, S.; Xue, P.; Han, X.; Zhang, C.; Yang, L.; Liu, L.; Wang, X.; Li, H.; Fu, J.; Zhou, Y. Exosomal MiR-130b-3p Targets SIK1 to Inhibit Medulloblastoma Tumorigenesis. *Cell Death Dis.* **2020**, *11*, 408. [CrossRef] [PubMed]
9. Zhu, L.; Sun, H.T.; Wang, S.; Huang, S.L.; Zheng, Y.; Wang, C.Q.; Hu, B.Y.; Qin, W.; Zou, T.T.; Fu, Y.; et al. Isolation and Characterization of Exosomes for Cancer Research. *J. Hematol. Oncol.* **2020**, *13*, 152. [CrossRef]
10. Zhang, Y.; Liu, Y.; Liu, H.; Tang, W.H. Exosomes: Biogenesis, Biologic Function and Clinical Potential. *Cell Biosci.* **2019**, *9*, 19. [CrossRef]
11. Li, Z.B.; Chen, X.; Yi, X. Tumor Promoting Effects of Exosomal MicroRNA-210 Derived from Lung Cancer Cells on Lung Cancer through the RUNX3/PI3K/AKT Signaling Pathway Axis. *J. Biol. Regul. Homeost. Agents* **2021**, *35*, 473–484. [CrossRef]
12. Skog, J.; Würdinger, T.; van Rijn, S.; Meijer, D.H.; Gainche, L.; Curry, W.T.; Carter, B.S.; Krichevsky, A.M.; Breakefield, X.O. Glioblastoma Microvesicles Transport RNA and Proteins That Promote Tumour Growth and Provide Diagnostic Biomarkers. *Nat. Cell Biol.* **2008**, *10*, 1470–1476. [CrossRef] [PubMed]
13. Wang, J.; Bo, X.; Yi, X.; Xiao, X.; Zheng, Q.; Ma, L.; Li, B. Exosome-Transferred LINC01559 Promotes the Progression of Gastric Cancer via PI3K/AKT Signaling Pathway. *Cell Death Dis.* **2020**, *11*, 723. [CrossRef]
14. Théry, C.; Zitvogel, L.; Amigorena, S. Exosomes: Composition, Biogenesis and Function. *Nat. Rev. Immunol.* **2002**, *2*, 569–579. [CrossRef]
15. Yang, X.; Zhang, Y.; Zhang, Y.; Zhang, S.; Qiu, L.; Zhuang, Z.; Wei, M.; Deng, X.; Wang, Z.; Han, J. The Key Role of Exosomes on the Pre-Metastatic Niche Formation in Tumors. *Front. Mol. Biosci.* **2021**, *8*, 703640. [CrossRef] [PubMed]
16. Kogure, A.; Yoshioka, Y.; Ochiya, T. Extracellular Vesicles in Cancer Metastasis: Potential as Therapeutic Targets and Materials. *Int. J. Mol. Sci.* **2020**, *21*, 4463. [CrossRef] [PubMed]
17. Aili, Y.; Maimaitiming, N.; Qin, H.; Ji, W.; Fan, G.; Wang, Z.; Wang, Y. Tumor Microenvironment and Exosomes in Brain Metastasis: Molecular Mechanisms and Clinical Application. *Front. Oncol.* **2022**, *12*, 5684. [CrossRef] [PubMed]
18. Kaczorowska, A.; Miękus, N.; Stefanowicz, J.; Adamkiewicz-Drożyńska, E. Selected Matrix Metalloproteinases (MMP-2, MMP-7) and Their Inhibitor (TIMP-2) in Adult and Pediatric Cancer. *Diagnostics* **2020**, *10*, 547. [CrossRef] [PubMed]
19. Xin, X.; Zeng, X.; Gu, H.; Li, M.; Tan, H.; Jin, Z.; Hua, T.; Shi, R.; Wang, H. CD147/EMMPRIN Overexpression and Prognosis in Cancer: A Systematic Review and Meta-Analysis. *Sci. Rep.* **2016**, *6*, 32804. [CrossRef]
20. Ivanov, D.P.; Al-Rubai, A.J.; Grabowska, A.M.; Pratten, M.K. Separating Chemotherapy-Related Developmental Neurotoxicity from Cytotoxicity in Monolayer and Neurosphere Cultures of Human Fetal Brain Cells. *Toxicol. In Vitro* **2016**, *37*, 88–96. [CrossRef] [PubMed]
21. Tian, Y.; Gong, M.; Hu, Y.; Liu, H.; Zhang, W.; Zhang, M.; Hu, X.; Aubert, D.; Zhu, S.; Wu, L.; et al. Quality and Efficiency Assessment of Six Extracellular Vesicle Isolation Methods by Nano-Flow Cytometry. *J. Extracell Vesicles* **2020**, *9*, 1697028. [CrossRef] [PubMed]
22. Sharma, T.; Schwalbe, E.C.; Williamson, D.; Sill, M.; Hovestadt, V.; Mynarek, M.; Rutkowski, S.; Robinson, G.W.; Gajjar, A.; Cavalli, F.; et al. Second-Generation Molecular Subgrouping of Medulloblastoma: An International Meta-Analysis of Group 3 and Group 4 Subtypes. *Acta Neuropathol.* **2019**, *138*, 309–326. [CrossRef] [PubMed]
23. Taylor, M.D.; Northcott, P.A.; Korshunov, A.; Remke, M.; Cho, Y.J.; Clifford, S.C.; Eberhart, C.G.; Parsons, D.W.; Rutkowski, S.; Gajjar, A.; et al. Molecular Subgroups of Medulloblastoma: The Current Consensus. *Acta Neuropathol.* **2012**, *123*, 465–472. [CrossRef]
24. Northcott, P.A.; Jones, D.T.W.; Kool, M.; Robinson, G.W.; Gilbertson, R.J.; Cho, Y.J.; Pomeroy, S.L.; Korshunov, A.; Lichter, P.; Taylor, M.D.; et al. Medulloblastomics: The End of the Beginning. *Nat. Rev. Cancer* **2012**, *12*, 818–834. [CrossRef] [PubMed]

25. Northcott, P.A.; Robinson, G.W.; Kratz, C.P.; Mabbott, D.J.; Pomeroy, S.L.; Clifford, S.C.; Rutkowski, S.; Ellison, D.W.; Malkin, D. Taylor, M.D.; et al. Medulloblastoma. *Nat. Rev. Dis. Prim.* **2019**, *5*, 11. [CrossRef]
26. Théry, C.; Witwer, K.W.; Aikawa, E.; Alcaraz, M.J.; Anderson, J.D.; Andriantsitohaina, R.; Antoniou, A.; Arab, T.; Archer, F. Atkin-Smith, G.K.; et al. Minimal Information for Studies of Extracellular Vesicles 2018 (MISEV2018): A Position Statement of the International Society for Extracellular Vesicles and Update of the MISEV2014 Guidelines. *J. Extracell Vesicles* **2018**, *7*, 1535750 [CrossRef]
27. Royo, F.; Théry, C.; Falcón-Pérez, J.M.; Nieuwland, R.; Witwer, K.W. Methods for Separation and Characterization of Extracellular Vesicles: Results of a Worldwide Survey Performed by the ISEV Rigor and Standardization Subcommittee. *Cells* **2020**, *9*, 1955 [CrossRef]
28. Théry, C.; Clayton, A.; Amigorena, S.; Raposo, G. Isolation and Characterization of Exosomes from Cell Culture Supernatants *Curr. Protoc. Cell Biol.* **2006**, *30*, 2–22. [CrossRef] [PubMed]
29. van Deun, J.; Mestdagh, P.; Agostinis, P.; Akay, Ö.; Anand, S.; Anckaert, J.; Martinez, Z.A.; Baetens, T.; Beghein, E.; Bertier, L.; et al. EV-TRACK: Transparent Reporting and Centralizing Knowledge in Extracellular Vesicle Research. *Nat. Methods* **2017**, *14*, 228–232 [CrossRef]
30. Baran, J.; Baj-Krzyworzeka, M.; Weglarczyk, K.; Szatanek, R.; Zembela, M.; Barbasz, J.; Czupryna, A.; Szczepanik, A.; Zembala, M Circulating Tumour-Derived Microvesicles in Plasma of Gastric Cancer Patients. *Cancer Immunol. Immunother.* **2010**, *59*, 841–850 [CrossRef]
31. Yamamoto, H.; Watanabe, Y.; Oikawa, R.; Morita, R.; Yoshida, Y.; Maehata, T.; Yasuda, H.; Itoh, F. BARHL2 Methylation Using Gastric Wash DNA or Gastric Juice Exosomal DNA Is a Useful Marker for Early Detection of Gastric Cancer in an H. Pylori -Independent Manner. *Clin. Transl. Gastroenterol.* **2016**, *7*, e184. [CrossRef] [PubMed]
32. Han, L.; Sheng, B.; Zeng, Q.; Yao, W.; Jiang, Q. Correlation between MMP2 Expression in Lung Cancer Tissues and Clinical Parameters: A Retrospective Clinical Analysis. *BMC Pulm. Med.* **2020**, *20*, 283. [CrossRef]
33. Kessenbrock, K.; Plaks, V.; Werb, Z. Matrix Metalloproteinases: Regulators of the Tumor Microenvironment. *Cell* **2010**, *141*, 52 [CrossRef] [PubMed]
34. Sier, C.F.M.; Zuidwijk, K.; Zijlmans, H.J.M.A.A.; Hanemaaijer, R.; Mulder-Stapel, A.A.; Prins, F.A.; Dreef, E.J.; Kenter, G.G. Fleuren, G.J.; Gorter, A. EMMPRIN-Induced MMP-2 Activation Cascade in Human Cervical Squamous Cell Carcinoma. *Int. J Cancer* **2006**, *118*, 2991–2998. [CrossRef]
35. Menck, K.; Scharf, C.; Bleckmann, A.; Dyck, L.; Rost, U.; Wenzel, D.; Dhople, V.M.; Siam, L.; Pukrop, T.; Binder, C.; et al Tumor-Derived Microvesicles Mediate Human Breast Cancer Invasion through Differentially Glycosylated EMMPRIN. *J. Mol Cell Biol.* **2015**, *7*, 143–153. [CrossRef]
36. Sun, J.; Hemler, M.E. Regulation of MMP-1 and MMP-2 Production through CD147/Extracellular Matrix Metalloproteinase Inducer Interactions. *Cancer Res.* **2001**, *61*, 2276–2281. [PubMed]
37. Fahs, A.; Hussein, N.; Zalzali, H.; Ramadan, F.; Ghamloush, F.; Tamim, H.; el Homsi, M.; Badran, B.; Boulos, F.; Tawil, A. et al. CD147 Promotes Tumorigenesis via Exosome-Mediated Signaling in Rhabdomyosarcoma. *Cells* **2022**, *11*, 2267. [CrossRef] [PubMed]
38. Colangelo, N.W.; Azzam, E.I. Extracellular Vesicles Originating from Glioblastoma Cells Increase Metalloproteinase Release by Astrocytes: The Role of CD147 (EMMPRIN) and Ionizing Radiation. *Cell Commun. Signal.* **2020**, *18*, 21. [CrossRef]
39. Chu, T.; Chen, X.; Yu, J.; Xiao, J.; Fu, Z. Extracellular Matrix Metalloproteinase Inducer Is a Negative Prognostic Factor of Pediatric Medulloblastoma. *Pathol. Oncol. Res.* **2011**, *17*, 705–711. [CrossRef]
40. Isaacson, K.J.; Martin Jensen, M.; Subrahmanyam, N.B.; Ghandehari, H. Matrix-Metalloproteinases as Targets for Controlled Delivery in Cancer: An Analysis of Upregulation and Expression. *J. Control. Release* **2017**, *259*, 62–75. [CrossRef]
41. Shimoda, M.; Khokha, R. Metalloproteinases in Extracellular Vesicles. *Biochim. Biophys. Acta Mol. Cell Res.* **2017**, *1864*, 1989–2000 [CrossRef] [PubMed]
42. Redzic, J.S.; Kendrick, A.A.; Bahmed, K.; Dahl, K.D.; Pearson, C.G.; Robinson, W.A.; Robinson, S.E.; Graner, M.W.; Eisenmesser E.Z. Extracellular Vesicles Secreted from Cancer Cell Lines Stimulate Secretion of MMP-9, IL-6, TGF-B1 and EMMPRIN. *PLoS ONE* **2013**, *8*, e71225. [CrossRef] [PubMed]
43. Hatanaka, M.; Higashi, Y.; Fukushige, T.; Baba, N.; Kawai, K.; Hashiguchi, T.; Su, J.; Zeng, W.; Chen, X.; Kanekura, T Cleaved CD147 Shed from the Surface of Malignant Melanoma Cells Activates MMP2 Produced by Fibroblasts. *Anticancer Res* **2014**, *34*, 7091–7096.
44. van Ommeren, R.; Garzia, L.; Holgado, B.L.; Ramaswamy, V.; Taylor, M.D. The Molecular Biology of Medulloblastoma Metastasis *Brain Pathol.* **2020**, *30*, 691–702. [CrossRef]
45. Whiteside, T.L. Tumor-Derived Exosomes and Their Role in Cancer Progression. In *Advances in Clinical Chemistry*; Academic Press Inc.: Cambridge, MA, USA, 2016; Volume 74. [CrossRef]
46. Angelucci, A.; D'Ascenzo, S.; Festuccia, C.; Gravina, G.L.; Bologna, M.; Dolo, V.; Pavan, A. Vesicle-Associated Urokinase Plasminogen Activator Promotes Invasion in Prostate Cancer Cell Lines. *Clin. Exp. Metastasis* **2000**, *18*, 163–170. [CrossRef] [PubMed]
47. Al-Nedawi, K.; Meehan, B.; Micallef, J.; Lhotak, V.; May, L.; Guha, A.; Rak, J. Intercellular Transfer of the Oncogenic Receptor EGFRvIII by Microvesicles Derived from Tumour Cells. *Nat. Cell Biol.* **2008**, *10*, 619–624. [CrossRef]

48. Özen, Ö.; Krebs, B.; Hemmerlein, B.; Pekrun, A.; Kretzschmar, H.; Herms, J. Expression of Matrix Metalloproteinases and Their Inhibitors in Medulloblastomas and Their Prognostic Relevance. *Clin. Cancer Res.* **2004**, *10*, 4746–4753. [CrossRef]
49. Mateo, E.C.; Motta, F.J.N.; Queiroz, R.G.P.; Scrileli, C.A.; Tone, L.G. Protein Expression of the Matrix Metalloproteinase (MMP-1, -2, -3, -9 and -14) in Ewing Family Tumors and Medulloblastoma of Pediatric Patients. *Pediatr. Ther.* **2013**, *3*, 1–5. [CrossRef]
50. al Halawani, A.; Mithieux, S.M.; Yeo, G.C.; Hosseini-Beheshti, E.; Weiss, A.S. Extracellular Vesicles: Interplay with the Extracellular Matrix and Modulated Cell Responses. *Int. J. Mol. Sci.* **2022**, *23*, 3389. [CrossRef]
51. Tóth, E.; Turiák, L.; Visnovitz, T.; Cserép, C.; Mázló, A.; Sódar, B.W.; Försönits, A.I.; Petővári, G.; Sebestyén, A.; Komlósi, Z.; et al. Formation of a Protein Corona on the Surface of Extracellular Vesicles in Blood Plasma. *J. Extracell Vesicles* **2021**, *10*, e12140. [CrossRef]
52. Palviainen, M.I.; Saraswat, M.; Varga, Z.; na Kitka, D.; Neuvonen, M.; Puhka, M.; Joenvä, S.; Renkonen, R.; Nieuwland, R.; Takatalo, M.; et al. Extracellular Vesicles from Human Plasma and Serum Are Carriers of Extravesicular Cargo-Implications for Biomarker Discovery. *PloS ONE* **2020**, *15*, e0236439. [CrossRef] [PubMed]
53. Albacete-Albacete, L. Extracellular Vesicles: An Emerging Mechanism Governing the Secretion and Biological Roles of Tenascin-C. *Front. Immunol.* **2021**, *12*, 1425. [CrossRef] [PubMed]
54. Jabłońska-Trypuć, A.; Matejczyk, M.; Rosochacki, S. Matrix Metalloproteinases (MMPs), the Main Extracellular Matrix (ECM) Enzymes in Collagen Degradation, as a Target for Anticancer Drugs. *J. Enzyme Inhib. Med. Chem.* **2016**, *31*, 177–183. [CrossRef]
55. Löffek, S.; Schilling, O.; Franzke, C.W. Series "Matrix Metalloproteinases in Lung Health and Disease" Edited by J. Müller-Quernheim and O. Eickelberg Number 1 in This Series: Biological Role of Matrix Metalloproteinases: A Critical Balance. *Eur. Respir. J.* **2011**, *38*, 191–208. [CrossRef] [PubMed]

Disclaimer/Publisher's Note: The statements, opinions and data contained in all publications are solely those of the individual author(s) and contributor(s) and not of MDPI and/or the editor(s). MDPI and/or the editor(s) disclaim responsibility for any injury to people or property resulting from any ideas, methods, instructions or products referred to in the content.

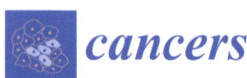

Review

The Role of Hypoxia and Cancer Stem Cells in Development of Glioblastoma

Tingyu Shi [1,2,†], Jun Zhu [3,†], Xiang Zhang [1,*] and Xinggang Mao [1,*]

1. Department of Neurosurgery, Xijing Hospital, Fourth Military Medical University, Xi'an 710032, China
2. Tangdu Hospital, Fourth Military Medical University, Xi'an 710024, China
3. State Key Laboratory of Cancer Biology, Institute of Digestive Diseases, Xijing Hospital, The Fourth Military Medical University, Xi'an 710032, China

* Correspondence: xzhang@fmmu.edu.cn (X.Z.); xgmao@fmmu.edu.cn (X.M.)
† These authors contributed equally to this work.

Simple Summary: As one of most malignant tumors in brain, glioblastoma (GBM) is lack of effective treatment and the prognosis of GBM patients is still very poor despite accumulated progresses. Hypoxia is an essential factor for the initiation and progression of GBM, especially for the glioma stem like cells (GSCs). Hypoxia induced many target genes which form a complicated molecular interacting network, influencing a lot of tumor behaviors by regulating key signal pathways. In addition, hypoxia has great impact on the interplayed niches of GCSs. Here, by systematically reviewing the role of hypoxia on the maintenance of GSCs and the development of GBM, and analyzing the related molecular mechanisms, we integrated the hypoxia related tumor features of GBM. This summary helps to deepen our knowledge of the tumorigenic mechanisms of GBM and can help to develop novel therapeutic strategies targeting hypoxia to improve the survival of GBM patients.

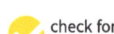

Citation: Shi, T.; Zhu, J.; Zhang, X.; Mao, X. The Role of Hypoxia and Cancer Stem Cells in Development of Glioblastoma. *Cancers* **2023**, *15*, 2613. https://doi.org/10.3390/cancers15092613

Academic Editors: Peter Hau, Annunziato Mangiola and Gianluca Trevisi

Received: 21 March 2023
Revised: 22 April 2023
Accepted: 3 May 2023
Published: 4 May 2023

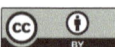

Copyright: © 2023 by the authors. Licensee MDPI, Basel, Switzerland. This article is an open access article distributed under the terms and conditions of the Creative Commons Attribution (CC BY) license (https://creativecommons.org/licenses/by/4.0/).

Abstract: Glioblastoma multiform (GBM) is recognized as the most malignant brain tumor with a high level of hypoxia, containing a small population of glioblastoma stem like cells (GSCs). These GSCs have the capacity of self-renewal, proliferation, invasion and recapitulating the parent tumor, and are major causes of radio-and chemoresistance of GBM. Upregulated expression of hypoxia inducible factors (HIFs) in hypoxia fundamentally contributes to maintenance and progression of GSCs. Therefore, we thoroughly reviewed the currently acknowledged roles of hypoxia-associated GSCs in development of GBM. In detail, we recapitulated general features of GBM, especially GSC-related features, and delineated essential responses resulted from interactions between GSC and hypoxia, including hypoxia-induced signatures, genes and pathways, and hypoxia-regulated metabolic alterations. Five hypothesized GSC niches are discussed and integrated into one comprehensive concept: hypoxic peri-arteriolar niche of GSCs. Autophagy, another protective mechanism against chemotherapy, is also closely related to hypoxia and is a potential therapeutic target for GBM. In addition, potential causes of therapeutic resistance (chemo-, radio-, surgical-, immuno-), and chemotherapeutic agents which can improve the therapeutic effects of chemo-, radio-, or immunotherapy are introduced and discussed. At last, as a potential approach to reverse the hypoxic microenvironment in GBM, hyperbaric oxygen therapy (HBOT) might be an adjuvant therapy to chemo-and radiotherapy after surgery. In conclusion, we focus on demonstrating the important role of hypoxia on development of GBM, especially by affecting the function of GSCs. Important advantages have been made to understand the complicated responses induced by hypoxia in GBM. Further exploration of targeting hypoxia and GSCs can help to develop novel therapeutic strategies to improve the survival of GBM patients.

Keywords: glioblastoma; stem cell; hypoxia; niche; autophagy; therapy

1. Introduction

Glioblastoma (GBM) is identified as one of the most malignant solid brain cancers, with an average annual incidence of about 4.45 per 100,000 population [1]. GBM patients present clinical manifestations of headache, weakness, vague vision, seizure and/or dizziness, depending on tumor location and degree of neurological impairment. The average diagnostic age of GBM patients is 64-years-old, with more females than males (6:4) [2]. With advancement of technology, novel imaging tools offer great assistance for oncologists in the diagnosis of GBM. Apart from conventional computed tomography (CT) and magnetic resonance imaging (MRI), dynamic contrast-enhanced (DCE) MRI, functional MRI, diffusion tensor imaging (DTI), magnetic resonance spectroscopy (MRS), diffusion-weighted imaging (DWI), single-photon emission computed tomography (SPECT), and positron emission tomography (PET) are all useful in clinical practice [3,4].

It has been proposed that GBMs have intrinsic cellular heterogeneity which consists of differentiated cells, quiescent cells, and glioblastoma stem cells (GSCs) [5]. Differentiated cells mainly contribute to tumorigenesis, proliferation, and invasion of glioblastoma. Quiescent cells are able to transdifferentiate into stem-like cells, and re-acquire self-renewal ability [6]. GSCs are recognized as reservoirs of tumor-initiating cells, accounting for therapeutic failure and GBM recurrence. The hypothesis of cancer stem cell (CSC) arises from human acute leukemia. Hematopoietic stem cells (HSCs) are a small population of multipotent cells with the potential of proliferation, self-renewal, differentiation, and regeneration of original tumors [7]. GSCs kept a certain degree of neural stem cell (NSC) features such as self-renewal and multi-differentiation potential [8]. NSC was first described in grown-up mammalians and mainly exists in two regions: one is the subventricular zone (SVZ) between the striatum and the lateral ventricle, and another is the subgranular zone (SGZ) within the dentate gyrus of the hippocampus [9,10].

Hypoxia plays a paramount important role in neuronal development which is a prerequisite for the neural crest cell migration [11]. Hypoxia mainly functions through hypoxia-inducible factors (HIFs, HIF1α, and HIF2α). In normoxia, HIF1α is hydroxylated and combined with a cancer suppressor Von Hippel-Lindau (VHL) to undergo ubiquitination process [12]. Under hypoxia, the HIF1α protein is speedily accumulated within cells and contributes to subsequent gene transactivation. HIF1α promotes glycolysis via upregulating critical enzymes of glycolytic pathway, such as HK2 (hexokinase 2) and pyruvate PDK1 (pyruvate dehydrogenase kinase 1). The literature has reported that HIF1α regulates stemness and differentiation of early NSC population via activating neural repressor Hes1 [13]. Suppression of HIF1α by meloxicam could exert antiproliferative efficacy in hepatocellular carcinoma (HCC) and lead to caspase-reliant apoptosis of HCC in hypoxia [14]. HIF2α is an intimate isoform of HIF1α [15]. Contrary to widespread expression of HIF1α in nearly all cells, HIF2α is selectively expressed in stem cells and endothelial cells of cancer. HIF1α shows high sensitivity towards oxygen concentration while HIF1β demonstrates constitutive expression regardless of oxygen concentration [16]. The HIF1α/HIF1β compound could translocate into the nucleus and further command genes that contain the hypoxia-response consensus sequence (HRE) [17].

Hypoxic areas in GBMs could be attributed to multiple factors such as upregulated cellular proliferation, insufficient oxygen diffusion, widespread tissue necrosis, broken blood-brain barrier, and aberrant tumor vascularization. Hypoxia is closely linked with the neoplastic biology of GBMs. Upregulated HIF expression in hypoxia promotes proliferation, infiltration, and self-renewal of GSC, ultimately leading to an enhanced level of therapeutic-resistance. However, the relationship between hypoxia and GSCs in the development of GBM is not clearly elaborated. Therefore, in our review, we recapitulate general features of GBM, describe GSC-related features, and delineate interactions between GSC and hypoxia. Given the importance of hypoxia for the initiation and progression of GBMs and GSCs, comprehensive study and discussion of these issues would give us more insights into the biological features of GBMs and provide novel avenues to develop promising treatments for GBMs targeting hypoxia and GSCs.

2. GSC and Hypoxia-Related Signatures

One of the central issues for studying GSCs is to identify the GSCs, primarily by using suitable molecular markers. It has been reported that CD9, CD133 (prominin-1), Olig2 integrin αβ, aldehyde dehydrogenase (ALDH), CD44, Sox2, Oct4, nestin, and the feature of side population (SP) can be used as signatures of GSCs [17–21] (Table 1). These markers are useful in the identification of stem cells, thus propelling relative studies. Via detecting expression of Oct4, Olig2, and nestin, it was reported that ING5 (a member of the epigenetic regulators ING family) could accelerate self-renewal of GSC, enhance its stem-cell pool and block its lineage differentiation [22]. When hypoxia is presented, many of these GSC markers are upregulated. Seidle et al. observed that SP-related genes are upregulated in hypoxia in three adherent glioma cells [23]. They also discovered that SP marker genes are highly expressed in both peri-vascular and hypoxic niches where both HIF1α and HIF2α are highly expressed [23]. However, whether all these cell markers can be applied precisely to identify stem cells remains controversial. Some $CD133^-$ cells also have the properties of GSCs and high plasticity of generating $CD133^+$ cells. Currently, the gold criterion to determine GSCs remains the competence of recapitulating original parent tumors under the condition of orthotopical transplantation. Therefore, further investigations are necessary to uncover intrinsic GSC features.

Table 1. GSC and hypoxia-regulated signatures, genes, and pathways.

Signature	Gene	Pathways	lncRNA	Protein
CD9	EGFR	DLK1	lncRNA H19	HILPDA (HIG2)
SP	TP53 mutation	Notch (CBF1)		
CD133	IDH mutation	VEGF		
Olig2	MCT4	JAK1//2-STAT3		
integrin αβ	PP2A	Wnt (TCF-1, LEF-1)		
ALDH	Klf4	avβ8-integrin-TGF-β1		
CD44	ABCB1			
Sox2	PTEN			
Oct4	PML			
nestin				

3. GSC and Hypoxia-Related Genes

GBMs can be further classified into four subtypes: mesenchymal, neural, proneural and classical subtypes. Neurofibromin 1 (NF1) deletion, chromosome 7 enrichment, platelet derived growth factor (PDGF) amplification, and tumor suppressor PTEN deficiency are discovered in these four types respectively [24]. In addition, p16 loss, epidermal growth factor receptor (EGFR) amplification, chromosome 22q loss, TP53 mutation, and CDKN2A loss are the most common and prominent signal alterations in GBMs [25] (Table 1). Among them, TP53 mutation is present in both primary and recurrent GBMs [26]. Recurrent GSC is able to accumulate temozolomide-associated mutations over primary GSC after chemo-therapy [26]. IDH1 is an oncogene which localizes in cytoplasm and peroxisome. IDH1 mutation is a symbol of early tumorigenesis, suppression of which could enhance sensitivity of GBM to chemotherapy. Glioma patients with IDH-mutation display better prognoses compared to those with IDH-wildtype. In the latest WHO classification, GBM only represents IDH-wildtype GBM, while IDH-mutant GBM, which was considered to account for 10% of GBMs in the past [27], is considered as a different subtype of diffuse glioma [28].

Considering the intimate relationship between GBMs and hypoxia, deep insight into genetic alterations of GBMs under hypoxic conditions is essential. Evidence has revealed that there is an intimate interplay between IDH1/2 and HIFs. Mutated IDH1/2 leads to elevated expression of oncometabolite R-2-hydroxyglutarate (2HG), which then decreases

HIF1α and HIF2α levels [29]. Interestingly, IDH mutation alone inhibits tumor growth while the combinatory effect of IDH1/2 and HIF promotes neoplastic growth, contributing to unfavorable prognosis in GBM patients. It is reported that expression of monocarboxylate transporter-4 (MCT4), protein phosphatase 2A (PP2A), Krupple-like 4 (Klf4), and ATP-binding cassette B1 (ABCB1) are upregulated under hypoxic conditions and lead to shorter survival spans of GBM patients [30–33]. It is acknowledged that HIF1α level increases after mammalian target of rapamycin (mTOR) is dysregulated [34]. Multiple genes participate in the above pathways, such as PTEN (phosphatase and tensin homolog), PML (promyelocytic leukemia), and EGFR [35,36].

4. GSC and Hypoxia-Related Pathways

Accumulated research showed that numerous signaling pathways are altered in GBM, such as PI3K/AKT/mTOR, MAPK, STAT3/bcl2, PI3K/RhoA/C, HIF/IDH1/2, VEGF, EGF, Wnt/βcatenin, and Notch [37–40] (Table 1). It has been indicated that ING5 (a member of the epigenetic regulators ING family) could increase the activity of PI3K/AKT via facilitating transcription of the calcium channel as well as the follicle stimulating hormone signaling gene, to maintain self-renewal of GSCs which partially causes resistance and recurrence of GBMs [22].

Under hypoxia, there are several alterations in GBM-related pathways. Grassi et al. reported that hypoxia could induce upregulation of Delta like non-canonical Notch ligand 1 (DLK1) in GBM, thus promoting colony formation of GBMs as well as gene expression of GSC markers [41]. A recent study showed that CBF1, a cardinal transcriptional modulator of Notch signaling pathway, could be activated by hypoxia to promote proliferation of GSCs and accelerate epithelial-to-mesenchyme transition (EMT), further enhancing chemoresistance of GBMs [42].

Vascular endothelial growth factor (VEGF) is a pro-angiogenic factor that mediates vascular permeability and angioedema. VEGFR2 is a receptor of VEGF. In hypoxia, both VEGF and VEGFR2 are up-regulated by HIF1α and overexpressed in GBM, accelerating tumor progression and invasion [43]. In addition, enhanced HIF1α expression could activate the JAK1//2-STAT3 pathway that closely associates with VEGF secretion, thus promoting self-renewal of GSCs [44]. Bevacizumab is a kind of anti-VEGF monoclonal antibody currently used as a second-line agent which shows efficiency in decreasing aberrant vascularization of GBM [45]. Brefeldin A is another inhibitor of VEGF in GBM [46]. However, anti-VEGF treatments inevitably lead to therapy resistance. An investigation indicated that resistance to anti-VEGF therapy in GBM is facilitated by elevation of regulatory T-cell (Treg), which might serve as potential targets with both immunologic and anti-VEGF effects [47].

The Wnt pathway has an intimate association with GSC features, being able to reduce CD133 and Nestin under both aerobic and anaerobic conditions. In hypoxia, HIF1α upregulates expression of both TCF-1 and LEF-1 to cooperate with Wnt signaling in GBM, reprograming GSC phenotype towards a more differentiated and less aggressive one. A study has revealed that hypoxia-induced Wnt activation could inhibit Notch pathway in primary GBM and enhance chemosensitivity of GBM cells towards temozolomide (TMZ) therapy [48].

Transforming growth factor β (TGFβ) is a downstream gene of HIF1α with two isoforms TGFβ1/β2. TGFβ plays significant roles in GBM progression and recurrence [49], and can promote GSC invasion in vitro [50]. Integrin αvβ8 is overexpressed in GSC and crucial for GSC self-renewal and GBM tumorigenesis. It was demonstrated that αvβ8 integrin mediates GBM progression via promoting TGFβ1-induced DNA replication, thus the αvβ8-integrin-TGFβ1 axis might function as a therapeutic target of GBM [51]. Dedifferentiation of non-stem cells into stem cells is known to be involved in EMT. Under hypoxia, GSCs could release TGFβ1 to promote EMT, leading to increased quantities of GSC and poor outcomes of GBM patients [49]. Interestingly, TGFβ is recognized as an upstream regulator of VEGF, and modulating VEGF and TGFβ signaling pathways collectively could effectively control neoplastic growth of GBMs [52].

Long noncoding RNA (lncRNA) H19 displays a tumorigenic role in GBMs under hypoxia. The research has highlighted that targeting lncRNA H19 might be a potential therapeutic strategy for GBMs [53]. Hypoxia-inducible and lipid droplet associated protein (HILPDA, also identified as HIG2) is inherently overexpressed in GBMs and enhanced by hypoxia, contributing to unfavorable prognosis of GBM patients [54].

5. GSC and Hypoxia-Related Metabolism

The "Warburg effect" refers to elevated levels of aerobic glycolysis in which pyruvate is transformed into lactate instead of entering Krebs cycle. Hypoxia could affect one-carbon metabolism of GSC via over-expression of aerobic glycolytic pathway enzymes such as LDHA (lactate dehydrogenase A), PFK1 (phosphofructokinase 1), and HK2, as well as down-regulation of vitamin B12 transporter protein TCN2 (Figure 1). TCN2 is indispensable in the process of GSC transformation into the highly malignant mesenchymal/CSC profile [55]. The IDH3α/cSHMT (cytosolic serine hydroxymethyltransferase) signaling axis is recognized as a novel regulatory target of one-carbon metabolism in GBM [56]. Epigenetic regulation via histone alteration, DNA methylation, and non-coding RNA could also mediate glycolytic metabolism in GBM [57]. Apart from glucose metabolism of GSCs, HIFs also play a vital role in the metabolism of amino acid. LAT1 is a transporter of branched chain amino acid (BCAA) while BCAT1 is a metabolic enzyme of BCAA. It was reported that HIF1α and HIF2α increase both mRNA and protein levels of LAT1 and BCAT1 in GBM under hypoxia [15]. In hypoxic condition, the major carbon fuel of GBM cells partially convert from glucose to glutamine [58]. α-ketoglutarate (αKG) is a medium metabolite in tricarboxylic acid (TCA) cycle. αKG and the associated amino acid glutamate are two key factors of GBM metabolic alterations [59]. It has been identified that Acyl-CoA-Binding protein could facilitate tumorigenesis of GBMs via promoting fatty acid oxidation [60]. In conclusion, hypoxia-related metabolism is essential for the initiation and progression of GBM, which is involved in complicated processes and deserves further investigation to obtain more insights of the GSC properties.

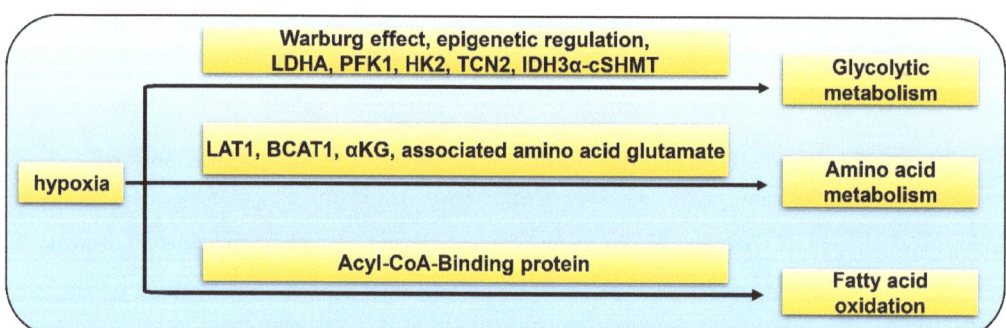

Figure 1. Hypoxia-related metabolism of GSC. Glycolytic metabolism: hypoxia promotes GSC glycolysis via Warburg effect, epigenetic regulation, LDHA, PFK1, HK2, TCN2, and IDH3α-cSHMT pathway; amino acid metabolism: hypoxia facilitates GSC glutamine metabolism by LAT1, BCAT1, αKG, and associated amino acid glutamate; fatty acid oxidation: hypoxia accelerates fatty acid metabolism through the Acyl-CoA-Binding protein.

6. GSC and Hypoxia-Related Vasculature

Vasculature plays a crucial role in GBM initiation and progression. There exist five potential mechanisms of GBM vascularization: angiogenesis, vasculogenesis, vessel mimicry, vessel co-option, and intussusception [61] (Figure 2). Angiogenesis in GBM could be attributed, to a large extent, to interplay between GSCs and endothelial cells via VEGFR, Notch, DLL-4, and nitric oxide (NO) signals. Recruitment of the bone marrow-originated endothelial progenitor cell (EPC) by SDF-1/CXCR-4 is the precondition of vasculogenesis [62]. During vascular mimicry, tumor cells constitute vascular channels which have no endothelial cells but are still able to transport erythrocytes. Proliferation of GBM was initiated by vessel co-option, followed by angiogenesis once tumor mass grew to a certain volume [63]. Intussusception is a type of vascular remodeling where a blood vessel divides into two. In vasculatures of GBMs, GSCs interact closely with adjacent cells. ECs release NO that diffuses into GSCs. GSCs generate pro-angiogenic VEGF-A to facilitate growth of ECs [64]. It has been testified that the PAX6/DLX5-WNT5A pathway might be an underlying regulator of interaction between GSC and EC in GBM [65]. Interplay between GSC and EC is important for GBM progression, which is affected by hypoxia. In spite of obvious vascularization, the microenvironment of a GBM is usually hypoxic which might be attributed to tortuous, poorly-organized, and insufficiently-perfused tumor vessels. Hypoxia increased expression of extracellular adenosine that activates the A_3 adenosine receptor (A_3 AR) to promote trans-differentiation of GSC into EC [66]. Hypoxia also induces fusion of GSC with EC through pseudo-endothelialization. Astrocytes mainly produce extracellular matrix (ECM) proteins such as proteoglycan, collagen, and laminin [67] (Figure 3). As important components of ECM, integrin α6, the receptor for laminin, is enriched in GSC, and promotes interactions between GSC and EC [68,69].

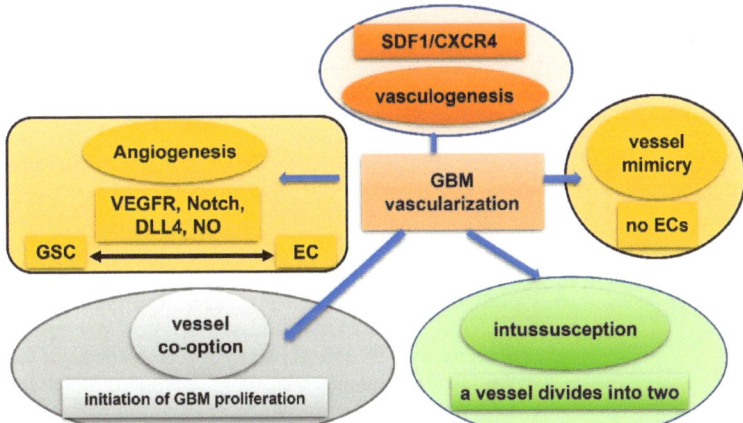

Figure 2. Five mechanisms of vascularization in glioblastoma. Angiogenesis: mainly attributed to interplay between GSCs and endothelial cells via VEGFR, Notch, DLL-4, and NO signals; vasculogenesis: bone marrow-derived endothelial progenitor cell (EPC) is recruited via SDF-1/CXCR-4 axis; vascular mimicry: tumor cells constitute vascular channels which have no endothelial cells but are still capable of transporting erythrocytes; vessel co-option: initiates proliferation of GBMs and is followed by angiogenesis; Intussusception: a blood vessel divides into two.

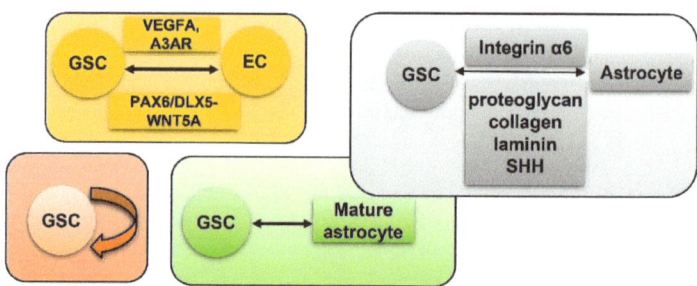

Figure 3. GSC and hypoxia-related vascularization. GSCs generate VEGFA and A_3 AR to facilitate proliferation of ECs. Meanwhile, GSC and EC interact via the PAX6/DLX5-WNT5A axis; astrocytes generate proteoglycan, collagen, laminin, and SHH to interact with GSC-produced Integrin α6 self-renewal of GSC; mature GBM cell could de-differentiate into GSC.

7. GSC and Hypoxia-Related Niches

Conventional therapies mainly target CSCs, but to some extent, surrounding niches also contribute to the malignancy of neoplasm [70]. The tumor microenvironment (TME) of GBM has attracted more attention in recent years, which generally includes dendritic cells, fibroblasts, vessels, macrophages, and cancer-draining lymph nodes. TME might assist self-renewal and stemness of GSCs, acting as novel therapeutic targets. Five niches are recognized and elucidated in detail in the current paper: peri-vascular niche, immune niche, hypoxia/necrotic niche, ECM niche, and peri-arteriolar niche [71]. The TME may contain more cell types that have impacts on GSCs. For example, astrocytes express Sonic hedgehog (SHH) and modulate the self-renewal of GSC and progression of GBM [72].

7.1. Peri-Vascular Niche of GSC

There is bidirectional crosstalk between a GSC and molecules from its peri-vascular niche such as endothelial cells (ECs), pericytes, astrocytes, and microglia/macrophages. The Notch ligand of EC cooperates with the Notch receptor of GSC to activate the Notch pathway, further promoting self-renewal of GSC [73]. Xin et al. reported that GBM-derived ECs can be detected in 46.9% of clinical samples, and EC markers were up-regulated in GSC cells, indicating that GSC might trans-differentiate into EC and vice versa [74].

7.2. Immune Niche of GSC

The immune niche of GBM consists of variance types of immune cells, among which macrophages are the most abundant cell types. Macrophages can be divided into M1 and M2 phenotypes [75]. The M1 subtype has the effect of killing tumor cells while the M2 subtype facilitates tumor survival by suppressing adaptive immunity of Th1 cells. Glioma infiltrating myeloid cell (GIM) belongs to the M2 phenotype, and promotes immune suppression of GBM and survival of GSC [76]. Tumor associated macrophages (TAMs) are immunosuppressive cells in GBMs, positively associated with tumor malignancy and negatively relating with patient survival [77]. Via releasing molecules such as macrophage colony-stimulating factor (M-CSF) and TGFβ, GSC is able to promote the M2-polarization of TAM [78] (Figure 4). In addition, GSC could recruit M2-polarized TAM to the hypoxic niche. Once microglia/macrophages are recruited by GSCs, they secrete TGFβ1 and IL10 to transfer into immunosuppressive cells [79]. The exact role of TAM in the immune niche of GSC demands further exploration. Chimeric antigen receptor T cell therapy of GBM has been a hot topic recently [80]. Effector T cells enhance sensitivity of GBM to lysis which could be reduced by HIF1α-dependent NANOG. It was reported that GSCs suppress proliferation of effector T cells via secretion of hypoxia-related galectin-3 [81]. CD8+ cytotoxic T lymphocyte (CTL) could sensitize GBM to conventional therapies [82]. Under hypoxia, cytotoxicity of CTL is impeded by hypoxia-induced interleukin-6-activated STAT3 pathways, leading to decreased survival of GBM patients [83]. Hypoxia also upregulates PD-L1 expression of activated T cells which suppress immunity of GBM.

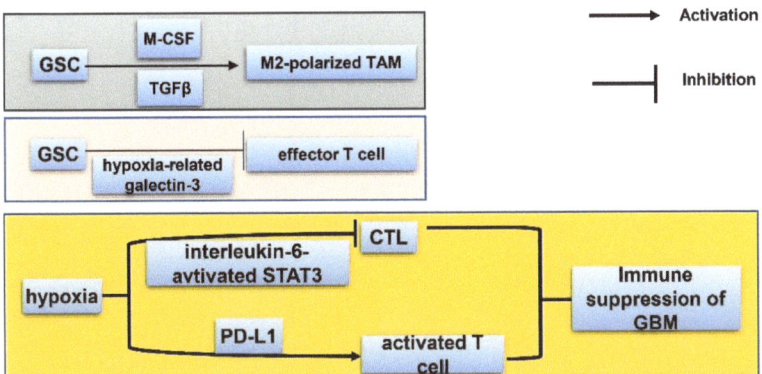

Figure 4. Immune niche of GSC. Via releasing macrophage colony-stimulating factor (M-CSF) and TGF-β, GSC could promote M2-polarization of TAM; by secreting hypoxia-related galectin-3, GSCs suppress proliferation of effector T cells; hypoxia enhances the PD-L1 level of activated T cells and induces interleukin-6-activated STAT3 to impede cytotoxicity of CTLs (cytotoxic T lymphocytes). The above described processes all contribute to immune suppression and decreased survival of GBM patients.

7.3. Hypoxia/Necrotic Niche of GSC

Apart from the GSC immune niche, the hypoxia/necrotic niche is identified as another niche of GSC, in which hypoxia facilitates proliferation and self-renewal of GSC by both induction of stem cell signatures and upregulation of HIF1α and VEGF [84]. Histologically, pseudopalisading necrosis (PPN), the hypoxic area in GBM surrounded by numerous intensively packed cancer cells, is a fundamental histologic hallmark of GBM [85]. Hypoxia gives rise to acidification which then upregulates HIF expression and promotes GSC maintenance [86]. Pharmacological inhibition of HSP90, a hypoxia-regulated chaperone protein, could downregulate HIF expression and decrease oncogenicity of GBM [86]. In addition, hypoxia also has a great impact on the immune niche of GBM by promoting M2-like macrophage polarization and producing an immunosuppressive microenvironment [87,88].

7.4. ECM Niche of GSC

The extracellular matrix (ECM) niche is generally deemed as a section of the peri-arteriolar and peri-vascular microenvironment, although some reports indicate that it is an independent niche [89,90]. It is suggested that the ECM niche is established by GSC itself in that GSC could deposit components of the ECM niche. In addition, this GSC niche also consists of extracellular vesicles, glycoprotein and proteoglycan, laminin, and tenascin-C (TNC) [91,92] (Figure 5). The former three factors are generated by ECs. Laminin is secreted by GSC-related EC and facilitates GBM progression. TNC is an underlying GSC signature expressed by differentiated GBM cells [92]. Anti-TNC aptamers could inhibit GBM progression [92,93]. Very interestingly, by comprehensively studying the complicated molecular interacting networks of hypoxia regulated genes (HRGs-MINW) in GBM, Mao et al. found that CEBPD is a master transcriptional factor for the HRGs-MINW, and ECM mediated activation of EGFR/PI3K is a main down-stream pathway [94], which lends credence to the importance of the ECM niche for GBM. Notably, ECM proteins are critical hypoxia induced targets, and fibronectin (FN1), a key component of ECM, and integrin interaction mediated EGFR phosphorylation is a key step for CEBPD induced GBM progression [94]. As described above, integrin α6 is a potential GSC marker and plays and important role for the tumorigenicity of GSC [68,69].

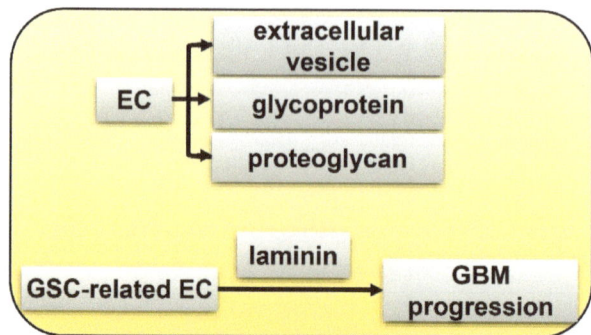

Figure 5. ECM (extracellular matrix) niche of GSC. EC generates extracellular vesicle, glycoprotein and proteoglycan; GSC-related EC secretes laminin to facilitate GBM progression.

7.5. Peri-Arteriolar Niche of GSC

Besides peri-vascular niche, peri-arteriolar area is another blood vessel related niche but it has different features. Structurally, five layers from the outer rim to the lumen constitute the walls of the arterioles in the GSC peri-arteriolar niche: tunica adventitia, tunica elastica externa, tunica media, tunica elastica interna, and endothelium. Peri-arteriolar GSC niche resembles that of HSC in the bone marrow in that five of the same factors, SDF-1α, CXCR4, OPN, CD44, and CatK, are identified in both niches [95]. Notably, hypoxia is also a remarkable feature of the Peri-arteriolar niche in GBM [96].

7.6. Interactions between the Five GSC Niches

There are intimate interplays between the five GSC niches mentioned above. TAM could trans-differentiate into EC, indicating that EC constitutes part of GSC immune niche [97]. It is obvious that microglia/macrophage is overlapped in both immune niche and peri-vascular niche. VEGF is expressed in both GSC and TAM, suggesting the existence of a pro-angiogenesis signaling pathway in GSC immune niche [97]. Hypoxia often presents in the development and metastasis of lymphocytes while oxygen-deficiency damages the proliferation and secretion of cytotoxic T lymphocytes [98]. Hypoxia improves the lytic ability of CD8$^+$ T cells and upregulates secretion of interferon-gamma by CD4$^+$ T cells in vitro [98] (Figure 6). In addition, hypoxia could activate the pSTAT pathway to promote expression of immunosuppressive cytokines such as CCL2 and CFS1, both of which suppress proliferation of T-cells and promote infiltration of macrophages, facilitating tumor invasion and progression [99]. More specifically, HIF1α inhibits the differentiation of Foxp3$^+$ Tregs by facilitating ubiquitination and degradation of Foxp3 in Th17 cells [100]. Meanwhile, the immune niche also has great impact on the HIF. Activated T cell receptor (TCR) enhances synthesis and stabilization of HIF1α in hypoxia. Moreover, CD4$^+$ type 1 Treg (Tr1), CD4$^+$ T helper 17 (Th17), and CD8$^+$ T cell in the immune niche of GBM could also stabilize HIF1α, implying a close association between the immune and hypoxic niches [101].

Formation of a GBM hypoxia/necrotic niche is possibly dependent on the peri-vascular niche, where tortuous vessels with insufficient perfusion are formed in the hypoxic necrosis areas in GBMs. Intriguingly, an upregulated level of HIF1α in GSCs results in enhancement of VEGF [102], which promotes malfunctional vessels. TAM could be activated by angiocrine-induced interleukin-6 (IL6) and subsequent argeinase-1 expression mediated by HIF2α, ultimately contributing to GBM progression [103]. Actually, peri-arteriolar niche, hypoxic niche, and immune niche might be the same type of GSC niche from three distinct viewpoints. Leukocyte-associated markers CD68, CD177, and MMP9 are expressed in the peri-arteriolar GSC niche where OPN is detected [104]. OPN co-localizes with CD68$^+$ macrophages [104]. Peri-arteriolar niche is intimately associated with hypoxia; the possible reason is that arterioles are transport vessels rather than exchange vessels, thereby peri hypoxic regions surrounding arterioles still form despite the oxygenated blood running along the arteriolar lumen. In addition, ECM niche is generally considered as part of peri-vascular niche, and plays essential roles in the interactions between GSC and immune niche [105].

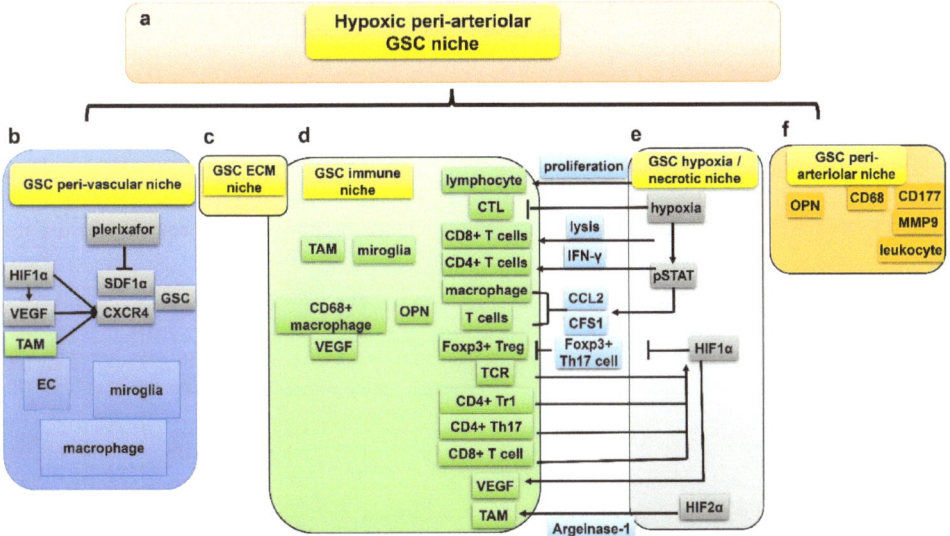

Figure 6. Five hypoxia-related GSC niches are closely associated and might be integrated into the hypoxic peri-arteriolar niche. (**a**) The integrated hypoxic peri-arteriolar niche is a combined concept from the inter-played 5 niches (**b–f**); (**b**) iInteraction between peri-vascular niche and hypoxia/necrotic niche via VEGF, SDF1α, CXCR4; (**c**) ECM niche (see details in Figure 5); (**d**) interaction between immune niche and hypoxia/necrotic niche via HIF1α, HIF2α, lymphocytes, CD8$^+$ T cells, interferon-γ, CD4$^+$ T cells, pSTAT pathway, CCL2, CFS1, macrophages, Foxp3$^+$ Tregs, Th17 cells, TCR, CD4$^+$ type1 Treg, and CD4$^+$ T helper 17; (**e**) GSC hypoxia/necrotic niche; (**f**) interaction between immune niche and peri-arteriolar niche via CD177, MMP9, OPN, and CD68$^+$ macrophages.

All five GSC niches are close to necrotic regions where VEGF and HIF1α are overexpressed. Upregulated VEGF and HIF1α further induce expression of SDF1α and CXCR4, both being critical for the maintenance of GSC stemness [106]. TAM also stimulates expression of SDF1α and CXCR4. Given the striking amounts of cell types and proteins overlapped in the five niches, they might be complementary and integrated as a comprehensive niche: the hypoxic peri-arteriolar niche of GSC, resembling HSC niche in the bone marrow [96].

Disrupting interactions between GSC and its protective niches might enhance anti-GBM therapeutic sensitivity. CXCR4 is a significant factor involved in the GSC niche. Lee et al. conducted a phase I clinical trial and demonstrated the safety of plerixafor, a reversible CXCR4 inhibitor, plus bevacizumab strategy in GBM [107].

8. GSC and Hypoxia-Related Autophagy

Another remarkable hypoxia induced response of GBM to obtain therapy resistance and tumorigenicity is autophagy [87,108]. Autophagy is a highly-conserved catabolic reaction during evolution, which is a downstream event of mTOR hyper-activation. When oxygen is sufficient, degradation of HIF1α lead to activation of mammalian target of rapamycin (mTOR) and inhibition of autophagy. Conversely, under hypoxia, autophagy is induced through abnormal activation of Notch, Wnt/β-catenin, Hedgehog signaling pathways, and autophagy-related 9 A (ATG9A) in GBM [109,110] (Figure 7). Autophagy modulates protein degradation and turnover of neuronal stem cells (NSCs). Upregulation of autophagy could promote self-renewal and expansion of GSCs. In hypoxic condition, autophagy is also closely related to dysregulated metabolism pathways in GSCs in that autophagy provides a source of energy for tumor cells [109]. Autophagy functions as a protective mechanism against chemotherapy in GBM. For instance, temozolomide (TMZ) resistance in GBM is partly attributed to induced autophagy. Fortunately, scientists have identified potential novel drugs targeting autophagy. Inhibition of autophagy enhances chemosensitivity of GSCs to TMZ by igniting ferroptosis [111]. Tocilizumab, an inhibitor of IL6 receptor, decreases autophagy and upregulates chemosensitivity of TMZ in GBM [112]. GBM patients treated with chloroquine (CQ), a kind of autophagy flux suppressant, display reduced chemoresistance and better survival [113]. Inhibitor of the MST4-ATG4B signaling axis suppresses autophagy, which then decreases the malignancy of GBM [114]. Taken together, autophagy increases hypoxia-induced chemoresistance of GBM while inhibitors of autophagy have the capacity to reverse this phenomenon, being a potential therapeutic target for GBM.

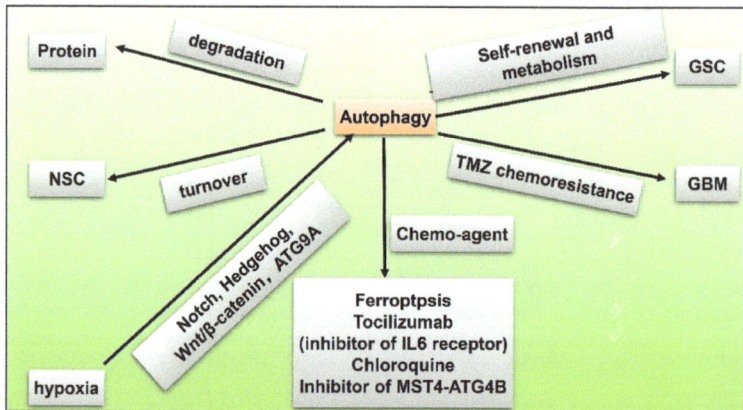

Figure 7. GSC and hypoxia-related autophagy. Hypoxia induces autophagy via activated Notch, Hedgehog, Wnt/β-catenin pathways, and autophagy-related 9 A (ATG9A) in GBM; autophagy modulates protein degradation; autophagy regulates turnover of NSCs; upregulated autophagy promotes self-renewal and metabolism of GSC; autophagy facilitates TMZ resistance in GBM; chemo agents such as ferroptosis, tocilizumab, chloroquine, and inhibitor of MST4-ATG4B axis suppress autophagy and reduce malignancy of GBM.

9. GSC and Hypoxia-Related Therapeutic Resistance

One of the essential reasons underlying the dismal prognosis of GBM patients is the intrinsic therapy-resistance feature of GBM cells. Despite the combination of surgical resection, chemo-and-radiotherapy, prognoses of GBM patients remain unfavorable with the median survival span around 14–16 months [115]. Actually, the majority of GBM patients show inevitable recurrence. Potential causes of therapeutic resistance in GBM need urgent investigation (Table 2). Due to the ability of GSCs to infiltrate proximate normal tissues and elevated levels of tumor vascularization, it is difficult to perform complete surgical resection for GBMs. Remanent tumor cells at the margin of post-surgery are more proliferative and aggressive. Frequent exposure to irradiation and subsequent activation of DNA-damage response resulted in alterations in cell cycle and cell cycle-related proteins, enhanced expression of Notch pathway, and production of insulin-like growth factor 1 (IGF1) in GSC, all of which at least contribute to GBM radio resistance [116]. TMZ-resistance in GBM correlates with increased levels of DNA double-strand break and p38-ERK1/2 axis [117]. There are other mechanisms of chemo-resistance in GBM, such as upregulated activation of COX2 [118] and elevated expression of multidrug resistance-associated protein

1 (MRP1) transporter in GSCs which could expel chemo-therapeutic drugs to extracellular medium [119].

Table 2. Causes of hypoxia-related therapeutic resistance in GSC.

Post-Surgical Recurrence	Radio Resistance	Chemo Resistance
GSC infiltrate proximate normal tissues	cell cycles alter	DNA double-strand break upregulates
tumor vascularization upregulates	cell cycle-related proteins alter	p38-ERK1/2 axis increases
diffusion around proximate tissues	expression of Notch increases	COX2 elevates
	GSC produces insulin-like growth factor 1 (IGF1)	multidrug resistance-associated protein 1 (MRP1)
	DNA-damage response activates via musashi-1	

10. GSC and Hypoxia-Related Chemotherapy

At present, TMZ is the only first-line effective chemo-agent for GBM, despite the plentiful clinical trials on chemotherapeutic agents currently under way. Interestingly, the efficacy of TMZ associates with activity of HIF1α [120]. Recent studies validated that combining TMZ with other molecules has clinical efficacy (Table 3). It has been widely recognized that promotor methylation of O6-methylguanine-DNA-methyltransferase (MGMT), a DNA repair enzyme, is a reliable marker for TMZ sensitivity of GBM treatment. There are other molecular mechanisms that can affect the TMZ sensitivity. Activation of epidermal growth factor receptor variant III (EGFRvIII) could enhance hypoxia-induced death in GBM [121]. Pretreatment with S-nitroso-N-acetylpenicillamine (SNAP) in GBM patients induces expression of HIF1α [122]. Based on these findings, recent studies revealed that TMZ, combined with either EGFRvIII or SNAP, could significantly prolong survival of patients with MGMT promoter methylated GBM [117]. Metformin (MET) is commonly utilized as an antidiabetic agent. It was suggested that TMZ plus MET could revert chemoresistance in hypoxic condition via suppression of the PI3K/mTOR pathway in GBM [37]. Bevacizumab plus biweekly temozolomide is well tolerated in recurrent GBM patients [123]. However, aberrant vasculature could increase post-bevacizumab regional hypoxia in refractory GBM patients [124]. In addition, several medicines or agents can influence the efficacy of TMZ. Imipramine, an anti-depressant agent, could stimulate phenotypical switch from GSCs to non-GSCs in hypoxia [125], and TMZ plus either imipramine or tranylcypromine, another anti-depressant, could reduce the cytotoxic effect of TMZ under hypoxia [126]. Decitabine (DAC), a DNA hypomethylating agent, could increase the cytotoxicity of TMZ in GBM [127]. N45, a kind of steroidal saponin with anti-neoplasm efficacy, could inhibit cellular proliferation through the hypoxia-associated ROS/PI3K/Akt pathway in TMZ-resistant GBM [128].

In addition to TMZ, there are multiple chemo-agents undergoing research. Tacrolimus (FK506) has capacity to increase chemosensitivity of GSC and reduce GBM tumor volume and hypoxia-induced surface markers (ki67, GFAP and nestin) in GSC [119]. Bortezomib (BTZ) could stabilize expression of HIF1α in a mice model [129], and Ursodeoxycholic acid (UDCA) combined with BTZ has a synergistic effect on treatment of GBM [130]. BAL101553 is an effective chemo-agent in targeting hypoxia-mediated angiogenesis of GBM, and EB1 might be a response-predictive marker of BAL101553 treatment [131]. Although bevacizumab attributes to regional hypoxia in recurrent GBM patients, the addition of anti-VEGF antibody bevacizumab to carmustine would not enhance incidence of hematologic toxicity, validating the safety of this combinatory therapy in treating GBM patients [132]. Evofosfamide (TH-302) plus bevacizumab (Bev) strategy is well tolerated in Bev-refractory GBM patients [133]. Here, Evofosfamide is activated in hypoxia to obtain the capacity of discharging the DNA-damaging Br-IPM (bromo-isophosphoramide mustard) moiety [134]. As an oncogenic driver of GBM, the expression of EGFR is upregulated during hypoxia, and the anti-EGFR antibody nimotuzumab exhibited beneficial effects for the survival of GBM patients [135]. Targeting HIFs is a promising chemo-therapeutic strategy in treating GBM. One issue to bear in mind is that strategies should be tailored to inhibit HIFs in a specific pattern while leaving non-neoplastic cells unaffected. Two categories of digitalis exhibited potential effects in treating GBM: digoxin and digitoxin. Digoxin is a heart glycoside involved in translational inhibition of both HIF1α and HIF2α [136]. It was identified that HIF-related digoxin is effective in targeting GBM under hypoxia. Digitoxin is a cardiac glycoside and a suppressant of HIF1α, which can target GSCs with high specificity [137]. In addition, Cetuximab and Topotecan have the potential to target GBM by reducing translation of HIF1α [138,139].

Table 3. Advances in hypoxia-related chemotherapy targeting GSC.

Chemo Agent	Function	Reference
TMZ	associates with HIF-1α and prolong survival span of GBM patients	(Lo Dico et al., 2018 [120]; Struve et al., 2020 [117])
TMZ plus EGFRvIII	EGFRvIII enhances hypoxia-induced death and cooperates with TMZ to prolong survival of patients with MGMT promoter methylated GBM	(Struve et al., 2020 [117]; Luger et al., 2020 [121])
TMZ plus SNAP	SNAP induces HIF-1α and cooperates with TMZ to benefit survival span of GBM patients with MGMT promoter methylated	(Tsai et al., 2019 [122])
TMZ plus metformin	reverts chemoresistance of GBM during hypoxia via inhibition of PI3K/mTOR pathway	(Lo Dico et al., 2019 [120])
Biweekly TMZ plus bevacizumab	well tolerated by refractory GBM patients but increases regional hypoxia	(Badruddoja et al., 2017 [123]; Gerstner et al., 2020 [124])
TMZ plus Decitabine	increases cytotoxicity of HIF-1α-related chemo-agent	(Gallitto et al., 2020 [127])
TMZ plus imipramine	reduces cytotoxic effect of TMZ under hypoxia	(Bielecka and Obuchowicz, 2017 [126])
TMZ plus tranylcypromine	reduces cytotoxic effect of TMZ under hypoxia	(Bielecka and Obuchowicz, 2017 [126])
N45	inhibits proliferation through hypoxia-associated ROS/PI3K/Akt pathway in TMZ-resistant GBM	(Zhang et al., 2020 [128])
Tacrolimus (FK506)	reduce GBM tumor volume and hypoxia-induce surface markers (ki67, GFAP and nestin) in GSC	(Torres et al., 2018 [119])
UDCA bortezomib plus BTZ	stabilizes expression of HIF-1α and a promising therapy for GBM patients	(Yao et al., 2020 [130])
BAL101553	targets hypoxia-mediated angiogenesis of GBM	(Bergès et al., 2020 [131])
Bevacizumab plus carmustine	not enhance incidence of hematologic toxicity but attributes to regional hypoxia in recurrent GBM	(Yerram et al., 2019 [132])
nimotuzumab	an anti-EGFR antibody that upregulates survival span of GBM patients	(Ronellenfitsch et al., 2018 [135])
Evofosfamide plus bevacizumab	activated during hypoxia and well tolerated by bevacizumab-regressive GBM patients	(Brenner et al., 2018 [133]; Takakusagi et al., 2018 [134])
amitriptyline	stimulates phenotypical switch from GSCs to non-GSCs	(Bielecka-Wajdman et al., 2017 [125])
digoxin	inhibits HIF-1α and HIF-2α to target GBM	(Patocka et al., 2020 [136])
digitoxin	suppresses HIF-1α to target GSCs	(Lee et al., 2017 [137])
Cetuximab	reduces translation of HIF-1α to target GBM	(Ferreira et al., 2020 [138])
Topotecan	reduces translation of HIF-1α to target GBM	(Bernstock et al., 2017 [139])

11. GSC and Hypoxia-Related Radiotherapy

Apart from chemotherapy, radiotherapy of GBM also obtained breakthroughs in recent years (Table 4), and a list of chemical agents or drugs are identified to have beneficial effects on radiotherapy. The flavonoid extracted from Eucommia ulmoides can increase the effect of GBM radiotherapy by downregulating the HIFa/MMP-2 pathway and inducing apoptosis during radiotherapy [140]. Olaparib is identified as a promising radiosensitizer that improves prognosis of GBM patients. A multicenter clinical trial revealed that Olaparib plus temozolomide and intensity modulated radiotherapy could improve patient prognosis while sparing healthy tissues and preserving neurocognitive functions in GBM patients [141].

Table 4. Advances in hypoxia-related radio-and-immune therapy targeting GSC.

Agent	Mechanism	Function	Reference
total flavonoid of Eucommia ulmoides	downregulates HIF-a/MMP-2 pathway and upregulates apoptosis	increase effect of GBM radiotherapy	(Wang et al., 2019 [140])
Olaparib	a promising radiosensitizer	improves prognosis of GBM patients	(Lesueur et al., 2019 [141])
Olaparib plus temozolomide	combined with intensity modulated radiotherapy	spares healthy tissues and preserves neurocognitive functions to improve prognosis of GBM patients	(Lesueur et al., 2019 [141])
nivolumab	a PD-1 inhibitor associates with PTEN mutation and MAPK enrichment	displays therapeutic efficacy of GBM	(Zhao et al., 2019 [35])
pembrolizumab	a PD-1 inhibitor associates with PTEN mutation and MAPK enrichment	displays therapeutic efficacy of GBM	(Hsu et al., 2020 [75])
nanoparticles	penetrates GBM niche and combines with chemo-, radio- and photodynamic therapies	displays therapeutic efficacy of GBM	(Yang et al., 2021 [142])

12. GSC and Hypoxia-Related Radio-, Immunotherapy

Immune therapy is one of the most promising ones for cancer, and has achieved great advances in several kinds of cancer [143]. However, to date, immune therapy is not successful in GBM treatment [82]. Plenty of studies were performed to find immunotherapeutic targeting of GSCs. GSCs secrete periostin (POSTN) to recruit cancer-supportive M2 phenotype of TAMs, which facilitates formation of immunosuppressive niche. Immune checkpoint inhibitor represents a kind of promising immunotherapy strategy in several kinds of tumors. Utilizing PD-1 inhibitors (nivolumab or pembrolizumab), a study indicated that therapeutic responses of GBM patients to anti-PD-1 immunotherapy correlate with specific molecular alterations such as PTEN mutation and MAPK enrichment. In general, manipulation of macrophage type between M1 and M2, and targeting immune checkpoint molecules, might act as a potential novel immunosuppressive strategy for GBM [35,75]. Targeting the microenvironment of GSCs with nanoparticles was reported to be effective in GBM immunotherapy. Distinct from the conventional delivery method, unique properties of nanoparticles enable successful penetration of drugs into GBM niche [142]. Nanoparticles could also be combined with chemo-radiotherapy, and photodynamic therapy. In the future, more individualized nanoplatforms ought to be designed to suit TME at distinct developing stages of GBM [142]. As described above, hypoxia plays important roles in regulating the immune niche of GBM [79,87,144], and might be promising therapeutic targets for immunotherapy.

13. GSC and Hyperbaric Oxygen Therapy

As a potential approach to reverse the hypoxic microenvironment in GBM, hyperbaric oxygen therapy (HBOT) is an innovative and effective adjuvant therapy to chemotherapy and irradiation in post-surgical GBM patients [145,146] (Table 5). HBOT enhances oxygen pressure in intratumoral, peritumoral, vascular tissues, and mitochondrial organelles, thus raising radio- and chemosensitivity of GBM cells [147]. Currently, there are two kinds of HBOT-radiotherapies: radiotherapy during HBOT; and radiation within 15 min after HBOT. Performing radiotherapy and HBOT simultaneously could prolong survival span of GBM patients. Only a small fraction of patients demonstrated severe side-effects such as conclusive seizure and radiation-correlated necrosis [148]. Nonetheless, conducting radiation during HBOT has not been used as a standard therapeutic modality, and potential reasons are: difficulties for radiation establishment; and underlying damage to surrounding normal tissues [149]. The rationale for performing radiation within 15 min subsequent to HBOT is that radiosensitivity of GBM peaks at exactly this time point. In addition, irradiation combined with chemical agents performed 15 min after HBOT caused no late toxicities in GBM patients [150]. A study indicated that performing radiation after HBOT could improve prognoses of GBM patients, with the 2-year overall survival (OS) and progression-free survival (PFS) rates reaching to 46.5% and 35.4%, respectively [151].

Table 5. Hyperbaric oxygen therapy (HBOT) in GSC.

Definition	Category	Benefit	Side-Effect	Difficulty	Reference
An adjuvant therapy to chemo-and-radio therapy in post-surgical GBM patients	radiotherapy during HBOT	prolong survival span of GBM patients	conclusive seizure and radiation-correlated necrosis	radiation establishment and underlying damage to normal tissues surrounded	(Chang, 1977 [148]; Ogawa et al., 2013 [149])
	radiation within 15 min after HBOT	improve prognoses of GBM patients, with progression-free survival rate reaching 46.5%	cause no late toxicities in GBM	requires more clinical validation	(Ogawa et al., 2012 [150]; Yahara et al., 2017 [151])

14. Conclusions

GBM is recognized as one of the most dismal brain tumors with unfavorable prognosis despite surgical resection, radio- and chemotherapy. GSCs are a small proportion of GBM cells which exhibit stem-like features such as self-renewal, invasion, and recapitulating the parent tumor, being major causes of GBM resistance. Hypoxia, tumor niches, and autophagy contribute to the maintenance and amplification of GSCs. Hypoxia plays a significant role, mainly mediated by HIF, in tumorigenesis of GBM including self-renewal of GSC, neovascularization, metabolism, IDH-mutation, Notch signaling pathway, and radio- and chemoresistance. Besides GSCs, the surrounding niches of GSCs also promote malignancy of GBM. Five niches are elucidated in this review: immune niche, peri-vascular niche, hypoxia/necrotic niche, peri-arteriolar niche, and extracellular matrix (ECM) niche. Interestingly, these five niches intimately interact with each other and might be integrated into a comprehensive category of niche: the hypoxic peri-arteriolar GSC niche. Autophagy, which can be boosted by hypoxia, is another protective mechanism against chemotherapy and is a potential therapeutic target for GBM. Other chemotherapeutic drugs, and novel adjuvant therapies such as HBOT, that can increase the effects of chemo- or radio-therapy and immunotherapy are also discussed in this paper. However, despite accumulated advantages, an effective treatment targeting hypoxia and GSCs is still lacking, mainly due to the fact that a lot of genes are induced by hypoxia which formed a complicated molecular interacting network affecting many biological processes [144]. Therefore, detailed mechanisms underlying hypoxia induced responses of GSC should be explored. The present paper summarized key features relevant to the GSC and hypoxia. Based on comprehensive understanding of these progresses, further laboratory work and clinical trials on hypoxia and GSCs can be developed to better prolong the survival span of GBM patients.

Author Contributions: Conceptualization, X.M. and X.Z.; writing—original draft preparation, T.S., J.Z.; writing—review and editing, X.M.; visualization, T.S., X.M.; supervision, X.Z.; project administration, X.M., X.Z.; funding acquisition, X.M. All authors have read and agreed to the published version of the manuscript.

Funding: This research was funded by National Natural Science Foundation of China (Grant No. 81972359). The APC was funded by Xijing Hospital, Fourth Military Medical University and National Natural Science Foundation of China (Grant No. 81972359).

Conflicts of Interest: The authors declare no conflict of interest.

References

1. Miller, K.D.; Ostrom, Q.T.; Kruchko, C.; Patil, N.; Tihan, T.; Cioffi, G.; Fuchs, H.E.; Waite, K.A.; Jemal, A.; Siegel, R.L.; et al. Brain and other central nervous system tumor statistics, 2021. *CA Cancer J. Clin.* **2021**, *71*, 381–406. [CrossRef]
2. Zhang, X.; Zhang, W.; Mao, X.G.; Cao, W.D.; Zhen, H.N.; Hu, S.J. Malignant Intracranial High Grade Glioma and Current Treatment Strategy. *Curr. Cancer Drug Targets* **2019**, *19*, 101–108. [CrossRef]
3. Park, J.E.; Kim, H.S.; Park, S.Y.; Jung, S.C.; Kim, J.H.; Heo, H.Y. Identification of Early Response to Anti-Angiogenic Therapy in Recurrent Glioblastoma: Amide Proton Transfer-weighted and Perfusion-weighted MRI compared with Diffusion-weighted MRI. *Radiology* **2020**, *295*, 397–406. [CrossRef]
4. Henderson, F., Jr.; Brem, S.; O'Rourke, D.M.; Nasrallah, M.; Buch, V.P.; Young, A.J.; Doot, R.K.; Pantel, A.; Desai, A.; Bagley, S.J.; et al. (18)F-Fluciclovine PET to distinguish treatment-related effects from disease progression in recurrent glioblastoma: PET fusion with MRI guides neurosurgical sampling. *Neuro Oncol. Pract.* **2020**, *7*, 152–157. [CrossRef]
5. Mao, X.G.; Zhang, X.; Zhen, H.N. Progress on potential strategies to target brain tumor stem cells. *Cell. Mol. Neurobiol.* **2009**, *29*, 141–155. [CrossRef]
6. Suva, M.L.; Rheinbay, E.; Gillespie, S.M.; Patel, A.P.; Wakimoto, H.; Rabkin, S.D.; Riggi, N.; Chi, A.S.; Cahill, D.P.; Nahed, B.V.; et al. Reconstructing and Reprogramming the Tumor-Propagating Potential of Glioblastoma Stem-like Cells. *Cell* **2014**, *157*, 580–594. [CrossRef]
7. Lee, G.H.; Hong, K.T.; Choi, J.Y.; Shin, H.Y.; Lee, W.W.; Kang, H.J. Immunosenescent characteristics of T cells in young patients following haploidentical haematopoietic stem cell transplantation from parental donors. *Clin. Transl. Immunol.* **2020**, *9*, e1124. [CrossRef]
8. Ho, N.T.T.; Rahane, C.S.; Pramanik, S.; Kim, P.S.; Kutzner, A.; Heese, K. FAM72, Glioblastoma Multiforme (GBM) and Beyond. *Cancers* **2021**, *13*, 1025. [CrossRef]
9. Valiyaveettil, D.; Malik, M.; Akram, K.S.; Ahmed, S.F.; Joseph, D.M. Prospective study to assess the survival outcomes of planned irradiation of ipsilateral subventricular and periventricular zones in glioblastoma. *Ecancermedicalscience* **2020**, *14*, 1021. [CrossRef]
10. Kumar, U. Immunolocalization of Gas7 in the Subgranular Zone of Mice Hippocampus. *Prague Med. Rep.* **2019**, *120*, 117–123. [CrossRef]
11. Niklasson, C.U.; Fredlund, E.; Monni, E.; Lindvall, J.M.; Kokaia, Z.; Hammarlund, E.U.; Bronner, M.E.; Mohlin, S. Hypoxia inducible factor-2alpha importance for migration, proliferation, and self-renewal of trunk neural crest cells. *Dev. Dyn.* **2021**, *250*, 191–236. [CrossRef]
12. Peng, S.; Zhang, J.; Tan, X.; Huang, Y.; Xu, J.; Silk, N.; Zhang, D.; Liu, Q.; Jiang, J. The VHL/HIF Axis in the Development and Treatment of Pheochromocytoma/Paraganglioma. *Front. Endocrinol.* **2020**, *11*, 586857. [CrossRef]
13. Večeřa, J.; Procházková, J.; Šumberová, V.; Pánská, V.; Paculová, H.; Lánová, M.K.; Mašek, J.; Bohačiaková, D.; Andersson, E.R.; Pacherník, J. Hypoxia/Hif1α prevents premature neuronal differentiation of neural stem cells through the activation of Hes1. *Stem Cell Res.* **2020**, *45*, 101770. [CrossRef]
14. Zhou, Y.; Dong, X.; Xiu, P.; Wang, X.; Yang, J.; Li, L.; Li, Z.; Sun, P.; Shi, X.; Zhong, J. Meloxicam, a Selective COX-2 Inhibitor, Mediates Hypoxia-Inducible Factor- (HIF-) 1α Signaling in Hepatocellular Carcinoma. *Oxidative Med. Cell. Longev.* **2020**, *2020*, 7079308. [CrossRef]
15. Zhang, B.; Chen, Y.; Shi, X.; Zhou, M.; Bao, L.; Hatanpaa, K.J.; Patel, T.; DeBerardinis, R.J.; Wang, Y.; Luo, W. Regulation of branched-chain amino acid metabolism by hypoxia-inducible factor in glioblastoma. *Cell. Mol. Life Sci. CMLS* **2021**, *78*, 195–206. [CrossRef]
16. Satija, S.; Kaur, H.; Tambuwala, M.M.; Sharma, P.; Vyas, M.; Khurana, N.; Sharma, N.; Bakshi, H.A.; Charbe, N.B.; Zacconi, F.C.; et al. Hypoxia-inducible factor (HIF): Fuel for cancer progression. *Curr. Mol. Pharmacol.* **2021**, *14*, 321–332. [CrossRef]

17. Kung-Chun Chiu, D.; Pui-Wah Tse, A.; Law, C.T.; Ming-Jing Xu, I.; Lee, D.; Chen, M.; Kit-Ho Lai, R.; Wai-Hin Yuen, V.; Wing-Sum Cheu, J.; Wai-Hung Ho, D.; et al. Hypoxia regulates the mitochondrial activity of hepatocellular carcinoma cells through HIF/HEY1/PINK1 pathway. *Cell. Death Dis.* **2019**, *10*, 934. [CrossRef]
18. Bosman, F.T.; Carneiro, F.; Hruban, R.H.; Theise, N.D. *WHO Classification of Tumours of the Digestive System*; WHO: Lyon, France, 2010.
19. Li, G.; Li, Y.; Liu, X.; Wang, Z.; Zhang, C.; Wu, F.; Jiang, H.; Zhang, W.; Bao, Z.; Wang, Y.; et al. ALDH1A3 induces mesenchymal differentiation and serves as a predictor for survival in glioblastoma. *Cell. Death Dis.* **2018**, *9*, 1190. [CrossRef]
20. Wang, C.; Wang, Z.; Chen, C.; Fu, X.; Wang, J.; Fei, X.; Yan, X.; Xu, R. A low MW inhibitor of CD44 dimerization for the treatment of glioblastoma. *Br. J. Pharmacol.* **2020**, *177*, 3009–3023. [CrossRef]
21. Ikushima, H.; Todo, T.; Ino, Y.; Takahashi, M.; Saito, N.; Miyazawa, K.; Miyazono, K. Glioma-initiating cells retain their tumorigenicity through integration of the Sox axis and Oct4 protein. *J. Biol. Chem.* **2011**, *286*, 41434–41441. [CrossRef]
22. Wang, F.; Wang, A.Y.; Chesnelong, C.; Yang, Y.; Nabbi, A.; Thalappilly, S.; Alekseev, V.; Riabowol, K. ING5 activity in self-renewal of glioblastoma stem cells via calcium and follicle stimulating hormone pathways. *Oncogene* **2018**, *37*, 286–301. [CrossRef]
23. Seidel, S.; Garvalov, B.K.; Wirta, V.; von Stechow, L.; Schanzer, A.; Meletis, K.; Wolter, M.; Sommerlad, D.; Henze, A.T.; Nister, M.; et al. A hypoxic niche regulates glioblastoma stem cells through hypoxia inducible factor 2 alpha. *Brain* **2010**, *133*, 983–995. [CrossRef]
24. Herting, C.J.; Chen, Z.; Pitter, K.L.; Szulzewsky, F.; Kaffes, I.; Kaluzova, M.; Park, J.C.; Cimino, P.J.; Brennan, C.; Wang, B.; et al. Genetic driver mutations define the expression signature and microenvironmental composition of high-grade gliomas. *Glia* **2017**, *65*, 1914–1926. [CrossRef]
25. Armocida, D.; Pesce, A.; Di Giammarco, F.; Frati, A.; Santoro, A.; Salvati, M. Long Term Survival in Patients Suffering from Glio-blastoma Multiforme: A Single-Center Observational Cohort Study. *Diagnostics* **2019**, *9*, 209. [CrossRef]
26. Orzan, F.; De Bacco, F.; Crisafulli, G.; Pellegatta, S.; Mussolin, B.; Siravegna, G.; D'Ambrosio, A.; Comoglio, P.M.; Finocchiaro, G.; Boccaccio, C. Genetic Evolution of Glioblastoma Stem-Like Cells From Primary to Recurrent Tumor. *Stem Cells* **2017**, *35*, 2218–2228. [CrossRef]
27. Van Noorden, C.J.F.; Hira, V.V.V.; van Dijck, A.J.; Novak, M.; Breznik, B.; Molenaar, R.J. Energy Metabolism in IDH1 Wild-Type and IDH1-Mutated Glioblastoma Stem Cells: A Novel Target for Therapy? *Cells* **2021**, *10*, 705. [CrossRef]
28. Louis, D.N.; Perry, A.; Wesseling, P.; Brat, D.J.; Cree, I.A.; Figarella-Branger, D.; Hawkins, C.; Ng, H.K.; Pfister, S.M.; Reifenberger, G.; et al. The 2021 WHO Classification of Tumors of the Central Nervous System: A summary. *Neuro Oncol.* **2021**, *23*, 1231–1251. [CrossRef]
29. Huang, J.; Yu, J.; Tu, L.; Huang, N.; Li, H.; Luo, Y. Isocitrate Dehydrogenase Mutations in Glioma: From Basic Discovery to Therapeutics Development. *Front. Oncol.* **2019**, *9*, 506. [CrossRef]
30. Voss, D.M.; Spina, R.; Carter, D.L.; Lim, K.S.; Jeffery, C.J.; Bar, E.E. Disruption of the monocarboxylate transporter-4-basigin interaction inhibits the hypoxic response, proliferation, and tumor progression. *Sci. Rep.* **2017**, *7*, 4292. [CrossRef]
31. Gao, D.; Nyalali, A.M.K.; Hou, Y.; Xu, Y.; Zhou, J.; Zhao, W.; Huang, B.; Li, F. 2,5-Dimethyl Celecoxib Inhibits Proliferation and Cell Cycle and Induces Apoptosis in Glioblastoma by Suppressing CIP2A/PP2A/Akt Signaling Axis. *J. Mol. Neurosci.* **2021**, *71*, 1703–1713. [CrossRef]
32. Wang, P.; Zhao, L.; Gong, S.; Xiong, S.; Wang, J.; Zou, D.; Pan, J.; Deng, Y.; Yan, Q.; Wu, N.; et al. HIF1α/HIF2α-Sox2/Klf4 promotes the malignant progression of glioblastoma via the EGFR-PI3K/AKT signalling pathway with positive feedback under hypoxia. *Cell. Death Dis.* **2021**, *12*, 312. [CrossRef]
33. Malmström, A.; Łysiak, M.; Åkesson, L.; Jakobsen, I.; Mudaisi, M.; Milos, P.; Hallbeck, M.; Fomichov, V.; Broholm, H.; Grunnet, K.; et al. ABCB1 single-nucleotide variants and survival in patients with glioblastoma treated with radiotherapy concomitant with temozolomide. *Pharm. J.* **2020**, *20*, 213–219. [CrossRef]
34. Huang, W.; Ding, X.; Ye, H.; Wang, J.; Shao, J.; Huang, T. Hypoxia enhances the migration and invasion of human glioblastoma U87 cells through PI3K/Akt/mTOR/HIF-1α pathway. *Neuroreport* **2018**, *29*, 1578–1585. [CrossRef]
35. Zhao, J.; Chen, A.X.; Gartrell, R.D.; Silverman, A.M.; Aparicio, L.; Chu, T.; Bordbar, D.; Shan, D.; Samanamud, J.; Mahajan, A.; et al. Immune and genomic correlates of response to anti-PD-1 immunotherapy in glioblastoma. *Nat. Med.* **2019**, *25*, 462–469. [CrossRef]
36. Iwanami, A.; Gini, B.; Zanca, C.; Matsutani, T.; Assuncao, A.; Nael, A.; Dang, J.; Yang, H.; Zhu, S.; Kohyama, J.; et al. PML mediates glioblastoma resistance to mammalian target of rapamycin (mTOR)-targeted therapies. *Proc. Natl. Acad. Sci. USA* **2013**, *110*, 4339–4344. [CrossRef]
37. Li, X.; Wu, C.; Chen, N.; Gu, H.; Yen, A.; Cao, L.; Wang, E.; Wang, L. PI3K/Akt/mTOR signaling pathway and targeted therapy for glioblastoma. *Oncotarget* **2016**, *7*, 33440–33450. [CrossRef]
38. Li, H.; Chen, L.; Li, J.J.; Zhou, Q.; Huang, A.; Liu, W.W.; Wang, K.; Gao, L.; Qi, S.T.; Lu, Y.T. miR-519a enhances chemosensitivity and promotes autophagy in glioblastoma by targeting STAT3/Bcl2 signaling pathway. *J. Hematol. Oncol.* **2018**, *11*, 70. [CrossRef]
39. Nicolas, S.; Abdellatef, S.; Haddad, M.A.; Fakhoury, I.; El-Sibai, M. Hypoxia and EGF Stimulation Regulate VEGF Expression in Human Glioblastoma Multiforme (GBM) Cells by Differential Regulation of the PI3K/Rho-GTPase and MAPK Pathways. *Cells* **2019**, *8*, 1397. [CrossRef]

40. Rajakulendran, N.; Rowland, K.J.; Selvadurai, H.J.; Ahmadi, M.; Park, N.I.; Naumenko, S.; Dolma, S.; Ward, R.J.; So, M.; Lee, L.; et al. Wnt and Notch signaling govern self-renewal and differentiation in a subset of human glioblastoma stem cells. *Genes Dev.* **2019**, *33*, 498–510. [CrossRef]
41. Grassi, E.S.; Pantazopoulou, V.; Pietras, A. Hypoxia-induced release, nuclear translocation, and signaling activity of a DLK1 intracellular fragment in glioma. *Oncogene* **2020**, *39*, 4028–4044. [CrossRef]
42. Maciaczyk, D.; Picard, D.; Zhao, L.; Koch, K.; Herrera-Rios, D.; Li, G.; Marquardt, V.; Pauck, D.; Hoerbelt, T.; Zhang, W.; et al. CBF1 is clinically prognostic and serves as a target to block cellular invasion and chemoresistance of EMT-like glioblastoma cells. *Br. J. Cancer* **2017**, *117*, 102–112. [CrossRef]
43. Kreuger, J.; Claesson-Welsh, L.; Olsson, A.-K.; Dimberg, A. VEGF receptor signalling—In control of vascular function. *Nat. Rev. Mol. Cell Biol.* **2006**, *7*, 359–371.
44. Almiron Bonnin, D.A.; Havrda, M.C.; Lee, M.C.; Liu, H.; Zhang, Z.; Nguyen, L.N.; Harrington, L.X.; Hassanpour, S.; Cheng, C.; Israel, M.A. Secretion-mediated STAT3 activation promotes self-renewal of glioma stem-like cells during hypoxia. *Oncogene* **2018**, *37*, 1107–1118. [CrossRef]
45. Vredenburgh, J.J.; Desjardins, A.; Herndon, J.E.; Marcello, J.; Reardon, D.A.; Quinn, J.A.; Rich, J.N.; Sathornsumetee, S.; Gururangan, S.; Sampson, J. Bevacizumab Plus Irinotecan in Recurrent Glioblastoma Multiforme. *J. Clin. Oncol.* **2007**, *25*, 4722–4729. [CrossRef]
46. Lu, F.I.; Wang, Y.T.; Wang, Y.S.; Wu, C.Y.; Li, C.C. Involvement of BIG1 and BIG2 in regulating VEGF expression and angiogenesis. *FASEB J. Off Publ. Fed. Am. Soc. Exp. Biol.* **2019**, *33*, 9959–9973. [CrossRef]
47. Long, Y.; Tao, H.; Karachi, A.; Grippin, A.J.; Jin, L.; Chang, Y.E.; Zhang, W.; Dyson, K.A.; Hou, A.Y.; Na, M.; et al. Dysregulation of Glutamate Transport Enhances Treg Function That Promotes VEGF Blockade Resistance in Glioblastoma. *Cancer Res.* **2020**, *80*, 499–509. [CrossRef]
48. Boso, D.; Rampazzo, E.; Zanon, C.; Bresolin, S.; Maule, F.; Porcù, E.; Cani, A.; Della Puppa, A.; Trentin, L.; Basso, G.; et al. HIF-1α/Wnt signaling-dependent control of gene transcription regulates neuronal differentiation of glioblastoma stem cells. *Theranostics* **2019**, *9*, 4860–4877. [CrossRef]
49. Lin, Y.T.; Wu, K.J. Epigenetic regulation of epithelial-mesenchymal transition: Focusing on hypoxia and TGF-β signaling. *J. Biomed. Sci.* **2020**, *27*, 39. [CrossRef]
50. Ye, X.Z.; Xu, S.L.; Xin, Y.H.; Yu, S.C.; Ping, Y.F.; Chen, L.; Xiao, H.L.; Wang, B.; Yi, L.; Wang, Q.L.; et al. Tumor-associated microglia/macrophages enhance the invasion of glioma stem-like cells via TGF-β1 signaling pathway. *J. Immunol.* **2012**, *189*, 444–453. [CrossRef]
51. Guerrero, P.A.; Tchaicha, J.H.; Chen, Z.; Morales, J.E.; Mccarty, N.; Wang, Q.; Sulman, E.P.; Fuller, G.; Lang, F.F.; Rao, G. Glioblastoma stem cells exploit the αvβ8 integrin-TGFβ1 signaling axis to drive tumor initiation and progression. *Oncogene* **2017**, *36*, 6568–6580. [CrossRef]
52. Mangani, D.; Weller, M.; Seyed Sadr, E.; Willscher, E.; Seystahl, K.; Reifenberger, G.; Tabatabai, G.; Binder, H.; Schneider, H. Limited role for transforming growth factor-β pathway activation-mediated escape from VEGF inhibition in murine glioma models. *Neuro Oncol.* **2016**, *18*, 1610–1621. [CrossRef]
53. Wu, W.; Hu, Q.; Nie, E.; Yu, T.; Wu, Y.; Zhi, T.; Jiang, K.; Shen, F.; Wang, Y.; Zhang, J.; et al. Hypoxia induces H19 expression through direct and indirect Hif-1α activity, promoting oncogenic effects in glioblastoma. *Sci. Rep.* **2017**, *7*, 45029. [CrossRef]
54. Mao, X.G.; Wang, C.; Liu, D.Y.; Zhang, X.; Wang, L.; Yan, M.; Zhang, W.; Zhu, J.; Li, Z.C.; Mi, C.; et al. Hypoxia upregulates HIG2 expression and contributes to bevacizumab resistance in glioblastoma. *Oncotarget* **2016**, *7*, 47808–47820. [CrossRef]
55. Zhang, K.; Xu, P.; Sowers, J.L.; Machuca, D.F.; Mirfattah, B.; Herring, J.; Tang, H.; Chen, Y.; Tian, B.; Brasier, A.R.; et al. Proteome Analysis of Hypoxic Glioblastoma Cells Reveals Sequential Metabolic Adaptation of One-Carbon Metabolic Pathways. *Mol. Cell. Proteom. MCP* **2017**, *16*, 1906–1921. [CrossRef]
56. May, J.L.; Kouri, F.M.; Hurley, L.A.; Liu, J.; Tommasini-Ghelfi, S.; Ji, Y.; Gao, P.; Calvert, A.E.; Lee, A.; Chandel, N.S.; et al. IDH3α regulates one-carbon metabolism in glioblastoma. *Sci. Adv.* **2019**, *5*, eaat0456. [CrossRef]
57. Dong, Z.; Cui, H. Epigenetic modulation of metabolism in glioblastoma. *Semin. Cancer Biol.* **2019**, *57*, 45–51. [CrossRef]
58. Colwell, N.; Larion, M.; Giles, A.J.; Seldomridge, A.N.; Sizdahkhani, S.; Gilbert, M.R.; Park, D.M. Hypoxia in the glioblastoma microenvironment: Shaping the phenotype of cancer stem-like cells. *Neuro Oncol.* **2017**, *19*, 887–896. [CrossRef]
59. Maus, A.; Peters, G.J. Erratum to: Glutamate and α-ketoglutarate: Key players in glioma metabolism. *Amino Acids* **2017**, *49*, 1143. [CrossRef]
60. Duman, C.; Yaqubi, K.; Hoffmann, A.; Acikgöz, A.A.; Korshunov, A.; Bendszus, M.; Herold-Mende, C.; Liu, H.K.; Alfonso, J. Acyl-CoA-Binding Protein Drives Glioblastoma Tumorigenesis by Sustaining Fatty Acid Oxidation. *Cell Metab.* **2019**, *30*, 274–289.e275. [CrossRef]
61. Javelot, H.; Michel, B.; Marquis, A.; Didelot, N.; Socha, M.; Javelot, T.; Petitpain, N. Acute withdrawal syndrome after discontinuation of a short analgesic treatment with tramadol. *Therapie* **2016**, *71*, 347–348. [CrossRef]
62. Zhou, W.; Guo, S.; Liu, M.; Burow, M.E.; Wang, G. Targeting CXCL12/CXCR4 Axis in Tumor Immunotherapy. *Curr. Med. Chem.* **2019**, *26*, 3026–3041. [CrossRef]
63. Ahir, B.K.; Engelhard, H.H.; Lakka, S.S. Tumor Development and Angiogenesis in Adult Brain Tumor: Glioblastoma. *Mol. Neurobiol.* **2020**, *57*, 2461–2478. [CrossRef]

64. Treps, L.; Perret, R.; Edmond, S.; Ricard, D.; Gavard, J. Glioblastoma stem-like cells secrete the pro-angiogenic VEGF-A factor in extracellular vesicles. *J. Extracell. Vesicles* **2017**, *6*, 1359479. [CrossRef]
65. Hu, B.; Wang, Q.; Wang, Y.A.; Hua, S.; Sauvé, C.G.; Ong, D.; Lan, Z.D.; Chang, Q.; Ho, Y.W.; Monasterio, M.M.; et al. Epigenetic Activation of WNT5A Drives Glioblastoma Stem Cell Differentiation and Invasive Growth. *Cell* **2016**, *167*, 1281–1295.e18 [CrossRef]
66. Rocha, R.; Torres, Á.; Ojeda, K.; Uribe, D.; Rocha, D.; Erices, J.; Niechi, I.; Ehrenfeld, P.; San Martín, R.; Quezada, C. The Adenosine A3 Receptor Regulates Differentiation of Glioblastoma Stem-Like Cells to Endothelial Cells under Hypoxia. *Int. J. Mol. Sci.* **2018**, *19*, 1228. [CrossRef]
67. Lathia, J.D.; Li, M.; Hall, P.E.; Gallagher, J.; Hale, J.S.; Wu, Q.; Venere, M.; Levy, E.; Rani, M.R.; Huang, P.; et al. Laminin alpha 2 enables glioblastoma stem cell growth. *Ann. Neurol.* **2012**, *72*, 766–778. [CrossRef]
68. Lathia, J.D.; Gallagher, J.; Heddleston, J.M.; Wang, J.; Eyler, C.E.; Macswords, J.; Wu, Q.; Vasanji, A.; McLendon, R.E.; Hjelmeland A.B.; et al. Integrin alpha 6 regulates glioblastoma stem cells. *Cell Stem Cell* **2010**, *6*, 421–432. [CrossRef]
69. Corsini, N.S.; Martin-Villalba, A. Integrin alpha 6: Anchors away for glioma stem cells. *Cell Stem Cell* **2010**, *6*, 403–404. [CrossRef]
70. Bikfalvi, A.; da Costa, C.A.; Avril, T.; Barnier, J.V.; Bauchet, L.; Brisson, L.; Cartron, P.F.; Castel, H.; Chevet, E.; Chneiweiss, H. et al. Challenges in glioblastoma research: Focus on the tumor microenvironment. *Trends Cancer* **2023**, *9*, 9–27. [CrossRef]
71. Verhaak, R.G.; Hoadley, K.A.; Purdom, E.; Wang, V.; Qi, Y.; Wilkerson, M.D.; Miller, C.R.; Ding, L.; Golub, T.; Mesirov, J.P. et al. Integrated Genomic Analysis Identifies Clinically Relevant Subtypes of Glioblastoma Characterized by Abnormalities in PDGFRA, IDH1, EGFR, and NF1. *Cancer Cell* **2010**, *17*, 98–110. [CrossRef]
72. Jeng, K.S.; Chang, C.F.; Lin, S.S. Sonic Hedgehog Signaling in Organogenesis, Tumors, and Tumor Microenvironments. *Int. J. Mol. Sci.* **2020**, *21*, 758. [CrossRef]
73. Zhu, T.S.; Costello, M.A.; Talsma, C.E.; Flack, C.G.; Crowley, J.G.; Hamm, L.L.; He, X.; Hervey-Jumper, S.L.; Heth, J.A.; Muraszko K.M. Endothelial Cells Create a Stem Cell Niche in Glioblastoma by Providing NOTCH Ligands That Nurture Self-Renewal of Cancer Stem-Like Cells. *Cancer Res.* **2011**, *71*, 6061–6072. [CrossRef]
74. Mei, X.; Chen, Y.S.; Chen, F.R.; Xi, S.Y.; Chen, Z.P. Glioblastoma stem cell differentiation into endothelial cells evidenced through live-cell imaging. *Neuro Oncol.* **2017**, *19*, 1109–1118. [CrossRef]
75. Hsu, S.P.C.; Chen, Y.C.; Chiang, H.C.; Huang, Y.C.; Huang, C.C.; Wang, H.E.; Wang, Y.S.; Chi, K.H. Rapamycin and hydroxy chloroquine combination alters macrophage polarization and sensitizes glioblastoma to immune checkpoint inhibitors. *J. Neuro Oncol.* **2020**, *146*, 417–426. [CrossRef]
76. Arcuri, C.; Fioretti, B.; Bianchi, R.; Mecca, C.; Tubaro, C.; Beccari, T.; Franciolini, F.; Giambanco, I.; Donato, R. Microglia-glioma cross-talk: A two way approach to new strategies against glioma. *Front. Biosci.* **2017**, *22*, 268–309. [CrossRef]
77. Singh, R.; Mishra, M.K.; Aggarwal, H. Inflammation, Immunity, and Cancer. *Mediat. Inflamm.* **2017**, *2017*, 6027305. [CrossRef]
78. Li, D.; Zhang, Q.; Li, L.; Chen, K.; Yang, J.; Dixit, D.; Gimple, R.C.; Ci, S.; Lu, C.; Hu, L.; et al. beta2-Microglobulin Maintains Glioblastoma Stem Cells and Induces M2-like Polarization of Tumor-Associated Macrophages. *Cancer Res.* **2022**, *82*, 3321–3334 [CrossRef]
79. Vitale, I.; Manic, G.; Coussens, L.M.; Kroemer, G.; Galluzzi, L. Macrophages and Metabolism in the Tumor Microenvironment *Cell Metab.* **2019**, *30*, 36–50. [CrossRef]
80. Kwok, D.; Okada, H. T-Cell based therapies for overcoming neuroanatomical and immunosuppressive challenges within the glioma microenvironment. *J. Neuro Oncol.* **2020**, *147*, 281–295. [CrossRef]
81. Peng, W.; Wang, H.Y.; Miyahara, Y.; Peng, G.; Wang, R.-F. Tumor-Associated Galectin-3 Modulates the Function of Tumor-Reactive T Cells. *Cancer Res.* **2008**, *68*, 7228–7236. [CrossRef]
82. Weenink, B.; French, P.J.; Sillevis Smitt, P.A.E.; Debets, R.; Geurts, M. Immunotherapy in Glioblastoma: Current Shortcomings and Future Perspectives. *Cancers* **2020**, *12*, 751. [CrossRef]
83. Tong, L.; Li, J.; Li, Q.; Wang, X.; Medikonda, R.; Zhao, T.; Li, T.; Ma, H.; Yi, L.; Liu, P.; et al. ACT001 reduces the expression of PD-L1 by inhibiting the phosphorylation of STAT3 in glioblastoma. *Theranostics* **2020**, *10*, 5943–5956. [CrossRef]
84. Boyd, N.H.; Tran, A.N.; Bernstock, J.D.; Etminan, T.; Jones, A.B.; Gillespie, G.Y.; Friedman, G.K.; Hjelmeland, A.B. Glioma stem cells and their roles within the hypoxic tumor microenvironment. *Theranostics* **2021**, *11*, 665–683. [CrossRef]
85. Boyd, N.H.; Walker, K.; Ayokanmbi, A.; Gordon, E.R.; Whetsel, J.; Smith, C.M.; Sanchez, R.G.; Lubin, F.D.; Chakraborty, A.; Tran A.N.; et al. Chromodomain Helicase DNA-Binding Protein 7 Is Suppressed in the Perinecrotic/Ischemic Microenvironment and Is a Novel Regulator of Glioblastoma Angiogenesis. *Stem Cells* **2019**, *37*, 453–462. [CrossRef]
86. Filatova, A.; Seidel, S.; Böğürcü, N.; Gräf, S.; Garvalov, B.K.; Acker, T. Acidosis Acts through HSP90 in a PHD/VHL-Independent Manner to Promote HIF Function and Stem Cell Maintenance in Glioma. *Cancer Res.* **2016**, *76*, 5845–5856. [CrossRef]
87. Xu, J.; Zhang, J.; Zhang, Z.; Gao, Z.; Qi, Y.; Qiu, W.; Pan, Z.; Guo, Q.; Li, B.; Zhao, S.; et al. Hypoxic glioma-derived exosomes promote M2-like macrophage polarization by enhancing autophagy induction. *Cell Death Dis.* **2021**, *12*, 373. [CrossRef]
88. Dong, F.; Qin, X.; Wang, B.; Li, Q.; Hu, J.; Cheng, X.; Guo, D.; Cheng, F.; Fang, C.; Tan, Y.; et al. ALKBH5 Facilitates Hypoxia Induced Paraspeckle Assembly and IL8 Secretion to Generate an Immunosuppressive Tumor Microenvironment. *Cancer Res* **2021**, *81*, 5876–5888. [CrossRef]
89. Mondal, A.; Kumari Singh, D.; Panda, S.; Shiras, A. Extracellular Vesicles As Modulators of Tumor Microenvironment and Disease Progression in Glioma. *Front. Oncol.* **2017**, *7*, 144. [CrossRef]

90. Walker, C.; Mojares, E.; Del Río Hernández, A. Role of Extracellular Matrix in Development and Cancer Progression. *Int. J. Mol. Sci.* **2018**, *19*, 3028. [CrossRef]
91. Reinhard, J.; Brösicke, N.; Theocharidis, U.; Faissner, A. The extracellular matrix niche microenvironment of neural and cancer stem cells in the brain. *Int. J. Biochem. Cell Biol.* **2016**, *81*, 174–183. [CrossRef]
92. Faissner, A.; Roll, L.; Theocharidis, U. Tenascin-C in the matrisome of neural stem and progenitor cells. *Mol. Cell. Neurosci.* **2017**, *81*, 22–31. [CrossRef]
93. Belter, A.; Gudanis, D.; Rolle, K.; Piwecka, M.; Gdaniec, Z.; Naskręt-Barciszewska, M.Z.; Barciszewski, J. Mature miRNAs form secondary structure, which suggests their function beyond RISC. *PLoS ONE* **2014**, *9*, e113848. [CrossRef]
94. Mao, X.G.; Xue, X.Y.; Lv, R.; Ji, A.; Shi, T.Y.; Chen, X.Y.; Jiang, X.F.; Zhang, X. CEBPD is a master transcriptional factor for hypoxia regulated proteins in glioblastoma and augments hypoxia induced invasion through extracellular matrix-integrin mediated EGFR/PI3K pathway. *Cell Death Dis.* **2023**, *14*, 269. [CrossRef]
95. Hira, V.V.V.; Van Noorden, C.J.F.; Carraway, H.E.; Maciejewski, J.P.; Molenaar, R.J. Novel therapeutic strategies to target leukemic cells that hijack compartmentalized continuous hematopoietic stem cell niches. *Biochim. Biophys. Acta Rev. Cancer* **2017**, *1868*, 183–198. [CrossRef]
96. Aderetti, D.A.; Hira, V.V.V.; Molenaar, R.J.; van Noorden, C.J.F. The hypoxic peri-arteriolar glioma stem cell niche, an integrated concept of five types of niches in human glioblastoma. *Biochim. Biophys. Acta Rev. Cancer* **2018**, *1869*, 346–354. [CrossRef]
97. Liebelt, B.D.; Shingu, T.; Zhou, X.; Ren, J.; Shin, S.A.; Hu, J. Glioma Stem Cells: Signaling, Microenvironment, and Therapy. *Stem Cells Int.* **2016**, *2016*, 7849890. [CrossRef]
98. Doedens, A.L.; Phan, A.T.; Stradner, M.H.; Fujimoto, J.K.; Nguyen, J.V.; Yang, E.; Johnson, R.S.; Goldrath, A.W. Hypoxia-inducible factors enhance the effector responses of CD8(+) T cells to persistent antigen. *Nat. Immunol.* **2013**, *14*, 1173–1182. [CrossRef]
99. An, Z.; Knobbe-Thomsen, C.B.; Wan, X.; Fan, Q.W.; Reifenberger, G.; Weiss, W.A. EGFR Cooperates with EGFRvIII to Recruit Macrophages in Glioblastoma. *Cancer Res.* **2018**, *78*, 6785–6794. [CrossRef]
100. Guo, X.Y.; Zhang, G.H.; Wang, Z.N.; Duan, H.; Xie, T.; Liang, L.; Cui, R.; Hu, H.R.; Wu, Y.; Dong, J.J.; et al. A novel Foxp3-related immune prognostic signature for glioblastoma multiforme based on immunogenomic profiling. *Aging* **2021**, *13*, 3501–3517. [CrossRef]
101. Kiyokawa, J.; Kawamura, Y.; Ghouse, S.M.; Acar, S.; Barçın, E.; Martínez-Quintanilla, J.; Martuza, R.L.; Alemany, R.; Rabkin, S.D.; Shah, K.; et al. Modification of Extracellular Matrix Enhances Oncolytic Adenovirus Immunotherapy in Glioblastoma. *Clin. Cancer Res. Off J. Am. Assoc. Cancer Res.* **2021**, *27*, 889–902. [CrossRef]
102. Brat, D.J.; Meir, E.G.V. Glomeruloid Microvascular Proliferation Orchestrated by VPF/VEGF: A New World of Angiogenesis Research. *Am. J. Pathol.* **2001**, *158*, 789–796. [CrossRef]
103. Wang, Q.; He, Z.; Huang, M.; Liu, T.; Wang, Y.; Xu, H.; Duan, H.; Ma, P.; Zhang, L.; Zamvil, S.S.; et al. Vascular niche IL-6 induces alternative macrophage activation in glioblastoma through HIF-2α. *Nat. Commun.* **2018**, *9*, 559. [CrossRef]
104. Wei, J.; Marisetty, A.; Schrand, B.; Gabrusiewicz, K.; Hashimoto, Y.; Ott, M.; Grami, Z.; Kong, L.Y.; Ling, X.; Caruso, H.; et al. Osteopontin mediates glioblastoma-associated macrophage infiltration and is a potential therapeutic target. *J. Clin. Investig.* **2019**, *129*, 137–149. [CrossRef]
105. Peng, P.; Zhu, H.; Liu, D.; Chen, Z.; Zhang, X.; Guo, Z.; Dong, M.; Wan, L.; Zhang, P.; Liu, G.; et al. TGFBI secreted by tumor-associated macrophages promotes glioblastoma stem cell-driven tumor growth via integrin alphavbeta5-Src-Stat3 signaling. *Theranostics* **2022**, *12*, 4221–4236. [CrossRef]
106. Ho, S.Y.; Ling, T.Y.; Lin, H.Y.; Liou, J.T.J.; Liu, F.C.; Chen, I.; Lee, S.W.; Hsu, Y.; Lai, D.M.; Liou, H.H. SDF-1/CXCR4 Signaling Maintains Stemness Signature in Mouse Neural Stem/Progenitor Cells. *Stem Cells Int.* **2017**, *2017*, 2493752. [CrossRef]
107. Lee, E.Q.; Duda, D.G.; Muzikansky, A.; Gerstner, E.R.; Kuhn, J.G.; Reardon, D.A.; Nayak, L.; Norden, A.D.; Doherty, L.; LaFrankie, D.; et al. Phase I and Biomarker Study of Plerixafor and Bevacizumab in Recurrent High-Grade Glioma. *Clin. Cancer Res. Off J. Am. Assoc. Cancer Res.* **2018**, *24*, 4643–4649. [CrossRef]
108. Jawhari, S.; Ratinaud, M.H.; Verdier, M. Glioblastoma, hypoxia and autophagy: A survival-prone 'menage-a-trois'. *Cell Death Dis.* **2016**, *7*, e2434. [CrossRef]
109. Ryskalin, L.; Gaglione, A.; Limanaqi, F.; Biagioni, F.; Familiari, P.; Frati, A.; Esposito, V.; Fornai, F. The Autophagy Status of Cancer Stem Cells in Gliobastoma Multiforme: From Cancer Promotion to Therapeutic Strategies. *Int. J. Mol. Sci.* **2019**, *20*, 3824. [CrossRef]
110. Abdul Rahim, S.A.; Dirkse, A.; Oudin, A.; Schuster, A.; Bohler, J.; Barthelemy, V.; Muller, A.; Vallar, L.; Janji, B.; Golebiewska, A.; et al. Regulation of hypoxia-induced autophagy in glioblastoma involves ATG9A. *Br. J. Cancer* **2017**, *117*, 813–825. [CrossRef]
111. Buccarelli, M.; Marconi, M.; Pacioni, S.; De Pascalis, I.; D'Alessandris, Q.G.; Martini, M.; Ascione, B.; Malorni, W.; Larocca, L.M.; Pallini, R.; et al. Inhibition of autophagy increases susceptibility of glioblastoma stem cells to temozolomide by igniting ferroptosis. *Cell Death Dis.* **2018**, *9*, 841. [CrossRef]
112. Xue, H.; Yuan, G.; Guo, X.; Liu, Q.; Zhang, J.; Gao, X.; Guo, X.; Xu, S.; Li, T.; Shao, Q.; et al. A novel tumor-promoting mechanism of IL6 and the therapeutic efficacy of tocilizumab: Hypoxia-induced IL6 is a potent autophagy initiator in glioblastoma via the p-STAT3-MIR155-3p-CREBRF pathway. *Autophagy* **2016**, *12*, 1129–1152. [CrossRef]
113. Julio Sotelo, E.B.; López-González, M.A. Adding Chloroquine to Conventional Treatment for Glioblastoma Multiforme: A Randomized, Double-Blind, Placebo-Controlled Trial. *Ann. Intern. Med.* **2006**, *144*, 337–343. [CrossRef]

114. Huang, T.; Kim, C.K.; Alvarez, A.A.; Pangeni, R.P.; Wan, X.; Song, X.; Shi, T.; Yang, Y.; Sastry, N.; Horbinski, C.M.; et al. MST4 Phosphorylation of ATG4B Regulates Autophagic Activity, Tumorigenicity, and Radioresistance in Glioblastoma. *Cancer Cell* **2017**, *32*, 840–855.e8. [CrossRef]
115. Pottoo, F.H.; Javed, M.N.; Rahman, J.U.; Abu-Izneid, T.; Khan, F.A. Targeted delivery of miRNA based therapeuticals in the clinical management of Glioblastoma Multiforme. *Semin. Cancer Biol.* **2020**, *69*, 391–398. [CrossRef]
116. Dixit, D.; Prager, B.C.; Gimple, R.C.; Poh, H.X.; Wang, Y.; Wu, Q.; Qiu, Z.; Kidwell, R.L.; Kim, L.J.Y.; Xie, Q.; et al. The RNA m6A Reader YTHDF2 Maintains Oncogene Expression and Is a Targetable Dependency in Glioblastoma Stem Cells. *Cancer Discov.* **2021**, *11*, 480–499. [CrossRef]
117. Struve, N.; Binder, Z.A.; Stead, L.F.; Brend, T.; Bagley, S.J.; Faulkner, C.; Ott, L.; Müller-Goebel, J.; Weik, A.S.; Hoffer, K.; et al. EGFRvIII upregulates DNA mismatch repair resulting in increased temozolomide sensitivity of MGMT promoter methylated glioblastoma. *Oncogene* **2020**, *39*, 3041–3055. [CrossRef]
118. Jalota, A.; Kumar, M.; Das, B.C.; Yadav, A.K.; Chosdol, K.; Sinha, S. A drug combination targeting hypoxia induced chemoresistance and stemness in glioma cells. *Oncotarget* **2018**, *9*, 18351–18366. [CrossRef]
119. Torres, Á.; Arriagada, V.; Erices, J.I.; Toro, M.; Rocha, J.D.; Niechi, I.; Carrasco, C.; Oyarzún, C.; Quezada, C. FK506 Attenuates the MRP1-Mediated Chemoresistant Phenotype in Glioblastoma Stem-Like Cells. *Int. J. Mol. Sci.* **2018**, *19*, 2697. [CrossRef]
120. Lo Dico, A.; Martelli, C.; Diceglie, C.; Lucignani, G.; Ottobrini, L. Hypoxia-Inducible Factor-1α Activity as a Switch for Glioblastoma Responsiveness to Temozolomide. *Front. Oncol.* **2018**, *8*, 249. [CrossRef]
121. Luger, A.L.; Lorenz, N.I.; Urban, H.; Divé, I.; Engel, A.L.; Strassheimer, F.; Dettmer, K.; Zeiner, P.S.; Shaid, S.; Struve, N.; et al. Activation of Epidermal Growth Factor Receptor Sensitizes Glioblastoma Cells to Hypoxia-Induced Cell Death. *Cancers* **2020**, *12*, 2144. [CrossRef]
122. Tsai, C.K.; Huang, L.C.; Wu, Y.P.; Kan, I.Y.; Hueng, D.Y. SNAP reverses temozolomide resistance in human glioblastoma multiforme cells through down-regulation of MGMT. *FASEB J. Off Publ. Fed. Am. Soc. Exp. Biol.* **2019**, *33*, 14171–14184. [CrossRef]
123. Badruddoja, M.A.; Pazzi, M.; Sanan, A.; Schroeder, K.; Kuzma, K.; Norton, T.; Scully, T.; Mahadevan, D.; Ahmadi, M.M. Phase II study of bi-weekly temozolomide plus bevacizumab for adult patients with recurrent glioblastoma. *Cancer Chemother. Pharmacol.* **2017**, *80*, 715–721. [CrossRef]
124. Gerstner, E.R.; Emblem, K.E.; Yen, Y.F.; Dietrich, J.; Jordan, J.T.; Catana, C.; Wenchin, K.L.; Hooker, J.M.; Duda, D.G.; Rosen, B.R.; et al. Vascular dysfunction promotes regional hypoxia after bevacizumab therapy in recurrent glioblastoma patients. *Neuro Oncol. Adv.* **2020**, *2*, vdaa157. [CrossRef]
125. Bielecka-Wajdman, A.M.; Lesiak, M.; Ludyga, T.; Sieroń, A.; Obuchowicz, E. Reversing glioma malignancy: A new look at the role of antidepressant drugs as adjuvant therapy for glioblastoma multiforme. *Cancer Chemother. Pharmacol.* **2017**, *79*, 1249–1256. [CrossRef]
126. Bielecka, A.M.; Obuchowicz, E. Antidepressant drugs can modify cytotoxic action of temozolomide. *Eur. J. Cancer Care* **2017**, *26*, e12551. [CrossRef]
127. Gallitto, M.; Cheng He, R.; Inocencio, J.F.; Wang, H.; Zhang, Y.; Deikus, G.; Wasserman, I.; Strahl, M.; Smith, M.; Sebra, R.; et al. Epigenetic preconditioning with decitabine sensitizes glioblastoma to temozolomide via induction of MLH1. *J. Neuro Oncol.* **2020**, *147*, 557–566. [CrossRef]
128. Zhang, S.; Lu, Y.; Li, H.; Ji, Y.; Fang, F.; Tang, H.; Qiu, P. A steroidal saponin form Paris vietnamensis (Takht.) reverses temozolomide resistance in glioblastoma cells via inducing apoptosis through ROS/PI3K/Akt pathway. *Biosci. Trends* **2020**, *14*, 123–133. [CrossRef]
129. Ludman, T.; Melemedjian, O.K. Bortezomib and metformin opposingly regulate the expression of hypoxia-inducible factor alpha and the consequent development of chemotherapy-induced painful peripheral neuropathy. *Mol. Pain* **2019**, *15*, 1744806919850043. [CrossRef]
130. Yao, Z.; Zhang, X.; Zhao, F.; Wang, S.; Chen, A.; Huang, B.; Wang, J.; Li, X. Ursodeoxycholic Acid Inhibits Glioblastoma Progression via Endoplasmic Reticulum Stress Related Apoptosis and Synergizes with the Proteasome Inhibitor Bortezomib. *ACS Chem. Neurosci.* **2020**, *11*, 1337–1346. [CrossRef]
131. Bergès, R.; Tchoghandjian, A.; Sergé, A.; Honoré, S.; Figarella-Branger, D.; Bachmann, F.; Lane, H.A.; Braguer, D. EB1-dependent long survival of glioblastoma-grafted mice with the oral tubulin-binder BAL101553 is associated with inhibition of tumor angiogenesis. *Oncotarget* **2020**, *11*, 759–774. [CrossRef]
132. Yerram, P.; Reiss, S.N.; Modelevsky, L.; Gavrilovic, I.T.; Kaley, T. Evaluation of toxicity of carmustine with or without bevacizumab in patients with recurrent or progressive high grade gliomas. *J. Neuro Oncol.* **2019**, *145*, 57–63. [CrossRef]
133. Brenner, A.; Zuniga, R.; Sun, J.D.; Floyd, J.; Hart, C.P.; Kroll, S.; Fichtel, L.; Cavazos, D.; Caflisch, L.; Gruslova, A.; et al. Hypoxia-activated evofosfamide for treatment of recurrent bevacizumab-refractory glioblastoma: A phase I surgical study. *Neuro Oncol.* **2018**, *20*, 1231–1239. [CrossRef]
134. Takakusagi, Y.; Kishimoto, S.; Naz, S.; Matsumoto, S.; Saito, K.; Hart, C.P.; Mitchell, J.B.; Krishna, M.C. Radiotherapy Synergizes with the Hypoxia-Activated Prodrug Evofosfamide: In Vitro and In Vivo Studies. *Antioxid. Redox Signal.* **2018**, *28*, 131–140. [CrossRef]
135. Ronellenfitsch, M.W.; Zeiner, P.S.; Mittelbronn, M.; Urban, H.; Pietsch, T.; Reuter, D.; Senft, C.; Steinbach, J.P.; Westphal, M.; Harter, P.N. Akt and mTORC1 signaling as predictive biomarkers for the EGFR antibody nimotuzumab in glioblastoma. *Acta Neuropathol. Commun.* **2018**, *6*, 81. [CrossRef]

36. Patocka, J.; Nepovimova, E.; Wu, W.; Kuca, K. Digoxin: Pharmacology and toxicology-A review. *Environ. Toxicol. Pharmacol.* **2020**, *79*, 103400. [CrossRef]
37. Lee, D.H.; Cheul Oh, S.; Giles, A.J.; Jung, J.; Gilbert, M.R.; Park, D.M. Cardiac glycosides suppress the maintenance of stemness and malignancy via inhibiting HIF-1α in human glioma stem cells. *Oncotarget* **2017**, *8*, 40233–40245. [CrossRef]
38. Ferreira, N.N.; Granja, S.; Boni, F.I.; Ferreira, L.M.B.; Reis, R.M.; Baltazar, F.; Gremião, M.P.D. A novel strategy for glioblastoma treatment combining alpha-cyano-4-hydroxycinnamic acid with cetuximab using nanotechnology-based delivery systems. *Drug. Deliv. Transl. Res.* **2020**, *10*, 594–609. [CrossRef]
39. Bernstock, J.D.; Ye, D.; Gessler, F.A.; Lee, Y.J.; Peruzzotti-Jametti, L.; Baumgarten, P.; Johnson, K.R.; Maric, D.; Yang, W.; Kögel, D.; et al. Topotecan is a potent inhibitor of SUMOylation in glioblastoma multiforme and alters both cellular replication and metabolic programming. *Sci. Rep.* **2017**, *7*, 7425. [CrossRef]
40. Wang, Y.; Tan, X.; Li, S.; Yang, S. The total flavonoid of Eucommia ulmoides sensitizes human glioblastoma cells to radiotherapy via HIF-α/MMP-2 pathway and activates intrinsic apoptosis pathway. *OncoTargets Ther.* **2019**, *12*, 5515–5524. [CrossRef]
41. Lesueur, P.; Lequesne, J.; Grellard, J.M.; Dugué, A.; Coquan, E.; Brachet, P.E.; Geffrelot, J.; Kao, W.; Emery, E.; Berro, D.H.; et al. Phase I/IIa study of concomitant radiotherapy with olaparib and temozolomide in unresectable or partially resectable glioblastoma: OLA-TMZ-RTE-01 trial protocol. *BMC Cancer* **2019**, *19*, 198. [CrossRef]
42. Yang, M.; Li, J.; Gu, P.; Fan, X. The application of nanoparticles in cancer immunotherapy: Targeting tumor microenvironment. *Bioact. Mater.* **2021**, *6*, 1973–1987. [CrossRef]
43. Zhang, Y.; Zhang, Z. The history and advances in cancer immunotherapy: Understanding the characteristics of tumor-infiltrating immune cells and their therapeutic implications. *Cell. Mol. Immunol.* **2020**, *17*, 807–821. [CrossRef]
44. Mao, X.G.; Xue, X.Y.; Wang, L.; Wang, L.; Li, L.; Zhang, X. Hypoxia Regulated Gene Network in Glioblastoma Has Special Algebraic Topology Structures and Revealed Communications Involving Warburg Effect and Immune Regulation. *Cell. Mol. Neurobiol.* **2019**, *39*, 1093–1114. [CrossRef]
45. Huang, L.; Boling, W.; Zhang, J.H. Hyperbaric oxygen therapy as adjunctive strategy in treatment of glioblastoma multiforme. *Med. Gas Res.* **2018**, *8*, 24–28. [CrossRef]
46. Alpuim Costa, D.; Sampaio-Alves, M.; Netto, E.; Fernandez, G.; Oliveira, E.; Teixeira, A.; Daniel, P.M.; Bernardo, G.S.; Amaro, C. Hyperbaric Oxygen Therapy as a Complementary Treatment in Glioblastoma-A Scoping Review. *Front. Neurol.* **2022**, *13*, 886603. [CrossRef]
47. Stępień, K.; Ostrowski, R.P.; Matyja, E. Hyperbaric oxygen as an adjunctive therapy in treatment of malignancies, including brain tumours. *Med. Oncol.* **2016**, *33*, 101. [CrossRef]
48. Chang, C.H. Hyperbaric oxygen and radiation therapy in the management of glioblastoma. *Natl. Cancer Inst. Monogr.* **1977**, *46*, 163–169.
49. Ogawa, K.; Kohshi, K.; Ishiuchi, S.; Matsushita, M.; Yoshimi, N.; Murayama, S. Old but new methods in radiation oncology: Hyperbaric oxygen therapy. *Int. J. Clin. Oncol.* **2013**, *18*, 364–370. [CrossRef]
50. Ogawa, K.; Ishiuchi, S.; Inoue, O.; Yoshii, Y.; Saito, A.; Watanabe, T.; Iraha, S.; Toita, T.; Kakinohana, Y.; Ariga, T.; et al. Phase II Trial of Radiotherapy After Hyperbaric Oxygenation With Multiagent Chemotherapy (Procarbazine, Nimustine, and Vincristine) for High-Grade Gliomas: Long-Term Results. *Int. J. Radiat. Oncol. Biol. Phys.* **2012**, *82*, 732–738. [CrossRef]
51. Yahara, K.; Ohguri, T.; Udono, H.; Yamamoto, J.; Tomura, K.; Onoda, T.; Imada, H.; Nishizawa, S.; Korogi, Y. Radiotherapy using IMRT boosts after hyperbaric oxygen therapy with chemotherapy for glioblastoma. *J. Radiat. Res.* **2017**, *58*, 351–356. [CrossRef]

Disclaimer/Publisher's Note: The statements, opinions and data contained in all publications are solely those of the individual author(s) and contributor(s) and not of MDPI and/or the editor(s). MDPI and/or the editor(s) disclaim responsibility for any injury to people or property resulting from any ideas, methods, instructions or products referred to in the content.

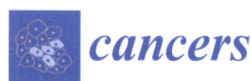

Article

Characterization and Optimization of the Tumor Microenvironment in Patient-Derived Organotypic Slices and Organoid Models of Glioblastoma

Vera Nickl [1,*], Juliana Eck [2], Nicolas Goedert [1], Julian Hübner [3], Thomas Nerreter [3], Carsten Hagemann [1], Ralf-Ingo Ernestus [1], Tim Schulz [1], Robert Carl Nickl [1], Almuth Friederike Keßler [1], Mario Löhr [1], Andreas Rosenwald [2], Maria Breun [1] and Camelia Maria Monoranu [4]

1 Department of Neurosurgery, University Hospital Würzburg, 97080 Würzburg, Germany
2 Institute of Pathology, University of Würzburg, 97080 Würzburg, Germany
3 Department of Hematology, University Hospital Würzburg, 97080 Würzburg, Germany
4 Department of Neuropathology, Institute of Pathology, University of Würzburg, 97080 Würzburg, Germany
* Correspondence: nickl_v@ukw.de

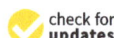

Simple Summary: Glioblastoma is the most common malignant brain tumor in adults, entailing a very short survival. New therapeutic strategies are desperately needed. Immunotherapeutic approaches seem promising, yet their breakthrough is hindered by interactions of the tumor with its immunological tumor environment. In order to understand these complex interactions, innovative glioblastoma models are needed. We aimed to investigate whether patient-derived tumor models are able to maintain the tumor's microenvironment signature and composition. Secondly, we added immune cells to our model in order to reflect a more realistic tumor microenvironment, which could be used for preclinical testing of novel immunotherapeutic approaches. Thus, we hope to contribute to the challenging task of advancing glioblastoma therapy.

Abstract: While glioblastoma (GBM) is still challenging to treat, novel immunotherapeutic approaches have shown promising effects in preclinical settings. However, their clinical breakthrough is hampered by complex interactions of GBM with the tumor microenvironment (TME). Here, we present an analysis of TME composition in a patient-derived organoid model (PDO) as well as in organotypic slice cultures (OSC). To obtain a more realistic model for immunotherapeutic testing, we introduce an enhanced PDO model. We manufactured PDOs and OSCs from fresh tissue of GBM patients and analyzed the TME. Enhanced PDOs (ePDOs) were obtained via co-culture with PBMCs (peripheral blood mononuclear cells) and compared to normal PDOs (nPDOs) and PT (primary tissue). At first, we showed that TME was not sustained in PDOs after a short time of culture. In contrast, TME was largely maintained in OSCs. Unfortunately, OSCs can only be cultured for up to 9 days. Thus, we enhanced the TME in PDOs by co-culturing PDOs and PBMCs from healthy donors. These cellular TME patterns could be preserved until day 21. The ePDO approach could mirror the interaction of GBM, TME and immunotherapeutic agents and may consequently represent a realistic model for individual immunotherapeutic drug testing in the future.

Keywords: glioblastoma; organoids; slice culture; tumormicroenvironment

Citation: Nickl, V.; Eck, J.; Goedert, N.; Hübner, J.; Nerreter, T.; Hagemann, C.; Ernestus, R.-I.; Schulz, T.; Nickl, R.C.; Keßler, A.F.; et al. Characterization and Optimization of the Tumor Microenvironment in Patient-Derived Organotypic Slices and Organoid Models of Glioblastoma. *Cancers* **2023**, *15*, 2698. https://doi.org/10.3390/cancers15102698

Academic Editors: Annunziato Mangiola and Gianluca Trevisi

Received: 24 March 2023
Revised: 23 April 2023
Accepted: 8 May 2023
Published: 10 May 2023

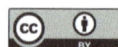

Copyright: © 2023 by the authors. Licensee MDPI, Basel, Switzerland. This article is an open access article distributed under the terms and conditions of the Creative Commons Attribution (CC BY) license (https:// creativecommons.org/licenses/by/ 4.0/).

1. Introduction

Glioblastoma (GBM) is the most malignant primary brain tumor with a median survival time of 14.6 months and a five-year survival rate of 6% [1]. Maximum standard therapy includes extensive surgery, if functionally possible, followed by radiotherapy combined with concomitant and adjuvant chemotherapy with temozolomide (TMZ) [2]. Lately chemotherapy has been modified with Lomustine for patients younger than 70 years and a methylated MGMT (O^6-methylguanine-methyltransferase)-promoter [3]. However, despite vigorous efforts in research during the last years introducing tumor treating fields [4] and anti-angiogenesis monoclonal VEGFR-antibodies [5], survival rates have not changed since 2005. During their limited life-span, patients suffer from neurological deficits such as hemiparesis, aphasia, seizures, and changes of personality, rendering the disease even more daunting. Relapse is certain and prognosis is even poorer in patients with a multifocal involvement [2,6] or an unmethylated MGMT-promoter [7,8]. New therapeutic approaches are desperately needed. In recent years, major progress has been made in developing new immunotherapeutic treatment options such as bispecific T-cell engagers (BiTes) [9,10], chimeric antigen receptors (CAR) T-cell therapies [11–13] or oncolytic viruses [14,15].

Immunotherapeutic therapies for solid tumors such as GBM are more challenging than for hematological tumors [16]. The solid tumor consists of complex cell–cell interactions of not only tumor cells, but also stromal, immune and vascular cells in addition to components of extracellular matrix. Together, these elements represent the tumor microenvironment (TME) [17]. Within the TME, regulatory T-cells (Tregs), tumor-associated macrophages (TAMs) or myeloid-derived suppressor cells (MDSCs) contribute to the immunosuppressive and exhausting character of tumors. Various pro-tumoral cell populations are, e.g., able to interact with inhibitory receptors as PD-1 (programmed cell death 1), CTLA4 (cytotoxic T-lymphocyte-associated antigen 4), TIM3 (T-cell immunoglobulin and mucin domain-containing protein 3), and LAG3 (lymphocyte activation gene 3) on T-cells and mediate immunosuppression and T-cell exhaustion [18]. Inhibiting these immune checkpoint receptors can lead to synergistic effects with immunotherapeutic approaches raising their functionality and rendering them more effective [19].

While the TME consists of only a small number of T-cells, TAMs represent up to 40% of the TME [20]. Macrophages are the most common infiltrating stromal components of the TME, generating an immunosuppressive environment [21]. Additionally, TAMs restrict the glycolytic flow which is important for cytotoxic T-cells [22] and diminish the effective anti-tumoral immune response. M1-macrophages (iNOS+) are induced via Interferon γ (IFNγ) and lipopolysaccharides, produce immunostimulating cytokines and, thus, express a tumor suppressive activity. M2-macrophages (CD163+), on the other hand, are, e.g., activated by interleukin 4 (IL4), dampen inflammatory reactions and promote immunoevasion of tumor cells as well as invasion and angiogenesis [23]. There are two main sources of macrophages in GBM: resident brain microglia and peripheral monocyte-derived macrophages (MDMs). MDMs are recruited from the bloodstream into the tumor through various chemokine signals [24]. Chemokine receptor CCR2 has emerged as a marker for MDMs in GBM, as it is expressed on peripheral monocytes but not on resident microglia [25]. CCR2 is a G-protein coupled receptor that binds to the chemokine CCL2, which is highly expressed in the GBM microenvironment [26]. CCL2-CCR2 signaling is critical for monocyte recruitment to the tumor site [27]. In GBM, CCR2+ macrophages have been shown to be predominantly MDMs, whereas CCR2- macrophages are primarily microglia [25]. CCR2+ macrophages have been associated with a more pro-tumoral phenotype, including enhanced angiogenesis, invasion, and immunosuppression [24].

TAMs produce IL4 and interleukin 10 (IL10) [28], leading to PD-1 expression and T-cell exhaustion [29]. Natural killer (NK) cells (CD7+) as a part of the innate immune system play a crucial role in fighting GBM as they are able to recognize surface antigens without prior sensibilization. The metabolic fitness of NK cells is not only influenced by extracellular vesicles, cytokines and chemokines, but also hypoxic gradients [30]. Myeloid-derived suppressor cells (MDSC), which are able to wipe out cytotoxic T-cells, can be eliminated by NK-cells leading to an antitumoral effect [31].

In a preclinical setting, these complex interactions of GBM, TME and therapeutic agents cannot be mirrored by GBM cell lines alone and antigen surface expression patterns cannot be assumed to be similar in GBM cell lines and intracerebral tumor tissue. Rupture of cell–cell-contacts during lysis, duration of cultivation and hypoxic gradients might be reasons for changes in these patterns [17]. Additionally, a robust TME including stromal, inflammatory and vascular cells as well as extracellular matrix is missing [32]. Recently, new ex vivo models have been introduced as alternatives to immortalized cell lines and advancement in drug testing [33–35]. Patient derived GBM-organoids (PDO) represent the histological features, cellular diversity, gene expression and mutational profiles of their corresponding parental tumors [35]. In addition, they can be generated quickly and reliable within two weeks from intraoperatively resected tissue [36]. Patient-derived organotypic slice cultures (OSCs) equally represent parental tumor patterns close to the in vivo tumor as OSCs contain not only tumor cells, but also components of the TME. Furthermore, the cellular architecture and tissue compartmentalization is maintained [34]. Freshly sliced this tissue is ready to use, but on the downside, slicing is a delicate method susceptible to deficiencies and depends on tissue quality [34]. Both ex vivo models have different advantages and can be used complementary in order to test new immunotherapeutic approaches ex vivo.

Therefore, the aim of the present study was to characterize the ex vivo TME in PDOs and OSCs in comparison to primary tissue (PT). In a second step, we introduced cellular TME components in PDOs by co-culture with PBMCs (peripheral blood mononuclear cells) and thus generated enhanced PDOs (ePDOs). We compared the capability of normal PDOs (nPDOs) and ePDOs to reflect the TME antigen expression patterns as seen in PT. This approach might hold potential as an ex vivo test system mirroring complex TME–tumor–therapy interactions, e.g., for immunotherapeutic approaches.

2. Methods

2.1. Tissue Samples

All patients were treated at the Department of Neurosurgery, University Hospital Würzburg, Germany, and gave written informed consent in accordance with the declaration of Helsinki, and as approved by the Institutional Review Board of the University of Würzburg (#22/20-me). The tumors were histologically assessed and graded on formalin fixed and paraffin embedded tissue sections by an experienced neuropathologist, according to the most recent criteria of the World Health Organization [37].

2.2. OSC

OSCs were prepared as previously described in Nickl et al.'s work [33]. After surgical tumor resection, the tissue was directly transferred to Hibernate A medium containing 1% Glutamax, 0.4% penicillin/streptomycin and 0.1% Amphotericin (HGPSA) (all from Gibco Carlsbad, CA, USA) and stored in ice. Next, the tumor tissue was carefully freed from necrosis and blood vessels and cut into approximately 2×0.5 cm pieces using scalpels. The pre-cut tumor was glued edgewise on a test tube with histoacryl glue and the tube filled with 38 °C molten agarose (Sigma-Aldrich, St. Louis, MO, USA). A -80 °C cooling block ensured rapid hardening of the agarose. The sample tube was clamped in the vibratome (Precisionary Instruments, Greenville, SC, USA) and 350 μm thick slices were cut using an advance of 3.5 mm/minutes and an oscillation of 6 Hz. The thin slices had to be carefully cut out with scalpels before they could be transferred with a wide pipette into the inserts with a semi-permeable membrane of 0.4 μm pore size (Greiner Bio-one, Frickenhausen, Germany) in a 24-well plate (Corning Costar, New York, NY, USA) containing brain slice medium (MEM supplemented with 25% normal horse serum, 25% Hank's Balanced salt solution (HBSS), 1% penicillin/streptomycin, 1% L-glutamine (all from Gibco, Carlsbad, CA, USA), vitamin C and 1% glucose (both from Sigma-Aldrich, St. Louis, MO, USA) at 35 °C, 5% CO_2 and 95% humidity. After standardized hematoxylin and eosin (HE) staining was performed for histology, the tumor content was assessed by an experienced neuropathologist. OSCs were fixed in 4% formalin (Carl Roth, Karlsruhe, Germany) for 24 h at 4 °C and then transferred to phosphate-buffered saline (PBS) (Sigma-Aldrich, St Louis, MO, USA) for immunohistochemical staining.

2.3. PDOs

PDOs were prepared according to Nickl et al.'s description [33]. For this purpose, fresh intraoperatively gained tumor tissue was temporarily stored on ice in Hibernate A medium. Necrotic areas and blood vessels were cleared and the tissue was minced carefully under the microscope into approximately 500 µm pieces with a scalpel. The tissue was then treated with RBC Lysis Buffer for 10 min and washed twice with Hibernate A medium. For incubation, tumor sections were transferred in PDO Medium consisting of 47.24% DMEM/F12, 47.25% Neurobasal, 0.02% B27 without Vitamin A (50×), 0.01% Glutamax, 0.01% N2, 0.01% NEAA, 0.004% penicillin/streptomycin, 0.001% β-Mercaptoethanol (all from Gibco, Carlsbad, CA, USA) and 0.00023% human insulin (Sigma Aldrich, St. Louis, MO, USA) to ultra-low attachment 6-well plates (Corning Costar, New York, NY, USA) and incubated at 37 °C, 5% CO_2 and 95% humidity on an orbital shaker at 120 rpm. After 2 weeks of cultivation, PDOs formed successfully and could be used for further experiments [35]. At the end of the experiments, PDOs were fixed in 4% formalin (Carl Roth, Karlsruhe, Germany) for 24 h at 4 °C and then transferred to phosphate-buffered saline (PBS) (Sigma-Aldrich, St. Louis, MO, USA) for immunohistochemical staining.

2.4. PBMC Preparation

PBMCs were isolated from healthy donors and cultured for ten days. The cells were then centrifuged (200 g, room temperature, 12 min) and diluted in 5 mL CTL medium containing 88% RPMI, 10% ml human serum, 1% Penicillin/Streptomycin, 1% Glutamax, 0.1% β-Mercaptoethanol (all from Gibco, Carlsbad, CA, USA). After a second centrifugation step (200 g, room temperature, 12 min) cells were brought to a concentration of 2×10^6/mL with CTL medium and incubated overnight with 150 U/mL IL2 (Miltenyi, Bergisch Gladbach, Germany) at 37 °C, 5% CO_2 and 95% humidity. After resuspending and counting the cells the next morning, they were washed in PBS (D8537; SigmaAldrich, St. Louis, MO, USA) at 500 g, room temperature, 5 min and brought to a concentration of 1×10^6/mL utilizing the PDO medium adding 150 U/mL IL2. PDOs and PBMCs were incubated at a ratio of 1:20 and a half medium change was performed every other day adding IL2 to a final concentration of 150 U/mL.

2.5. Immunohistochemistry

For immunohistochemistry, tissue was cut into 2 µm-slices, deparaffinized in xylene and hydrated in a graded series of alcohols. Heat-induced retrieval was either performed for 8 (CD4, CD8, CD45, CD68, CD163, FOXP3) or 10 (CD14, CCR2, TIM3) minutes with citrate buffer (pH = 6.0) or for 4 min with citrate buffer (pH = 7.0) (CD86). Alternatively, heat induced retrieval was performed in Tris-EDTA buffer (pH = 6.1) for 3 (CD7, CD25) or 10 (PD1) minutes or Tris-EDTA buffer (pH = 9.0) for 5 min (LAG3). After blocking with 30% hydrogen peroxide (PanReac Applichem, ITW Reagents, Darmstadt, Germany), slides were treated with 10% normal goat serum (Invitrogen, Waltham, MA, USA) for CCR2. Subsequently, the primary antibody was applied over night at 4 °C (CCR2, LAG3, PD1 and TIM3) or 1 h at room temperature (CD4, CD7, CD8, CD14, CD25, CD45, CD68, CD86, CD163 and FOXP3) (CD4 (396202, BioLegend, San Diego, CA, USA, clone: A17070D, dilution: 1:200), CD7 (M7255, Dako, clone: CBC37, dilution: 1:500), CD8 (372902, BioLegend, clone: C8/144B, dilution: 1:80), CD14 (ab183322, abcam, clone: SP192, dilution; 1:800), CD25 (MA5-12680, Thermo Fisher, Waltham, MA, USA clone: IL2R.1, dilution: 1:40), CD45 (M0701, Dako, clone: 1B11+PD7/26, dilution: 1:2000), CD68 (KiM1P, was gifted, dilution: 1:1000), CD86 (MA5-32078, Thermo Fisher, clone: SJ20-00, dilution: 1:400), CD163 (NCL-CD163, Leica, clone: 10D6, dilution: 1:800), CCR2 (ab209236, abcam, clone: EPR20261, dilution: 1:400), FOXP3 (ab20034, abcam, clone: 236A/E7, dilution: 1:400), LAG3 (PA5-97917, Thermo Fisher, clone: 29-450AA, dilution: 1:1000), PD1 (ab52587, abcam, clone: NAT105, dilution: 1:400), TIM3 (MA5-32841, Thermo-Fisher, clone: E5, dilution: 1:800)). Slides were then incubated with the secondary antibody for 20 min and labeled (HiDef Detection™ HRP 2-step Polymer Detection System, Cell Marque, Rocklin, CA, USA).

Diaminobenzadine (N-Histofine DAB 2V, Nichisei Biosciences inc., Chuo, Tokyo, Japan) was applied for 5 min (CCR2), 7 min (CD68, LAG3 and PD1) or 10 min (CD4, CD7, CD8, CD14, CD25, CD45, CD86, CD163, FOXP3, TIM3) and after rinsing with water, cell nuclei were counterstained using hemalum solution acid and mounted. Tonsil tissue was used as a positive control.

For the PT as well as the OSCs, five representative areas of view per slide were photographed using microscope (Olympus BX50), camera (Olympus DP27) and software (Olympus cellSense Entry, all Shinjuku, Tokyo, Japan) with standardized settings at 40× magnification. The whole PDO was photographed and analyzed. We detected positive staining intensity via the batch processing function of the open source program Fiji [38] by applying a specialized macro. Finally, we calculated the absolute and relative expression of all antigens for each PDOs/OSCs. All analyses were monitored and counterchecked by an experienced neuropathologist.

2.6. Statistical Analysis

Analyses were performed using IBM SPSS Statistics 27 (SPSS Worldwide, Chicago, IL, USA). For patients' characteristics we performed descriptive statistics, displaying either absolute and relative numbers or mean with range (minimum/maximum) wherever suitable. Data was examined for Gaussian distribution by Kolmogorov–Smirnov testing before testing for significance was conducted. We performed ANOVA for equally distributed data and the Friedmann's test for non-equally distributed data in order to determine significant differences in the antigen-expression patterns during the course of time in PDOs and OSCs. Differences in antigen expression patterns in PT, nPDOs and ePDOs were calculated using t-test. Effect size was calculated by Pearson's correlation coefficient r. Data was regarded as significant if $\alpha < 0.05$. Whenever percentages are given, they refer to the total cell count.

3. Results

3.1. Characterization of Patient Cohort

To establish the described ex vivo GBM models, tumor samples of 13 GBM IDH wildtype, CNS WHO grade 4 patients were utilized (Table 1). Patients were between 33 and 80 years old with a median age of 63.4 years and had a KPS between 70 and 100 with a median KPS of 86. A methylated MGMT promoter in tumor cells was found in 8 patients whereas 5 patients had an unmethylated MGMT promoter (cut off 10%).

Table 1. Clinical parameters of glioblastoma samples and the models they were utilized for ID = identification number; GBM = glioblastoma; ODG = oligodendroglioma; KPS = Karnofsky performance score; MGMT = O6-methylguanine-DNA methyltransferase; IDH = isocitrate dehydrogenase; ATRX = α thalassemia/mental retardation syndrome X-linked; OSC = organotypic slice cultures; nPDO = normal patient derived organoids; ePDO = enhanced patient-derived organoids; N/A = not analyzed.

ID	Sex	Age [Years]	Histology	KPS	Ki67 [%]	MGMT Promoter Methylation	MGMT Promoter Methylation [%]	IDH1 Mutation	IDH2 Mutation	ATRX Expression	Experiment
1	m	74	GBM	90	20	no	4	0	0	1	OSC
2	w	55	GBM	80	20	yes	22	0	0	1	nPDO
3	w	56	GBM	70	25	yes	25	0	0	1	nPDO
4	w	59	GBM	90	30	yes	44	0	0	1	nPDO
5	m	74	GBM	80	20	no	N/A	0	0	1	OSC, nPDO
6	m	68	GBM	80	30	yes	24	0	0	1	OSC, nPDO
7	w	73	GBM	90	25	yes	57	0	0	1	OSC, nPDO
8	m	64	GBM	80	40	no	4	0	0	1	OSC, nPDO
9	m	80	GBM	90	20	no	N/A	0	0	1	nPDO

Table 1. Cont.

ID	Sex	Age [Years]	Histology	KPS	Ki67 [%]	MGMT Promoter Methylation	MGMT Promoter Methylation [%]	IDH1 Mutation	IDH2 Mutation	ATRX Expression	Experiment
10	w	69	GBM	90	25	yes	71	0	0	1	nPDO
11	w	64	GBM	90	20	no	8	0	0	1	ePDO
12	w	70	GBM	80	50	yes	64	0	0	1	ePDO
13	m	33	GBM	100	20	yes	5	0	0	1	ePDO

3.2. TME Expression in PT

We investigated the antigen expression patterns of cellular TME components in PT and found low abundance of CD7+ cells (0.7%). T lymphocytes were also found in low levels, especially cytotoxic CD8+ T-cells (0.6%). CD4+ T helper cells could be detected in higher numbers (2.2%). Regulatory T-cells were not present (CD25+, FOXP3+). In general, the most abundant cell type in PT were myeloid cells. CD14+ monocytes represented 20.6% and among CD68+ macrophages (30.5%), M1-macrophages (iNOS+), whose presence was rather low (1.2%), M2-macrophages (CD163+), which displayed the largest TAM fraction (16.7%) and CCR2+ peripheral macrophages (3.8%) were found. TIM3 (16.1%) showed the highest expression of all inhibitory receptors, followed by LAG3 (2.5%) and PD1 (2.0%). Data are shown in Figure 1.

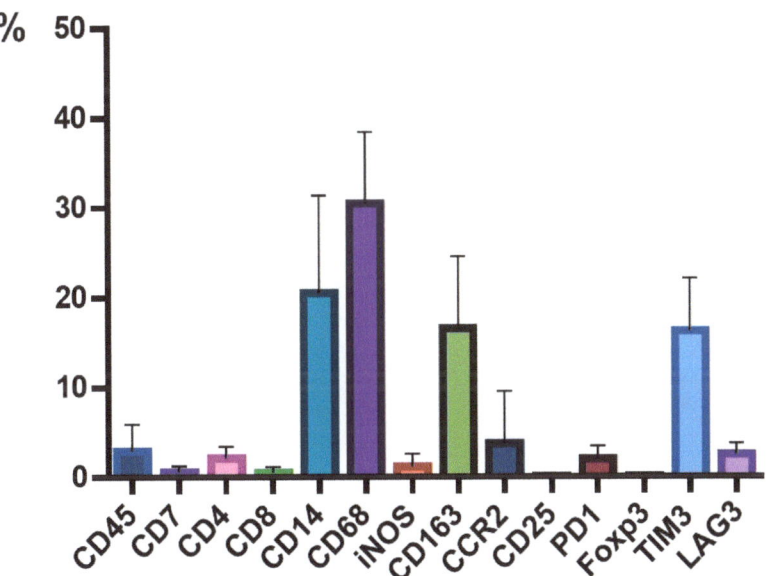

Figure 1. Relative expression of tumor microenvironment (TME) cells in primary tissue (PT). n = 10 patients. The relative expression of antigen patterns in GBM is given in [%]; PT is displayed in bar plots; whiskers indicate standard deviation.

3.3. TME Expression in PDOs

There were significant differences in the CD4+ count when comparing PT (2.2%) to PDOs at day 14 (0.6%) ($p = 0.04$). While CD8+ represented 0.6% in PT, none were detectable in PDOs at day 14. CD14+ monocytes decreased significantly from PT (20.6%) after 14 days of culture (7.5%) ($p = 0.03$). In contrast, CD68+ macrophages increased from 30.5% at PT to 34.7% in PDOs at day 7, but dropped significantly from day 7 to 22.8% at day 14 ($p = 0.001$).

iNOS+ M1 macrophages dropped from 1.2% in PT to 0.7% at day 14 in PDOs, as well as M2 macrophages from 16.7% in PT to 8.4% in PDOs at day 14. CCR2+ peripheral macrophages declined from PT (3.8%) to day 14 (0.7%). CD25+ regulatory T-cells were sparsely present in PT, but absent in PDOs at day 14. Concerning the checkpoint protein expression pattern PD1 and LAG3 expression declined significantly until day 14 in PDOs compared to PT (both $p = 0.03$). TIM3 and FOXP3 expression dropped, but not significantly. Data are shown in Figure 2. However, even though the absolute count of immune cells decreased in PDOs until day 14 compared to PT, the relative distribution of the TME components did not change. An example of a representative immunohistochemical staining is provided in Figure 3.

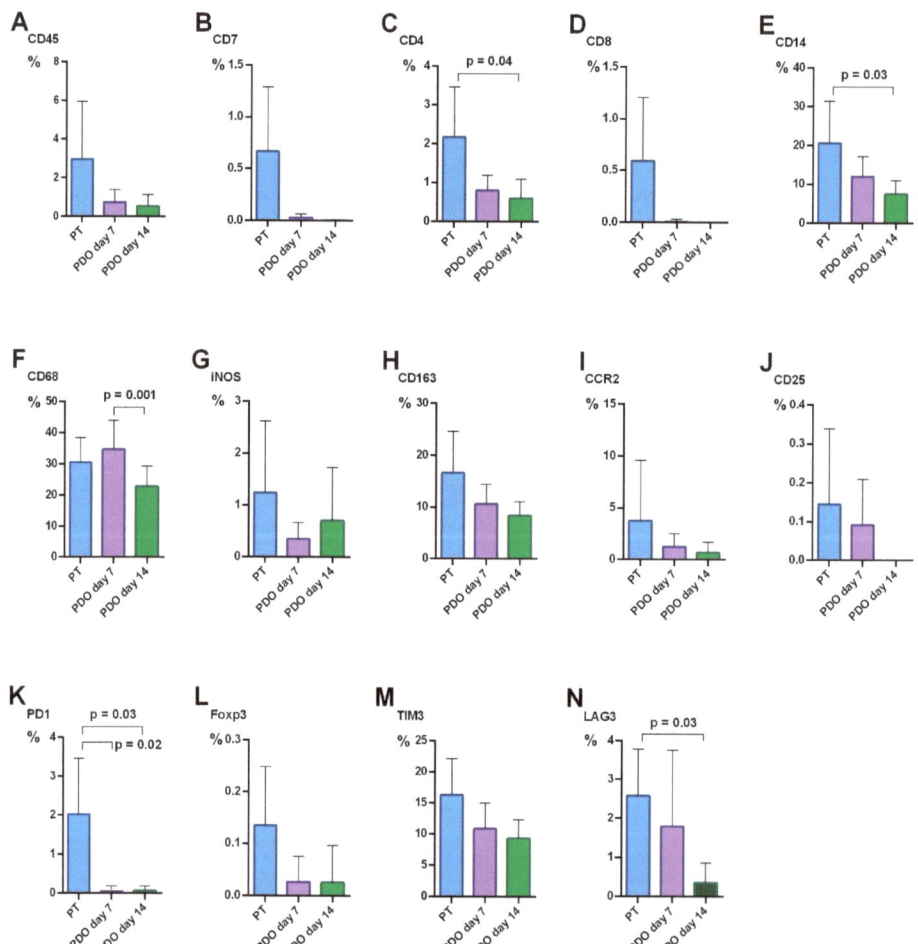

Figure 2. Alteration of TME cell presence over time in PT and in patient-derived organoids (PDOs) at day 7 and 14 of culture. n = 9 patients. The relative expression of cellular TME components [%] was quantified in PT (blue) and at day 7 (violet) and day 14 (green) of PDO culture: (**A**) CD45, (**B**) CD7, (**C**) CD4, (**D**) CD8, (**E**) CD14, (**F**) CD68, (**G**) iNOS, (**H**) CD163, (**I**) CCR2, (**J**) CD25, (**K**) PD1, (**L**) FOXP3, (**M**) TIM3, (**N**) LAG3; Whiskers indicate standard deviation; significant differences are indicated.

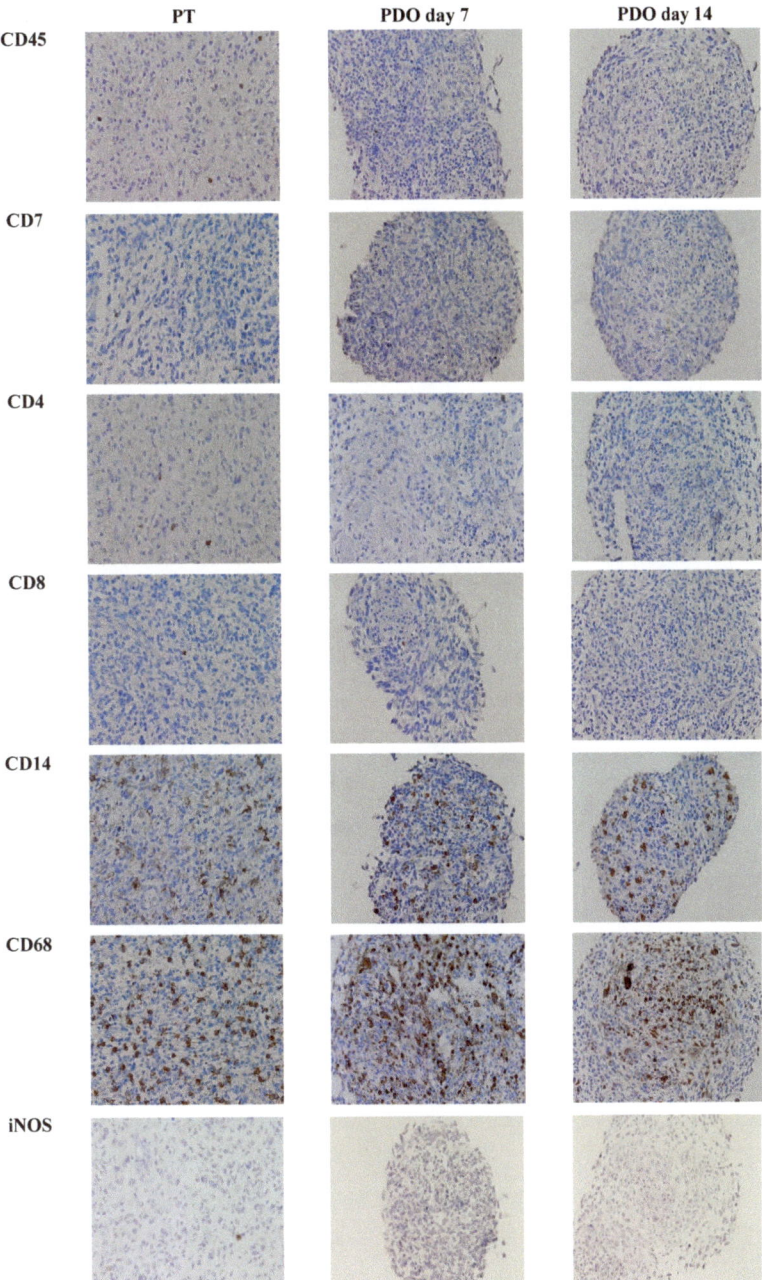

Figure 3. Cont.

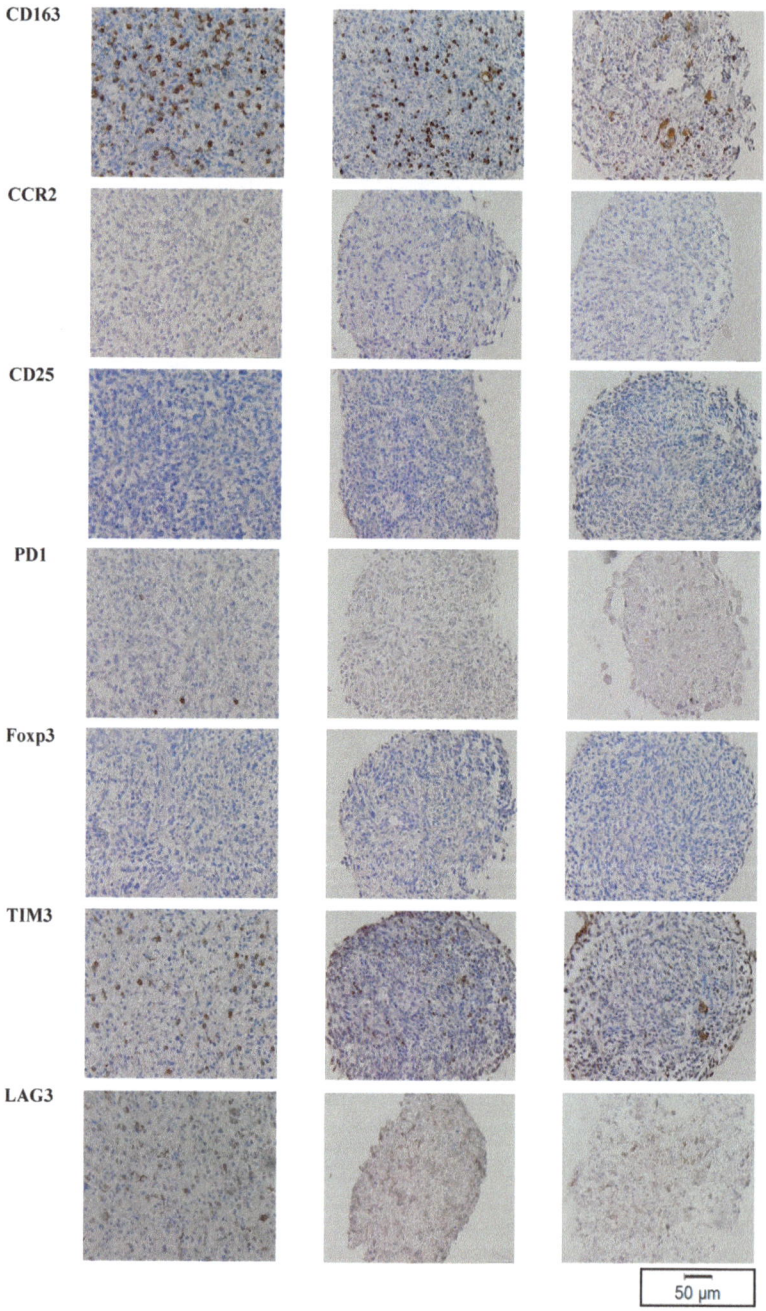

Figure 3. Example of representative immunohistochemical images for the TME composition in PT and in PDO day 7 and PDO day 14 (patient 6, Scale bar: 50 µm, magnification 40×).

3.4. TME Expression in OSC

As PDOs did not reflect the cellular antigen expression patterns to the same extent as PT after longer culture times, we strived for a different ex vivo model. We investigated the

TME expression in n = 5 OSCs. OSCs could be cultured up to day 9. Thus, we investigated antigen expression patterns from day 0 (equivalent to PT) to day 9. Surprisingly, OSCs were able to retain TME expression patterns to a higher extent. We did not find any significant alterations up to day 9. CD45+ cells declined (3.8% at day 0, 0.6% at day 9), as well as CD7+ cells and CD4+ cells. The monocytic marker CD14 decreased (16.8% at day 0, 7.7% at day 9), while macrophage markers CD68, CD163 and CCR2 were still expressed at comparable levels (CD68: 14.7% at day 0, 17.7% at day 9; CD163: 14.2% at day 0, 14.2% at day 9; CCR2: 1.5% at day 0, 0% at day 9, respectively). Interestingly, the M1-macrophage marker iNOS completely vanished (0.7% at day 0.0% at day 9). At the end of the culture, regulatory T cells were absent as both CD25 and FOXP3 were not expressed at day 8 or day 9. PD1, TIM3 and LAG3 expressions were initially at a very low level, but dropped further during culture. Data are shown in Figure 4. An example of a representative immunohistochemical staining is provided in Figure 5.

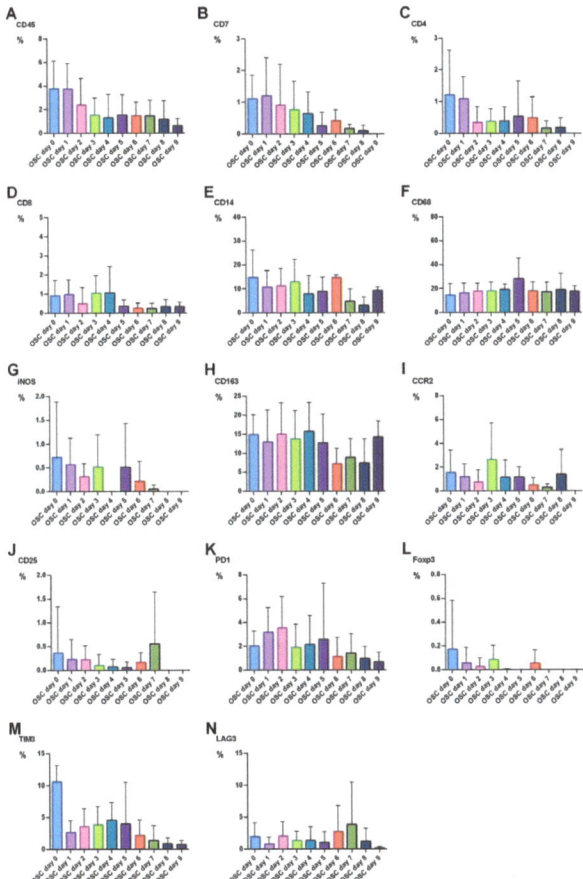

Figure 4. Alteration of TME cell marker abundance over time in organotypic slice culture (OSC) on day 1 to day 9 of culture. n = 5 patients. The relative expression of cellular TME components [%] was quantified from day 0 to day 9 of culture: (**A**) CD45, (**B**) CD7, (**C**) CD4, (**D**) CD8, (**E**) CD14, (**F**) CD68, (**G**) iNOS, (**H**) CD163, (**I**) CCR2, (**J**) CD25, (**K**) PD1, (**L**) FOXP3, (**M**) TIM3, (**N**) LAG3. No significant differences between day 0 and day 9 could be shown in antigen expression; Whiskers indicate standard deviation; significant differences are indicated.

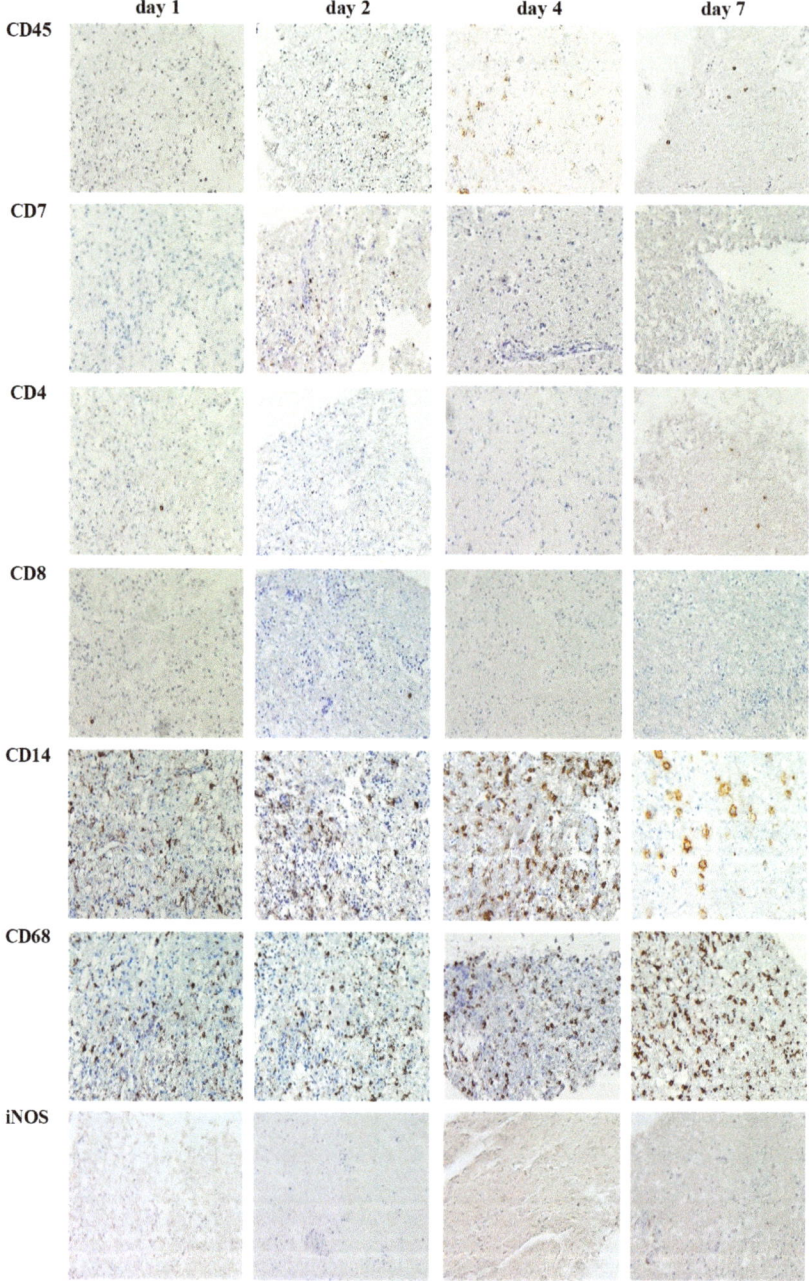

Figure 5. Cont.

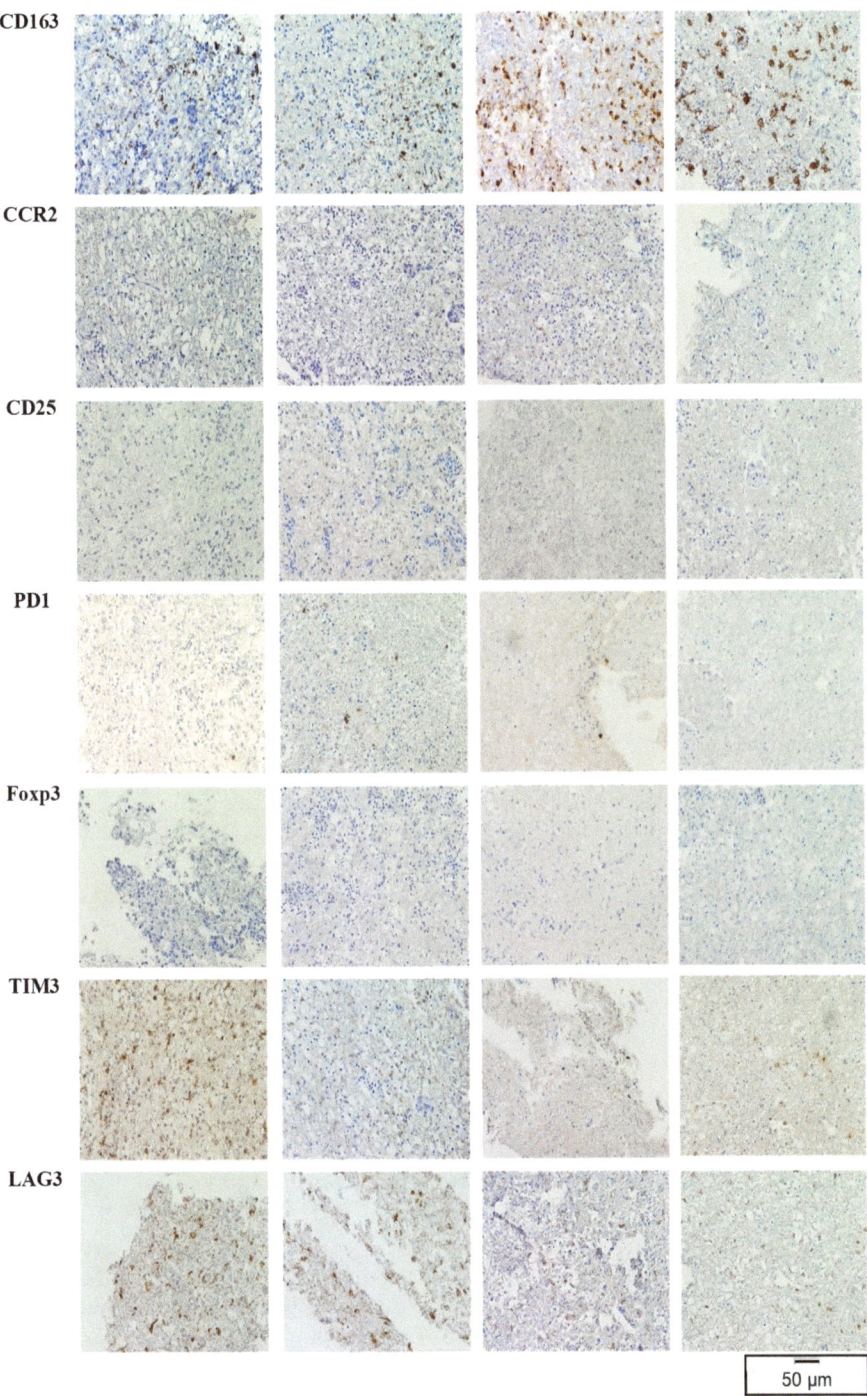

Figure 5. Example of representative immunohistochemical images for the TME composition in OSCs on day 1, day 2, day 4 and day 7 of culture (patient 5, Scale bar: 50 μm, magnification 40×).

3.5. TME Expression in ePDOs

Since OSCs could not be cultured for longer than nine days, we aimed to enhance the TME in PDOs by co-culturing them with PBMCs. Compared to PDOs, more tumor material was required to generate OSCs. In addition, PDOs stayed stable in culture over several months. However, the organoids did not reflect TME expression patterns as cellular components deteriorated rapidly during culture. Thus, we aimed at enhancing PDOs to better reflect cellular TME patterns and depict a model for immunotherapeutic testing.

In contrast to nPDOs, ePDOs were not affected by significant alterations in TME expression patterns until day 21 when comparing to PT (CD45+, CD4+, CD8+, CD7+ and CD68+ cells). Interestingly, iNOS+, CD14+ and CD163+ cells were practically not detectable in ePDOs after 21 days of culture, despite being present in the corresponding PT. Data are shown in Figure 6. An example of a representative immunohistochemical staining for is provided in Figure 7. Overall, ePDOs were able to reflect TME expression patterns significantly better than nPDOs.

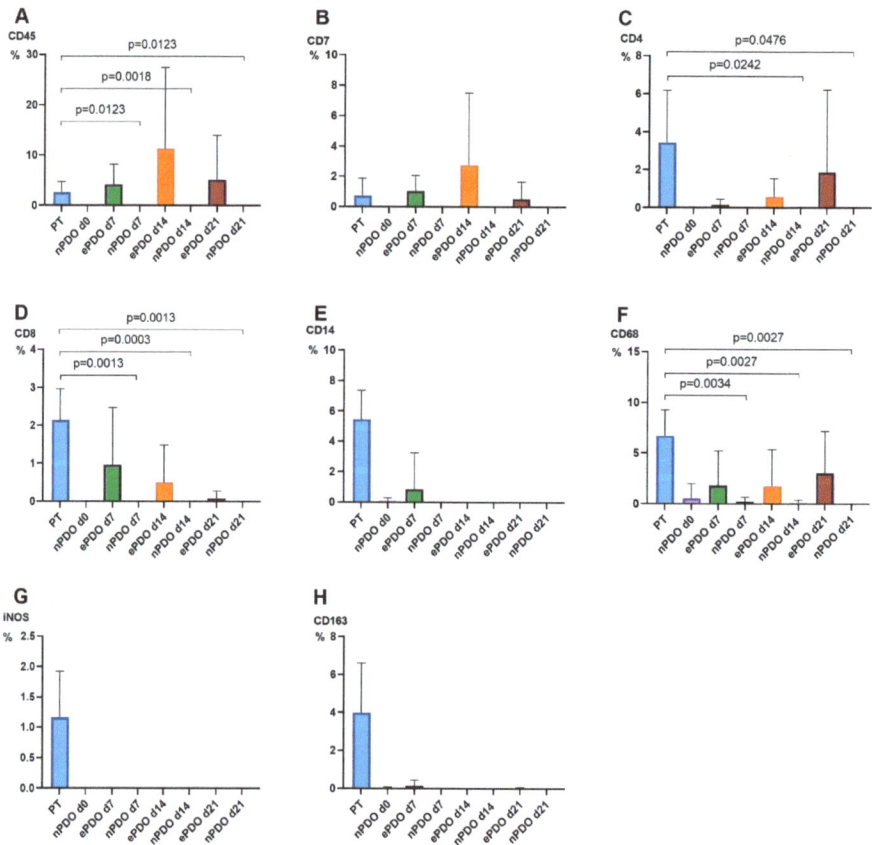

Figure 6. Expression of cellular TME markers in normal PDOs (nPDOs) and enhanced PDOs (ePDOs) at day 0, 7, 14 and 21 compared to PT. n = 3 patients. The relative expression of cellular TME components [%] was quantified in PT (blue) and at day 7 (green), day 14 (orange) and day 21 (red) of PDO culture in nPDOs and ePDOs: (**A**) CD45, (**B**) CD7, (**C**) CD4, (**D**) CD8, (**E**) CD14, (**F**) CD68, (**G**) iNOS, (**H**) CD163; Whiskers indicate standard deviation; significant differences are indicated.

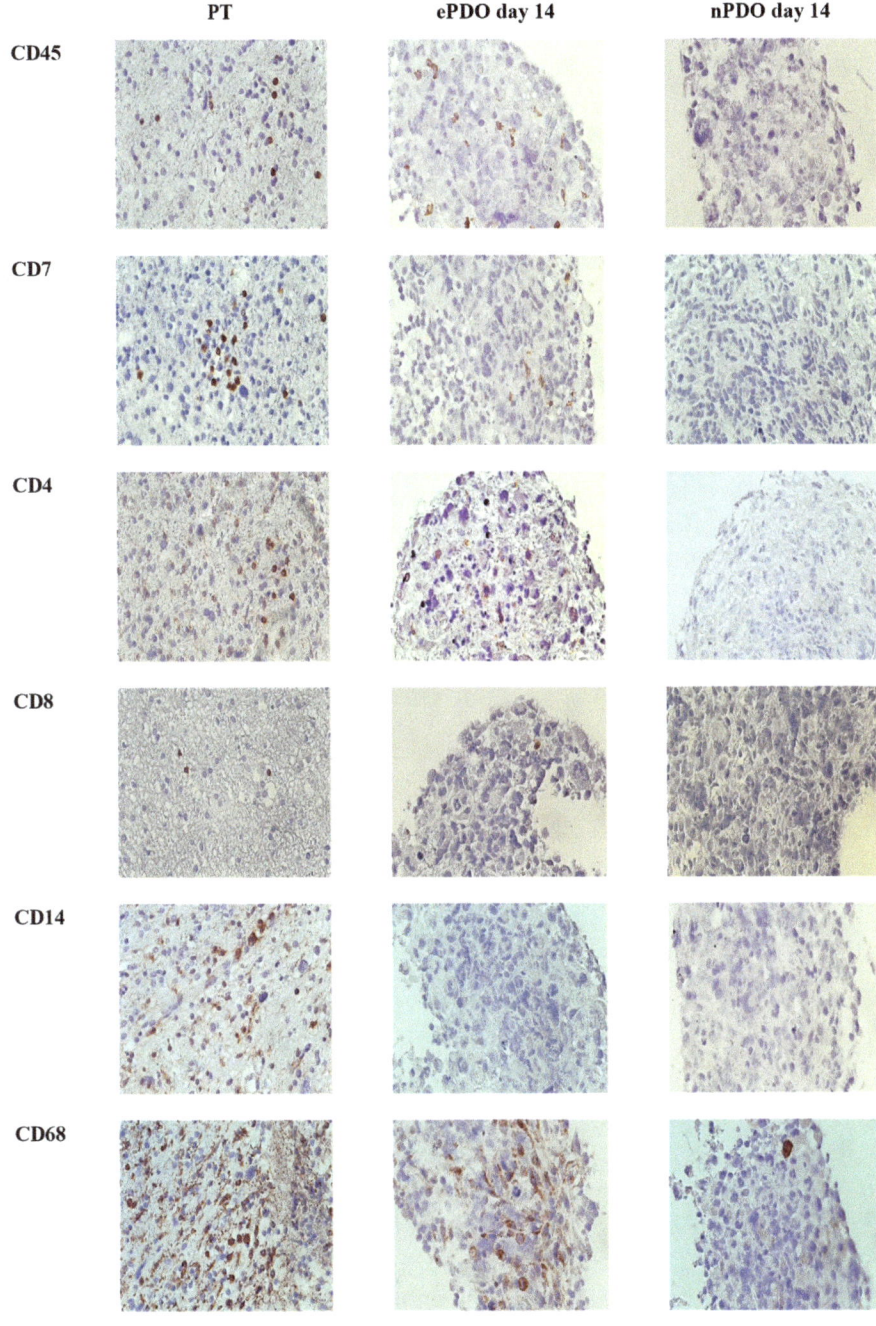

Figure 7. *Cont.*

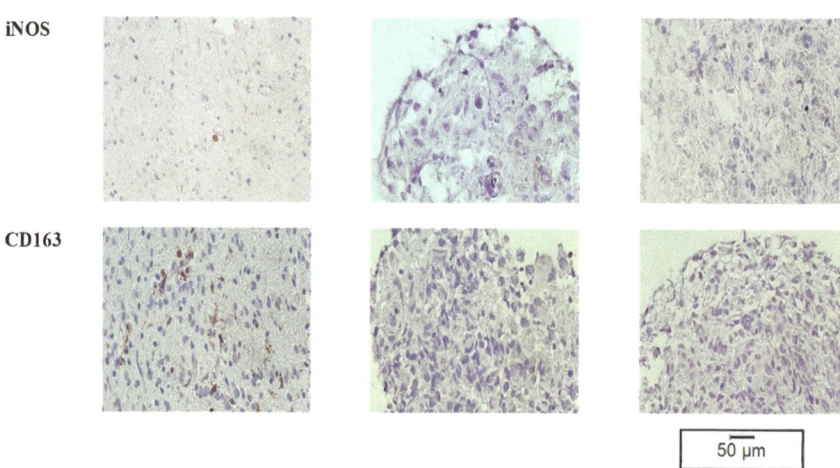

Figure 7. Example of representative immunohistochemical images for the TME in PT, in ePDO and nPDO (patient 13, Scale bar: 50 μm, magnification 40×).

4. Discussion

GBM is one of the most challenging solid tumors to treat, especially in relapse. Here we presented analysis of TME expression markers in two 3D ex vivo patient-derived models (PDOs and OSCs) as well as a time and cost-effective way to incorporate TME cells in PDOs

We showed that the TME was not sustained in PDOs and deteriorated after a short time of culture. In contrast, the TME was maintained in OSCs, albeit on low cellular count level. Unfortunately, OSCs could not be cultured longer than 9 days, rendering this model impractical for immunotherapeutic testing over a longer period of time. We found an efficient solution by co-culturing PDOs with PBMCs from healthy donors. Cellular TME patterns could be perseverd until day 21, which enables longer experimental setups.

Monocytes and macrophages were not as strongly represented in the ePDO model. As we did not stimulate macrophages *per se* using IL13 and IL4, but used PBMCs after ten days of culture with supplementation of IL2, lymphocytes were preselected over macrophages

According to recent studies [39–41], macrophages and microglia exhibit several important functions in glioblastoma organoids. Both are known to produce cytokines, such as tumor necrosis factor (TNF)-α, interleukin 1 (IL1), and interleukin 6 (IL6), which can impact GBM cell behavior and contribute to tumor growth, angiogenesis, and invasion. Moreover macrophages and microglia can modulate stress levels and cell viability in glioblastoma organoids by producing factors such as TGF-β and reactive oxygen species (ROS), as well as through phagocytosis of GBM cells. Furthermore, macrophages and microglia can interact with other cells of the TME and the tumor itself through various mechanisms, including cell-to-cell contact and secreted factors. These interactions can influence GBM behavior such as migration, invasion, and therapy response, by modulating signaling pathways and immune responses within the organoids. Importantly, GBM organoids have also been used to investigate the dynamic changes in macrophage and microglia populations upon treatment. For instance, studies have shown that radiotherapy, a common treatment for GBM can impact the composition and function of macrophages and microglia in GBM organoids which may have implications for the response of GBM to therapy and the development of therapy resistance. These studies highlight the significant role of macrophages and microglia in GBM organoids, specifically in terms of cytokine production, modulation of stress levels and cell viability, interactions with other cells, and dynamic changes upon treatment Further research in this area could provide valuable insights into the complex interplay between immune cells and GBM cells in organoid models, with potential implications for the development of novel therapeutic strategies for GBM.

The interaction of GBM and TME is mutual. We did not evaluate how tumor metabolism is influenced by incorporating PBMCs in the ePDOs nor did we analyze whether the phenotype of immune cells is changed after incubation with PDOs. Thus, we cannot make a statement about possible alterations due to co-culturing with GBM cells and the impact of the tumor on the differentiation of immune cells and vice versa. This would be an interesting aspect to study in order to characterize GBM-TME interactions closer and to investigate possible therapeutic approaches that could enhance the efficacy of immunotherapy in GBM.

As a next step, the ePDO model could be tested with various immunotherapeutic approaches in order to mimic the reality of the GBM-TME interactions even better. Manufacturing is technically feasible and cost-effective. In the future, ePDOs could be applied to draw a sophisticated conclusion whether therapies should be further explored and evaluated for a clinical setting.

5. Conclusions

We evaluated cellular TME antigen expression patterns using two different ex vivo tumor models and found that PDOs were not able to sustain the cellular TME, while OSCs were able to maintain TME cell types at a low expression level. However, we did not manage to culture OSCs longer than nine days, which renders this model sufficient but impractical for testing novel immunological approaches. Thus, we aimed for an optimized 3D ex vivo model that could serve for testing new therapeutic strategies in preclinical settings. By co-culturing PDOs with PBMCs, we showed that cellular TME expression patterns could be preserved for 21 days. This optimized PDO model can be efficiently generated, is easy to maintain and can serve as an excellent ex vivo approach to mirror the complex interactions of GBM and TME in the future.

Author Contributions: V.N., M.L. and C.M.M. participated in the design of the study. V.N., J.E. and N.G. performed the experiments. V.N., J.E. and N.G. performed the data analysis and interpretation with help of C.M.M. V.N., A.F.K., T.S., R.C.N., M.B., J.H., T.N. and M.L. provided the samples. V.N. and C.M.M. coordinated the work. V.N. and C.M.M. drafted the manuscript with the help of and critical revision by A.R., T.S., R.C.N., A.F.K., M.B., C.H., M.L. and R.-I.E. All authors have read and agreed to the published version of the manuscript.

Funding: This research was funded by the Interdisciplinary Center of Clinical Research (IZKF, B-450) Würzburg, Bavarian Center of Cancer Research (BZKF) and the publication supported by Open Access Publishing Fund of the University of Würzburg.

Institutional Review Board Statement: This study was approved by the Institutional Review Board of the University Hopsital of Würzburg (#22/20-me) on 15 October 2020.

Informed Consent Statement: Written informed consent has been obtained from the patients to publish this paper.

Data Availability Statement: Data are available upon request.

Acknowledgments: We would like to thank Michaela Hartmann, Dagmar Hemmerich, Petra Herud, Elisabeth Kaufmann and Siglinde Kühnel for technical support.

Conflicts of Interest: The authors declare no conflict of interest.

References

1. Robert Koch Institut. Zentrum Für Krebsregisterdaten. Available online: https://www.krebsdaten.de/Krebs/DE/Home/homepage_node.html (accessed on 23 April 2023).
2. Stupp, R.; Mason, W.P.; van den Bent, M.J.; Weller, M.; Fisher, B.; Taphoorn, M.J.B.; Belanger, K.; Brandes, A.A.; Marosi, C.; Bogdahn, U.; et al. Radiotherapy plus concomitant and adjuvant temozolomide for glioblastoma. *N. Engl. J. Med.* 2005, *352*, 987–996. [CrossRef] [PubMed]
3. Herrlinger, U.; Tzaridis, T.; Mack, F.; Steinbach, J.P.; Schlegel, U.; Sabel, M.; Hau, P.; Kortmann, R.-D.; Krex, D.; Grauer, O.; et al. Lomustine-temozolomide combination therapy versus standard temozolomide therapy in patients with newly diagnosed glioblastoma with methylated MGMT promoter (CeTeG/NOA-09): A randomised, open-label, phase 3 trial. *Lancet* 2019, *393*, 678–688. [CrossRef] [PubMed]
4. Rehman, A.A.; Elmore, K.B.; Mattei, T.A. The effects of alternating electric fields in glioblastoma: Current evidence on therapeutic mechanisms and clinical outcomes. *Neurosurg. Focus* 2015, *38*, E14. [CrossRef] [PubMed]
5. Diaz, R.J.; Ali, S.; Qadir, M.G.; De La Fuente, M.I.; Ivan, M.E.; Komotar, R.J. The role of bevacizumab in the treatment of glioblastoma. *J. Neurooncol.* 2017, *133*, 455–467. [CrossRef] [PubMed]
6. Patil, C.G.; Yi, A.; Elramsisy, A.; Hu, J.; Mukherjee, D.; Irvin, D.K.; Yu, J.S.; Bannykh, S.I.; Black, K.L.; Nuño, M.; et al. Prognosis of patients with multifocal glioblastoma: A case-control study. *J. Neurosurg.* 2012, *117*, 705–711. [CrossRef] [PubMed]
7. Esteller, M.; Garcia-Foncillas, J.; Andion, E.; Goodman, S.N.; Hidalgo, O.F.; Vanaclocha, V.; Baylin, S.B.; Herman, J.G. Inactivation of the DNA-repair gene MGMT and the clinical response of gliomas to alkylating agents. *N. Engl. J. Med.* 2000, *343*, 1350–1354. [CrossRef]
8. Rivera, A.L.; Pelloski, C.E. Diagnostic and prognostic molecular markers in common adult gliomas. *Expert. Rev. Mol. Diagn.* 2010, *10*, 637–649. [CrossRef]
9. Einsele, H.; Borghaei, H.; Orlowski, R.; Subklewe, M.; Roboz, G.J.; Zugmaier, G.; Kufer, P.; Iskander, K.; Kantarjian, H.M. The BiTE (bispecific T-cell engager) platform: Development and future potential of a targeted immuno-oncology therapy across tumor types. *Cancer* 2020, *126*, 3192–3201. [CrossRef]
10. Choi, B.D.; Suryadevara, C.M.; Gedeon, P.C.; Herndon, J.E., 2nd; Sanchez-Perez, L.; Bigner, D.D.; Sampson, J.H. Intracerebral delivery of a third generation EGFRvIII-specific chimeric antigen receptor is efficacious against human glioma. *J. Clin. Neurosci.* 2014, *21*, 189–190. [CrossRef]
11. Ahmed, N.; Brawley, V.; Hegde, M.; Bielamowicz, K.; Kalra, M.; Landi, D.; Robertson, C.; Gray, T.L.; Diouf, O.; Wakefield, A.; et al. HER2-Specific Chimeric Antigen Receptor-Modified Virus-Specific T Cells for Progressive Glioblastoma: A Phase 1 Dose-Escalation Trial. *JAMA Oncol.* 2017, *3*, 1094–1101. [CrossRef]
12. O'Rourke, D.M.; Nasrallah, M.P.; Desai, A.; Melenhorst, J.J.; Mansfield, K.; Morrissette, J.J.D.; Martinez-Lage, M.; Brem, S.; Maloney, E.; Shen, A.; et al. A single dose of peripherally infused EGFRvIII-directed CAR T cells mediates antigen loss and induces adaptive resistance in patients with recurrent glioblastoma. *Sci. Transl. Med.* 2017, *9*, eaaa0984. [CrossRef]
13. Brown, C.E.; Badie, B.; Barish, M.E.; Weng, L.; Ostberg, J.R.; Chang, W.C.; Naranjo, A.; Starr, R.; Wagner, J.; Wright, C.; et al. Bioactivity and Safety of IL13Ralpha2-Redirected Chimeric Antigen Receptor CD8+ T Cells in Patients with Recurrent Glioblastoma. *Clin. Cancer Res.* 2015, *21*, 4062–4072. [CrossRef] [PubMed]
14. Monie, D.D.; Bhandarkar, A.R.; Parney, I.F.; Correia, C.; Sarkaria, J.N.; Vile, R.G.; Li, H. Synthetic and systems biology principles in the design of programmable oncolytic virus immunotherapies for glioblastoma. *Neurosurg. Focus* 2021, *50*, E10. [CrossRef] [PubMed]
15. Estevez-Ordonez, D.; Chagoya, G.; Salehani, A.; Atchley, T.J.; Laskay, N.M.; Parr, M.S.; Elsayed, G.A.; Mahavadi, A.K.; Rahm, S.P.; Friedman, G.K.; et al. Immunovirotherapy for the Treatment of Glioblastoma and Other Malignant Gliomas. *Neurosurg. Clin. N. Am.* 2021, *32*, 265–281. [CrossRef] [PubMed]
16. Henze, J.; Tacke, F.; Hardt, O.; Alves, F.; Al Rawashdeh, W. Enhancing the Efficacy of CAR T Cells in the Tumor Microenvironment of Pancreatic Cancer. *Cancers* 2020, *12*, 1389. [CrossRef]
17. Tang, H.; Qiao, J.; Fu, Y.X. Immunotherapy and tumor microenvironment. *Cancer Lett.* 2016, *370*, 85–90. [CrossRef]
18. Tian, Y.; Li, Y.; Shao, Y.; Zhang, Y. Gene modification strategies for next-generation CAR T cells against solid cancers. *J. Hematol. Oncol.* 2020, *13*, 54. [CrossRef]
19. Poorebrahim, M.; Melief, J.; de Coaña, Y.P.; Wickström, S.L.; Cid-Arregui, A.; Kiessling, R. Counteracting CAR T cell dysfunction. *Oncogene* 2021, *40*, 421–435. [CrossRef]
20. Charles, N.A.; Holland, E.C.; Gilbertson, R.; Glass, R.; Kettenmann, H. The brain tumor microenvironment. *Glia* 2012, *60*, 502–514. [CrossRef]
21. Raguraman, R.; Parameswaran, S.; Kanwar, J.R.; Khetan, V.; Rishi, P.; Kanwar, R.K.; Krishnakumar, S. Evidence of Tumour Microenvironment and Stromal Cellular Components in Retinoblastoma. *Ocul. Oncol. Pathol.* 2019, *5*, 85–93. [CrossRef]
22. Vitale, I.; Manic, G.; Coussens, L.M.; Kroemer, G.; Galluzzi, L. Macrophages and Metabolism in the Tumor Microenvironment. *Cell Metab.* 2019, *30*, 36–50. [CrossRef] [PubMed]
23. Buonfiglioli, A.; Hambardzumyan, D. Macrophages and microglia: The cerberus of glioblastoma. *Acta Neuropathol. Commun.* 2021, *9*, 54. [CrossRef] [PubMed]
24. Roesch, S.; Rapp, C.; Dettling, S.; Herold-Mende, C. When Immune Cells Turn Bad-Tumor-Associated Microglia/Macrophages in Glioma. *Int. J. Mol. Sci.* 2018, *19*, 436. [CrossRef] [PubMed]

15. Bungert, A.D.; Urbantat, R.M.; Jelgersma, C.; Bekele, B.M.; Mueller, S.; Mueller, A.; Felsenstein, M.; Dusatko, S.; Blank, A.; Ghori, A.; et al. Myeloid cell subpopulations compensate each other for Ccr2-deficiency in glioblastoma. *Neuropathol. Appl. Neurobiol.* **2023**, *49*, e12863. [CrossRef]
16. Ransohoff, R.M. Chemokines and chemokine receptors: Standing at the crossroads of immunobiology and neurobiology. *Immunity* **2009**, *31*, 711–721. [CrossRef] [PubMed]
17. Sielska, M.; Przanowski, P.; Wylot, B.; Gabrusiewicz, K.; Maleszewska, M.; Kijewska, M.; Zawadzka, M.; Kucharska, J.; Vinnakota, K.; Kettenmann, H.; et al. Distinct roles of CSF family cytokines in macrophage infiltration and activation in glioma progression and injury response. *J. Pathol.* **2013**, *230*, 310–321. [CrossRef]
18. Vanichapol, T.; Chutipongtanate, S.; Anurathapan, U.; Hongeng, S. Immune Escape Mechanisms and Future Prospects for Immunotherapy in Neuroblastoma. *Biomed. Res. Int.* **2018**, *2018*, 1812535. [CrossRef]
19. Tahmasebi, S.; Elahi, R.; Esmaeilzadeh, A. Solid Tumors Challenges and New Insights of CAR T Cell Engineering. *Stem. Cell Rev. Rep.* **2019**, *15*, 619–636. [CrossRef]
20. Navin, I.; Lam, M.T.; Parihar, R. Design and Implementation of NK Cell-Based Immunotherapy to Overcome the Solid Tumor Microenvironment. *Cancers* **2020**, *12*, 3871. [CrossRef]
21. Parihar, R.; Rivas, C.; Huynh, M.; Omer, B.; Lapteva, N.; Metelitsa, L.S.; Gottschalk, S.M.; Rooney, C.M. NK Cells Expressing a Chimeric Activating Receptor Eliminate MDSCs and Rescue Impaired CAR-T Cell Activity against Solid Tumors. *Cancer Immunol. Res.* **2019**, *7*, 363–375. [CrossRef]
22. Martinez, M.; Moon, E.K. CAR T Cells for Solid Tumors: New Strategies for Finding, Infiltrating, and Surviving in the Tumor Microenvironment. *Front. Immunol.* **2019**, *10*, 128. [CrossRef] [PubMed]
23. Nickl, V.; Schulz, E.; Salvador, E.; Trautmann, L.; Diener, L.; Kessler, A.F.; Monoranu, C.M.; Dehghani, F.; Ernestus, R.-I.; Löhr, M.; et al. Glioblastoma-Derived Three-Dimensional Ex Vivo Models to Evaluate Effects and Efficacy of Tumor Treating Fields (TTFields). *Cancers* **2022**, *14*, 5177. [CrossRef] [PubMed]
24. Merz, F.; Gaunitz, F.; Dehghani, F.; Renner, C.; Meixensberger, J.; Gutenberg, A.; Giese, A.; Schopow, K.; Hellwig, C.; Schäfer, M.; et al. Organotypic slice cultures of human glioblastoma reveal different susceptibilities to treatments. *Neuro. Oncol.* **2013**, *15*, 670–681. [CrossRef] [PubMed]
25. Jacob, F.; Salinas, R.D.; Zhang, D.Y.; Nguyen, P.T.T.; Schnoll, J.G.; Wong, S.Z.H.; Thokala, R.; Sheikh, S.; Saxena, D.; Prokop, S.; et al. A Patient-Derived Glioblastoma Organoid Model and Biobank Recapitulates Inter- and Intra-tumoral Heterogeneity. *Cell* **2020**, *180*, 188–204.e22. [CrossRef]
26. Jacob, F.; Ming, G.-L.; Song, H. Generation and biobanking of patient-derived glioblastoma organoids and their application in CAR T cell testing. *Nat. Protoc.* **2020**, *15*, 4000–4033. [CrossRef]
27. Louis, D.N.; Perry, A.; Wesseling, P.; Brat, D.J.; Cree, I.A.; Figarella-Branger, D.; Hawkins, C.; Ng, H.K.; Pfister, S.M.; Reifenberger, G.; et al. The 2021 WHO Classification of Tumors of the Central Nervous System: A summary. *Neuro-Oncology* **2021**, *23*, 1231–1251. [CrossRef]
28. Feldheim, J.; Kessler, A.F.; Schmitt, D.; Wilczek, L.; Linsenmann, T.; Dahlmann, M.; Monoranu, C.M.; Ernestus, R.-I.; Hagemann, C.; Löhr, M. Expression of activating transcription factor 5 (ATF5) is increased in astrocytomas of different WHO grades and correlates with survival of glioblastoma patients. *OncoTargets Ther.* **2018**, *11*, 8673–8684. [CrossRef]
29. Sabate-Soler, S.; Nickels, S.L.; Saraiva, C.; Berger, E.; Dubonyte, U.; Barmpa, K.; Lan, Y.J.; Kouno, T.; Jarazo, J.; Robertson, G.; et al. Microglia integration into human midbrain organoids leads to increased neuronal maturation and functionality. *Glia* **2022**, *70*, 1267–1288. [CrossRef]
30. Klein, E.; Hau, A.-C.; Oudin, A.; Golebiewska, A.; Niclou, S.P. Glioblastoma Organoids: Pre-Clinical Applications and Challenges in the Context of Immunotherapy. *Front. Oncol.* **2020**, *10*, 604121. [CrossRef]
31. Xuan, W.; Lesniak, M.S.; James, C.D.; Heimberger, A.B.; Chen, P. Context-Dependent Glioblastoma-Macrophage/Microglia Symbiosis and Associated Mechanisms. *Trends Immunol.* **2021**, *42*, 280–292. [CrossRef]

Disclaimer/Publisher's Note: The statements, opinions and data contained in all publications are solely those of the individual author(s) and contributor(s) and not of MDPI and/or the editor(s). MDPI and/or the editor(s) disclaim responsibility for any injury to people or property resulting from any ideas, methods, instructions or products referred to in the content.

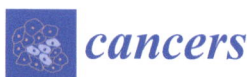

Article

Classification of Brainstem Gliomas Based on Tumor Microenvironment Status

Xiong Xiao [1], Xiaoou Li [1], Yi Wang [1], Changcun Pan [1], Peng Zhang [1], Guocan Gu [1], Tian Li [1], Zhuang Jiang [1], Yang Zhang [1,*] and Liwei Zhang [1,2,3,*]

[1] Department of Neurosurgery, Beijing Tiantan Hospital, Capital Medical University, Beijing 100070, China; neurocomputing@163.com (X.X.); leexiaou@163.com (X.L.); wydeqingsu@163.com (Y.W.); pcctt2010@163.com (C.P.); zhang_roc@163.com (P.Z.); gugc2018@163.com (G.G.); lt_ttyy@163.com (T.L.); jzq116@126.com (Z.J.)
[2] China National Clinical Research Center for Neurological Diseases, Beijing 100070, China
[3] Beijing Neurosurgical Institute, Beijing Tiantan Hospital, Capital Medical University, Beijing 100070, China
* Correspondence: zhangyang@bjtth.org (Y.Z.); zhangliweittyy@163.com (L.Z.); Tel.: +86-10-59976516 (Y.Z.); +86-10-59976514 (L.Z.)

Simple Summary: The tumor microenvironment (TME) is vital in tumor biology, impacting tumor recurrence, prognosis, and treatment response. Brainstem gliomas (BSGs) are challenging gliomas that originate in the brainstem and have distinct clinical and genomic profiles from other brain gliomas. However, the inter-tumor heterogeneity of the TME in BSGs and its correlation with clinical and biological characteristics remain unknown, hindering the development of novel BSG therapies. In this study, we utilized transcriptional data from a BSG cohort and employed established signatures to assess the TME status and classify BSGs accordingly. Subsequently, we found an association between the TME classification and patient prognosis as well as the tumor phenotype. Furthermore, we explored key genes or radiomics features that can determine classification and potentially facilitate clinical applications. This research aims to enhance our understanding of TME heterogeneity in BSGs and to provide insights for improving diagnosis and treatment.

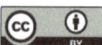

Citation: Xiao, X.; Li, X.; Wang, Y.; Pan, C.; Zhang, P.; Gu, G.; Li, T.; Jiang, Z.; Zhang, Y.; Zhang, L. Classification of Brainstem Gliomas Based on Tumor Microenvironment Status. *Cancers* **2023**, *15*, 4224. https://doi.org/10.3390/cancers15174224

Academic Editors: Annunziato Mangiola and Gianluca Trevisi

Received: 17 July 2023
Revised: 15 August 2023
Accepted: 21 August 2023
Published: 23 August 2023

Copyright: © 2023 by the authors. Licensee MDPI, Basel, Switzerland. This article is an open access article distributed under the terms and conditions of the Creative Commons Attribution (CC BY) license (https://creativecommons.org/licenses/by/4.0/).

Abstract: The inter-tumor heterogeneity of the tumor microenvironment (TME) and how it correlates with clinical profiles and biological characteristics in brainstem gliomas (BSGs) remain unknown, dampening the development of novel therapeutics against BSGs. The TME status was determined with a list of pan-cancer conserved gene expression signatures using a single-sample gene set enrichment analysis (ssGSEA) and was subsequently clustered via consensus clustering. BSGs exhibited a high inter-tumor TME heterogeneity and were classified into four clusters: "immune enriched, fibrotic", "immune-enriched, non-fibrotic", "fibrotic", and "depleted". The "fibrotic" cluster had a higher proportion of diffuse intrinsic pontine gliomas ($p = 0.041$), and "PA-like" tumors were more likely to be "immune-enriched, fibrotic" ($p = 0.044$). The four TME clusters exhibited distinct overall survival ($p < 0.001$) and independently impacted BSG outcomes. A four-gene panel as well as a radiomics approach were constructed to identify the TME clusters and achieved high accuracy for determining the classification. Together, BSGs exhibited high inter-tumor heterogeneity in the TME and were classified into four clusters with distinct clinical outcomes and tumor biological properties. The TME classification was accurately identified using a four-gene panel that can potentially be examined with the immunohistochemical method and a non-invasive radiomics method, facilitating its clinical application.

Keywords: brainstem glioma; tumor microenvironment; classification; survival

1. Introduction

Brainstem gliomas (BSGs) are a group of gliomas originating in the brainstem [1] that exhibit distinct clinical characteristics and molecular features from gliomas located in the cerebrum [1,2]. In particular, nearly half of the BSGs are diffuse intrinsic pontine gliomas (DIPGs) that represent the deadliest brain cancers in children with very low median survival of less than 12 months [3,4]. Due to the vital functions of the brainstem, surgical resection is quite challenging [5]. Meanwhile, radiotherapy usually provides limited benefits to patients' survival [6,7]. Additionally, Temozolomide-based chemotherapy has not proven effective in DIPGs, due to their common lack of hyper-methylation in gene O-6-Methylguanine-DNA methyltransferase [8]. The recent success of immunotherapy in hematopoietic malignancies and a variety of solid tumors have stimulated the development of novel immunotherapeutic approaches in treating BSGs, and some have generated encouraging results [9–12]. Immunotherapy in theory provides a promising treatment option for BSGs due to its ability to precisely target tumor cells while causing minimal disruption to normal neural structures [13]. However, there is no immunotherapeutic approach that has proven clinically effective against BSGs. Therefore, novel therapeutics are urgently needed for this type of brain tumor.

A comprehensive understanding of the tumor microenvironment (TME) in BSGs will facilitate the development of novel therapeutic approaches against BSGs, since TME plays a pivotal role in tumorigenesis and tumor progression [14] and engages key molecular pathways determining the response to therapeutics such as radiation and immunotherapies [15–17]. Several studies have revealed DIPG as an immune-cold tumor, exhibiting reduced infiltration of immune cells and a lower expression of immunosuppressive molecules relative to glioblastoma (GBM) [13]. These findings are consistent with previous reports that DIPG is innately resistant to an immune checkpoint blockade [12] and also suggest their unique TME features from gliomas in the other part of the brain. Meanwhile, recent advances in the TME investigation have promoted the development of a series of TME classification models for a variety of malignancies [15,18–20]. Based on inter-tumoral variations in TME components, these models provided clinicians with a useful tool for predicting therapeutic repones and patients' survival, as well as facilitating the development of novel therapeutics [15,18–20]. In gliomas, a three-subtype TME model suggests that its IS3 subtype would have a better response to mRNA-based anti-tumor vaccination [19]. However, as a unique group of gliomas, the TME classification for BSGs has not been reported.

BSGs are also a heterogeneous group of neoplastic disorders, as evidenced by reports detailing variations in patient demographics, clinical features, imaging characteristics, and molecular biology [1,2,21–23]. It is widely known that BSGs are divided into DIPGs and non-DIPGs, or H3K27M-mutant and H3K27-wildtype, according to their imaging and genomics findings [2]. Choux et al. defined a four-subtype classification based on tumors' locations and growth patterns, which proved useful in surgical case selections [21]. A five-subtype multimodality imaging-based radiological classification can help in selecting optimal treatment strategies for pediatric DIPGs [24]. We previously grouped BSGs into four subtypes according to their methylation status, and each type represented distinct clinical profiles and genomic landscapes [2]. We uncovered gene sets that were enriched in the methylation cluster H3-Medulla, involving immune-related pathways such as interferon-gamma/alpha signaling, the IL-10 pathway, and the CTLA-4 pathway [2]. However, the direct correlation of TME with clinical profiles and biological characteristics of BSGs was not examined in the study [2] or reported previously. Moreover, whether BSGs also exhibit inter-tumor heterogeneity in TME and how significant that heterogeneity is remain elusive.

Recently, Bagaev et al. utilized a list of gene expression signatures (GESs) that encompass four key features of TME to classify cancer: anti-tumor immune response, pro-tumor immune response, angiogenesis/fibrosis, and malignant cell properties [15]. The authors identified a pattern of TME subtypes, which persist across various types of cancers and are associated with immunotherapy response. However, the investigation did not include gliomas. Herein, we exploited these GESs to classify BSGs and revealed rather high inter-tumor heterogeneity in the TME among BSGs. As such, BSGs are grouped into four TME clusters with distinct clinical outcomes and differential tumor biological features. Furthermore, the TME classification system has independent prognostic value and can be identified using a four-gene panel, potentially with the routine immunohistochemical (IHC) method or by a non-invasive radiomics approach.

2. Materials and Methods

2.1. Patient Inclusion and RNA Sequencing

A total of 98 BSG cases were included in this study (Figure S1). Among them, 75 patients had RNA sequencing (RNA-seq) profiles that were published in our previous study [2], and RNA-seq profiles of 23 cases were firstly included in this study. The follow-up information of all these patients was updated as of December 2022. The demographic variables and mutation information, as well as other clinical variables, were extracted from the previously published literature [2]. The study was approved by the Institute Review Board (IRB) of Beijing Tiantan Hospital. Informed consent was waived by the IRB because of the retrospective nature and previously obtained consent in the previous study.

RNA-seq was performed on the Illumina HiSeq X Ten platform by Genetron Health (Beijing, China) [2]. Alignment was carried out using either STAR or hisat2, while gene expression profiling was performed using Cufflinks. The presence of batch effects between the expression profiles of the two RNA sequencing batches was evaluated using the Umap method (R package umap v0.2.7.0). If significant batch effects were observed, Combat_seq was employed to mitigate them (Figure S2) [25]. Following this step, the raw count data were transformed into transcripts per million (TPM) values for further analysis.

2.2. TME Status Estimation and Clustering

A list of GESs that encompass four key features of TME: anti-tumor immune response, pro-tumor immune response, angiogenesis/fibrosis, and malignant cell properties [15] were utilized to estimate the TME status of BSGs with the method of single-sample gene set enrichment analysis (ssGSEA). The results of ssGSEA were subjected to consensus clustering using the R package ConsensusClusterPlus (v1.51.1). The clustering was conducted by employing partitioning around the medoid and determining the distances between samples based on the Euclidean distance method. The optimal number of clusters was identified by analyzing the consensus cumulative distribution function (CDF) plot and its delta area plot (Figure S3). A heatmap was generated using the R package Pheatmap (v1.0.12) to depict the distribution of the ssGSEA results of the GESs among the clusters.

2.3. Estimation of Tumor Biological Features and Radiosensitivity

R package PROGENy (version 1.20.0) was used to evaluate the activity of 14 pathways commonly implicated in tumors based on RNA-seq profiles [26]. Radiosensitivity was estimated using the radiosensitivity index and radiotherapy risk signature [27,28], both inversely correlated with survival time after radiotherapy.

2.4. Identification of Key Genes Determining TME Clusters

Given that the TME classification is formed by two orthogonal properties: immune (immune-enriched vs. immune-depleted) and fibrosis (fibrotic vs. non-fibrotic) [15], we first examined the differential gene expression between the two immune-enriched clusters ("immune-enriched, fibrotic" and "immune-enriched, non-fibrotic") and the two immune depleted clusters ("fibrotic" and "depleted") through the R package limma (v3.15), and genes with FDR < 0.05 and |Log2FoldChange| > 3 were chosen for further analyses. Subsequently, we performed the binary least absolute shrinkage and selection operator (LASSO) regression analysis on these genes, and those with non-zero coefficients were selected as key genes. An "immune-enriched" score was subsequently generated based on the expression levels and coefficients of key genes, using the formula score = $\sum (\beta_i \times Exp_i)$ where β_i represents the corresponding regression coefficient of a gene, and Exp_i represents the TPM value of the gene. With the same approach, the key genes and according "fibrotic" score were established, respectively.

The established "immune-enriched" and "fibrotic" scores were further validated in BSG cases in five external datasets, namely the Pacific Pediatric Neuro-Oncology Consortium (PNOC) dataset, the Children's Brain Tumor Tissue Consortium (CBTTC) dataset, the Pediatric Cancer Genome Project (PCGP), the Real-time Clinical Genomics (RTCG) dataset, and our other unpublished RNA-seq dataset comprising 19 BSGs (Figure S1). All the included cases were first stratified as the high- and low-expression groups based on the scores from ssGSEA on GESs related to the immune-enriched or fibrosis properties. Receiver operating characteristic (ROC) curves were plotted, and the area under the curve (AUC) was calculated to demonstrate the accuracies of the "immune-enriched" and "fibrotic" scores in discriminating between the according high- and low-expression groups.

2.5. Multiplex Immunofluorescence Staining

In order to validate whether the key genes have differential expressions between the corresponding clusters, a total of 31 cases with available formalin-fixed paraffin-embedded samples were subjected to multiplex immunofluorescence staining. An OPALTM 7-color manual immunofluorescence staining kit (NEL811001KT, Akoya Bioscience, Marlborough, MA, USA) was used to perform multiplex immunofluorescence staining detection on paraffin-embedded tissues. After deparaffinization and hydration, an optimized program for each antigen was applied to the slides (Tables S1 and S2). Slides were scanned on the Vectra system (Vectra Polaris 1.0.7, Akoya Bioscience, Marlborough, MA, USA) and analyzed using the Inform software (2.4.6, Akoya Bioscience, Marlborough, MA, USA). The positive rate of each marker was defined as the number of positive cells' nuclei divided by the total number of nuclei in the section or the positive area divided by the total tissue area if the antigen was distributed in intercellular space. The counting of positive cells and the calculation of the staining area were performed by two neuropathologists, and the results were subsequently cross-validated.

2.6. Generation of Radiomics Models for Identifying TME Clusters

A total of 88 cases with available magnetic resonance imaging (MRI) data were included in the analysis. The T1-weighted, T2-weighted, and T1-weighted contrast sequences were previously published, and they were retrieved for this study [29]. The delineation of the tumor contour on each sequence was carried out by an experienced neurosurgeon using Slicer (version 5.2.1) and subsequently confirmed by another neurosurgeon. The extraction of radiomics features from the original images and images subjected to wavelet filtering and Laplacian of Gaussian filter was performed using Pyradiomics (version 3.0.1) [30]. Thus, a total of 3390 radiomics features were extracted.

Two predictive models were developed for the two TME properties: immune-enriched and fibrotic. The included cases were randomly divided into a training set and a test set using a 6:4 ratio. Within the training set, the radiomics features were compared between cases with high and low expression in the according TME property using Wilcoxon rank sum tests. Only features with a p-value < 0.05 were retained. Secondly, retained features were further selected using a random forest algorithm, resulting in no more than 10 features. Thirdly, the support vector machines (SVM) algorithm with the eps-regression type and a radial kernel based on these selected features were used to develop prediction models for the TME properties. The R package e1071 (version 1.7) was used for the analysis. ROCs were plotted, and AUCs were calculated to assess the model accuracy for the discrimination.

2.7. Statistical Analysis

Statistical analyses were performed using R (version 4.1.2). For continuous variables following a normal distribution, means and standard deviations were used for description, and t tests or ANOVAs were used for intergroup comparison. For continuous variables following a non-normal distribution, quartiles were used for description, and the Mann-Whitney U test or Kruskal-Wallis test was used for intergroup comparisons. Frequencies and percentages were calculated for categorical variables, and chi-square tests were used for intergroup comparisons. For pairwise comparisons between subgroups, *p* values were corrected via the Benjamini–Hochberg method. Overall survival was estimated and compared using the Kaplan-Meier method, and risk factors for prognosis were determined with univariate and multivariate Cox regression (R package survminer v0.4.9).

3. Results

3.1. BSGs Are Grouped into Four Clusters Based on TME Status

BSGs are a group of heterogeneous malignancies located in the brainstem, with distinct genetic mutations from gliomas in the other part of the brain [1,2]. Herein, we aimed to understand their heterogeneity in TME through the classification of BSGs utilizing a list of pan-cancer-conserved GESs that encompass four key features of TME: anti-tumor immune response, pro-tumor immune response, angiogenesis/fibrosis, and malignant cell properties [15]. A total of 98 BSG cases were included for the classification (Figure S1), resulting in four TME clusters: "immune-enriched, fibrotic (IEF)", "immune-enriched, non-fibrotic (IENF)", "fibrotic (F)", and "depleted (D)" (Figures 1a and S3).

The "fibrotic" cluster was characterized by the highest expression of genes related to angiogenesis/fibrosis, whereas it exhibited relatively low activity in the immune response (Figure 1b). The "immune-enriched, fibrotic" cluster showed increased activity in the angiogenesis/fibrosis and immune response, while the "depleted" cluster displayed the lowest levels of these TME properties (Figure 1b). Additionally, the "immune-enriched, non fibrotic" cluster displayed relatively increased activity in the immune response, whereas it exhibited a lower level of angiogenesis/fibrosis than the "immune-enriched, fibrotic" and "fibrotic" clusters (Figure 1b). In terms of malignant cell characteristics, the "fibrotic" BSGs exhibited the highest tumor proliferation rate, while the "fibrotic" and "immune enriched, fibrotic" clusters showed enhanced epithelial–mesenchymal transition (EMT) activity compared to the other clusters (Figure 1b). These results are consistent with the previous findings on the other malignancies [15], suggesting the TME classification is also conserved in BSGs.

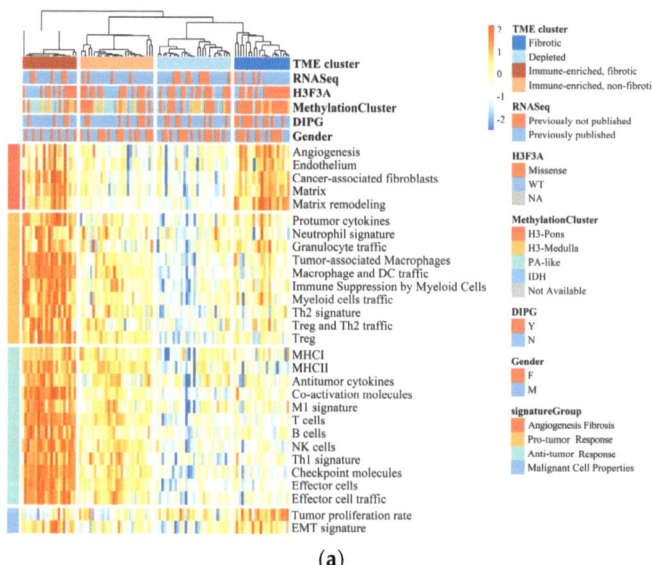

(a)

Figure 1. *Cont.*

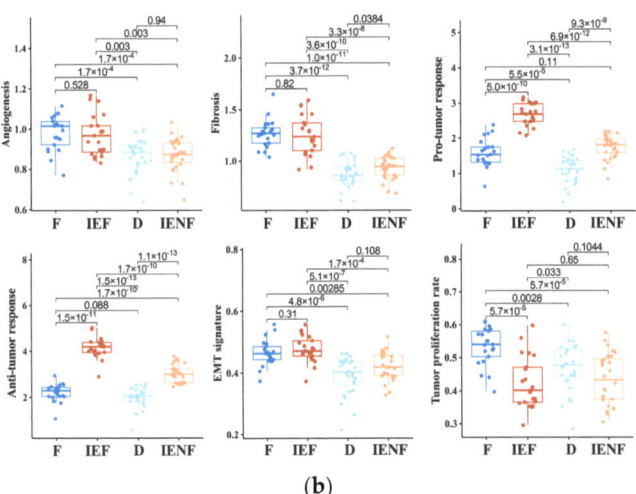

(b)

Figure 1. BSGs are grouped into four clusters based on their TME status. (**a**) A heatmap for results of consensus clustering based on the TME-related GESs among 98 BSG cases; (**b**) comparison of activities between clusters in key components of the pan-cancer TME GESs; the activities were measured as scores of the according GESs. F: fibrotic; IEF: immune-enriched, fibrotic; D: depleted; IENF: immune-enriched, non-fibrotic.

3.2. The TME Clusters Are Correlative with BSG Clinical and Molecular Features

We next correlated the clinical characteristics and molecular features of BSGs with the TME clusters (Figure 2). We observed that diffuse intrinsic pontine gliomas (DIPGs) accounted for nearly half of the fibrotic cluster; the proportion was significantly higher than that observed in the other clusters (Figure 2b, $p = 0.041$). Since a younger age, tumors located in the pons, the methylation cluster of H3-Pons, and WHO grade 4 tumors are highly correlated with the DIPG type [2,3], and they were also enriched in this cluster (Figure 2a,c,e,f). On the other hand, the fibrotic cluster constituted 35.5% of all DIPG tumors and represented the most common TME type in DIPG (Figure S4A). We also observed that the PA-like tumors were enriched in the "immune-enriched, fibrotic" cluster (Figure 2, $p = 0.044$), leading to a higher proportion of benign tumors (WHO grade 1) in this cluster (Figure 2, $p = 0.003$), since the PA-like tumors mainly comprise piloctyic astrocytoma and ganglioglioma [2]. Additionally, 42.9% of PA-like tumors exhibited the "immune-enriched, fibrotic" property (Figure S4B). Together, we observed the enrichment of DIPGs in the "fibrotic" type and the PA-like tumors in the "immune-enriched, fibrotic" cluster, thereby revealing the TME property for these two BSG types.

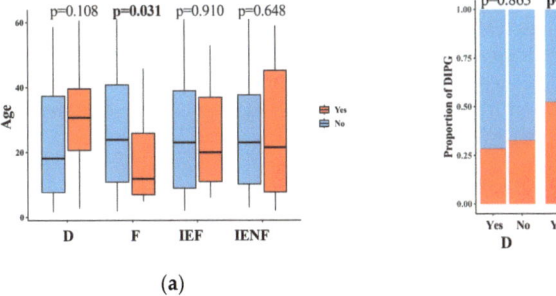

(a) (b)

Figure 2. *Cont.*

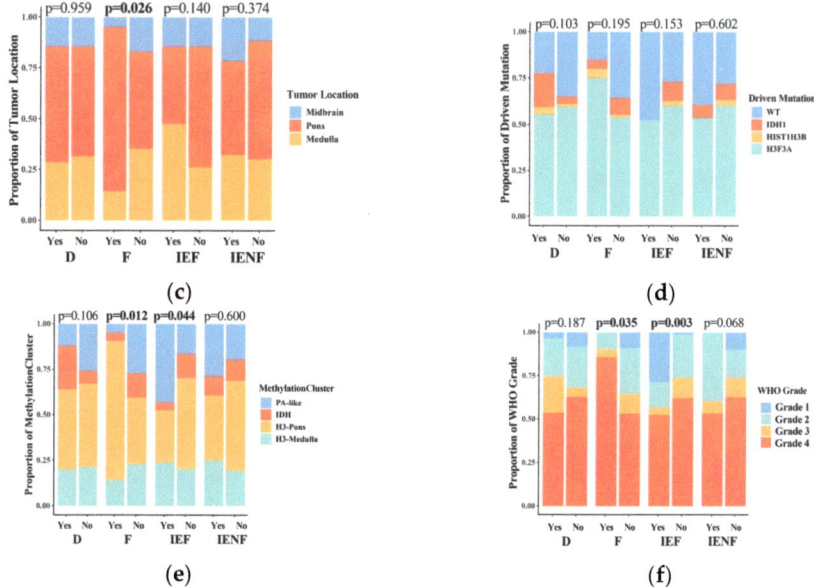

Figure 2. The TME clusters are correlated with the clinical and molecular features of BSGs. Comparisons between clusters in patients' ages (**a**); in proportions of DIPG (**b**), tumor locations (**c**), driver mutations (**d**), methylation clusters (**e**), and WHO grades (**f**). F: fibrotic; IEF: immune-enriched fibrotic; D: depleted; IENF: immune-enriched, non-fibrotic; bold font: $p < 0.05$.

3.3. The TME Clusters Predict Outcomes in BSG Patients

We next investigated the prognostic value of the TME classification system. With a medial follow-up time of 18.8 months, the four TME clusters exhibited distinct overall survival ($p < 0.001$, Figure 3a). Specifically, the "fibrotic" cluster displayed the poorest outcome with a median survival of 8.3 months, whereas the "depleted" cluster showed a better prognosis relative to the "fibrotic" cluster, with a median survival of 21.4 months. Both of the two immune-enriched clusters exhibited more favorable outcomes; the median survival is 34.0 and 50.8 months, respectively, in the "immune-enriched, fibrotic" and "immune-enriched, non-fibrotic" clusters.

The TME clusters, driver mutations, WHO grades, tumor locations, and DIPG diagnoses had an impact on patients' survival, as indicated by univariate Cox regression (Table S3). These variables were included in the multivariate Cox regression analysis, except for driver mutations, which have already been incorporated with WHO grades [31]. Demographic variables and "whether received radiotherapy/chemotherapy or not" were also included as they were potential factors for patients' survival [6,32]. As shown in Figure 3b, the TME classification emerged as an independent factor associated with overall survival along with the WHO grade, DIPG, received radiotherapy, and common prognosticators for BSGs [1,6,31,32]. Furthermore, a nomogram was constructed by integrating these variables and it showed relatively satisfactory accuracy in predicting the outcomes of malignant BSGs (Figure 3c).

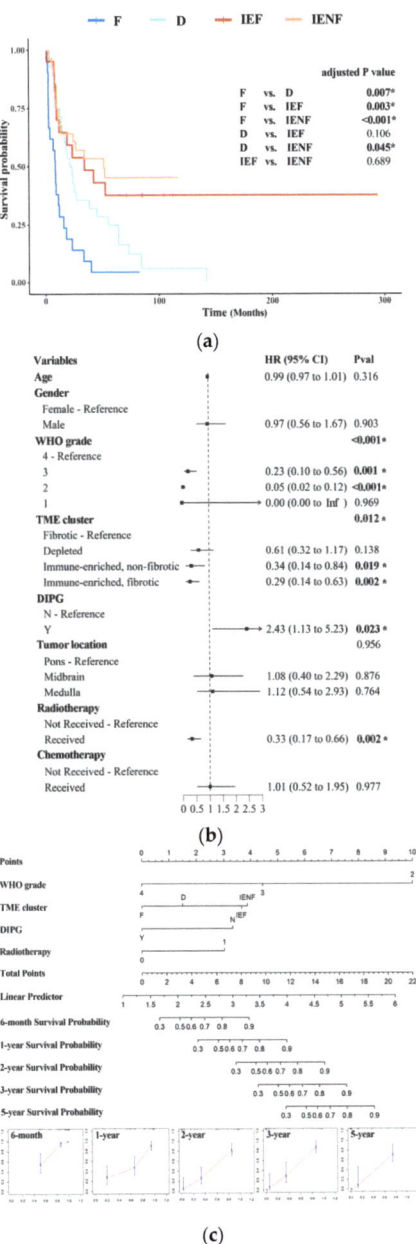

Figure 3. The TME clusters predict outcomes in BSG patients. (**a**) The Kaplan–Meier analysis showing the survival differences among the TME clusters; (**b**) the multivariate Cox regression showing variables including DIPG diagnosis, the TME clusters, received radiotherapy, and WHO grades as independent risk factors for prognosis; (**c**) a nomogram based on WHO grades, DIPG diagnosis, received radiotherapy, and the TME clusters. F: fibrotic; IEF: immune-enriched, fibrotic; D: depleted; IENF: immune-enriched, non-fibrotic; * $p < 0.05$.

3.4. The TME Clusters Exhibit Distinct Molecular Pathway Activity and Radiation Sensitivity

We next explored molecular mechanisms underlying the distinct outcomes exhibited by the four clusters. As suggested previously (Figure 1), the "fibrotic" cluster exhibited the highest level of angiogenesis, tumor cell proliferation, and EMT activity, which correlate with its worst-outcome phenotype. Meanwhile, this cluster also exhibited relatively high activity in the molecular pathways related to PI3K, hypoxia, TGF-β, and WNT (Figure 4a). Abnormal activations of these pathways are typical hallmarks of glioma [33–36], contributing to glioma progression and malignant phenotypes, such as proliferation, stem cell property, invasion, and angiogenesis [33,35–37]. In particular, the pathways of TGF-β and WNT are highly correlated with the process of fibrosis [33,35], and both pathways activities are elevated in the two fibrotic clusters, "fibrotic" and "immune-enriched, fibrotic", suggesting that these pathways would be intrinsic mechanisms for the fibrotic phenotype in glioma, thus requiring further exploration.

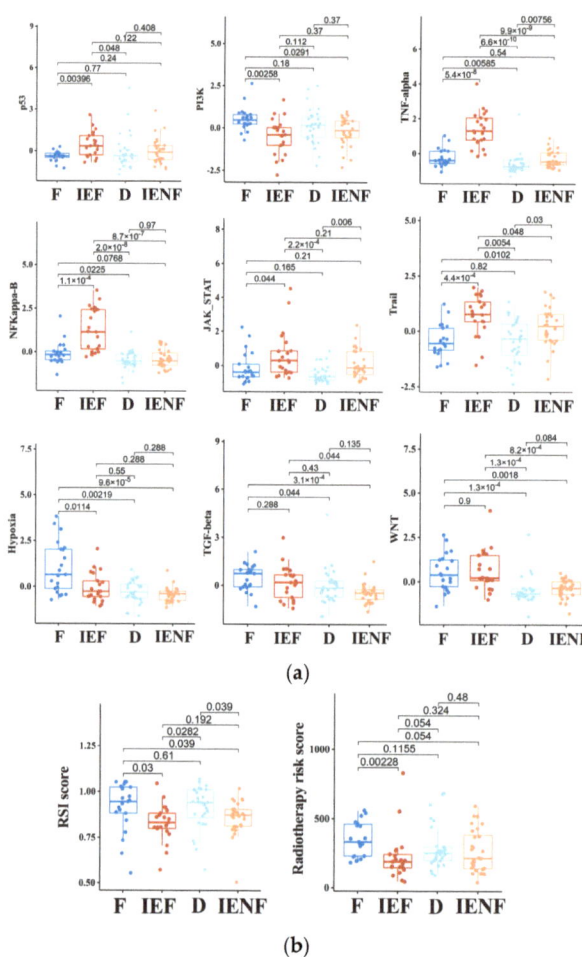

Figure 4. The TME clusters exhibit distinct molecular pathway activity and radiation sensitivity. (**a**) Comparisons of activities between clusters in the PROGENy pathways that are commonly implicated in tumors; (**b**) comparisons of radiosensitivity between clusters and the lower scores correlating with better outcomes following radiotherapy. F: fibrotic; IEF: immune-enriched, fibrotic; D: depleted; IENF: immune-enriched, non-fibrotic.

In contrast, we observed that the two immune-enriched clusters, "immune-enriched, fibrotic (IEF)" and "immune-enriched, non-fibrotic (IENF)", showed relatively high activities in the pathways related to the anti-tumor immune response (TNF-α), tumor inflammation (NF-κB and JAK-STATs), and apoptosis (Trail), as compared with the other clusters, thus providing molecular clues for their better outcomes (Figure 4a).

Since radiotherapy is a standard treatment for most BSGs [1], we next asked whether these clusters exhibited a difference in sensitivity to radiation, thus leading to their distinct outcomes. Therefore, we utilized two independent radiation-resistant signatures, both of which have shown high accuracy in predicting radiotherapeutic outcomes in glioma [27,28]. As a result, we observed that the "fibrotic" cluster showed a relatively high resistance score as compared with the two immune-enriched clusters (Figure 4b), reflecting that the "fibrotic" cluster is more resistant to radiotherapy. With respect to mechanisms underlying radiation resistance, the TP53 pathway is the core mechanism involved in radiation response, and its activity was consistently decreased in the cluster (Figure 4a). Furthermore, other pathways such as hypoxia, WNT, TGF-β, and PI3K are reportedly linked to glioma radio-resistance by modulating the TP53 pathway [33,38–40], and their activities were also elevated in the cluster (Figure 4a), indicating an intertwined effect of these pathways on the BSG radiotherapy response.

3.5. A Four-Gene Panel Determines the TME Classification

For the better clinical application of the TME classification system, we tried to identify a few key genes that can distinguish among the clusters and be examined using routine clinical assays as well. Since the classification is formed by two orthogonal axes, the immune (immune-enriched vs. immune-depleted) and fibrosis (fibrotic vs. non-fibrotic) [15], we first identified the differential gene expression related to the immune and fibrosis axes, respectively (Figure S6).

We next utilized the method of LASSO regression on filtered genes for dimensionality reduction and determining the key genes associated with each axis (Figure S6). As a result, we revealed that CD3E was a key gene overexpressed in the "immune-enriched" clusters, whereas COL3A1, CA9, and MMP1 were relatively highly expressed in the "fibrotic" clusters. Based on the coefficients computed from the LASSO regression, two signatures were constructed: fibrotic score = COL3A1 × 0.0010181389 + MMP1 × 0.0257429451 + CA9 × 0.0005309276; immune-enriched score = CD3E × 0.01988081.

The expression of the four-gene panel can classify the BSG into four TME clusters (Figure 5a,b). The panel exhibited rather high accuracy for classification with the value of AUC (area under the receiver operating characteristic curve) as 0.9813 and 0.9009 for the immune and fibrotic axes, respectively. This performance was also validated in another five external BSG datasets (Figures 5c and S5), further indicating the high accuracy of the panel for TME classification.

Finally, we exploited the IHC method to assay the expression of the four key genes in tumor tissues for validating and examining the possibility of using routine clinical assays for the determination of TME classification. As a result, the expression of the four genes was significantly elevated in the according clusters (Figure 5d,e), suggesting the reliability of these key genes and their potential as IHC markers for TME classification.

3.6. Radiomics Features Related to TME Clusters

After the selection via the methods of the Mann–Whitney U test and random forest selection, a list of 10 radiomic features emerged as the most important indicators for identifying the immune-enriched or fibrotic clusters (Figure 6a,b). Interestingly, most of the fibrosis-related features correlated with increased texture complexity, and the majority of immune-related features reflected high variation in the gray level, implying underlying links between the TME clusters and MRI features. SVM models integrating these features were successfully built for identifying the "immune-enriched" and "fibrotic" clusters, respectively. The two models demonstrated a rather high accuracy in identification according to clusters in the training, test, and external datasets (Figure 6c). Therefore, the TME clusters can be identified with non-invasive MRI analysis, which would facilitate the wide clinical application of TME classification.

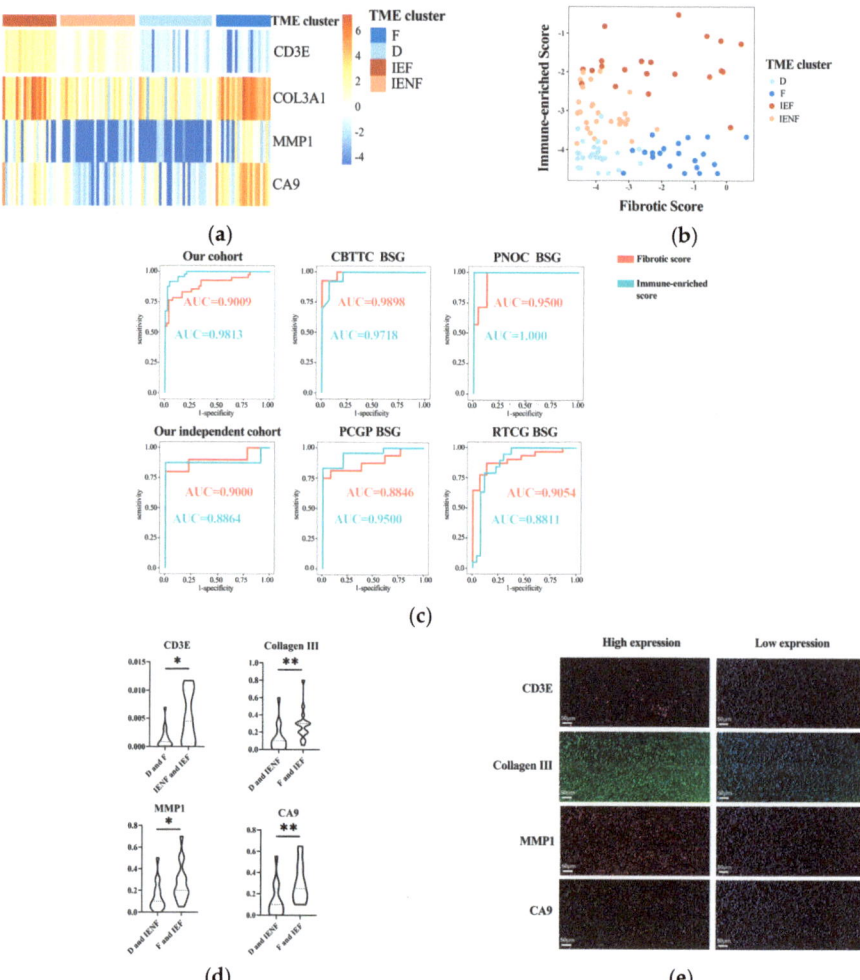

Figure 5. A four-gene panel determines the TME classification. (**a**) A heatmap showing distinct expression of the four genes among the TME clusters; (**b**) the immune-enriched or fibrotic scores based on the four-genes' expressions showing good discrimination ability for the TME clusters; (**c**) ROC curves showing high accuracy of the immune-enriched or fibrotic scores for identifying the according clusters in six independent cohorts; (**d**) differences of four genes' expressions between the TME clusters observed using multidimensional fluorescence staining; (**e**) representative multidimensional fluorescence staining images of four genes' expressions: CD3E in red, Collagen III in green, MMP1 in tangerine, and CA9 in gold. * $p < 0.05$; ** $p < 0.01$; F: fibrotic; IEF: immune-enriched, fibrotic; D: depleted; IENF: immune-enriched, non-fibrotic.

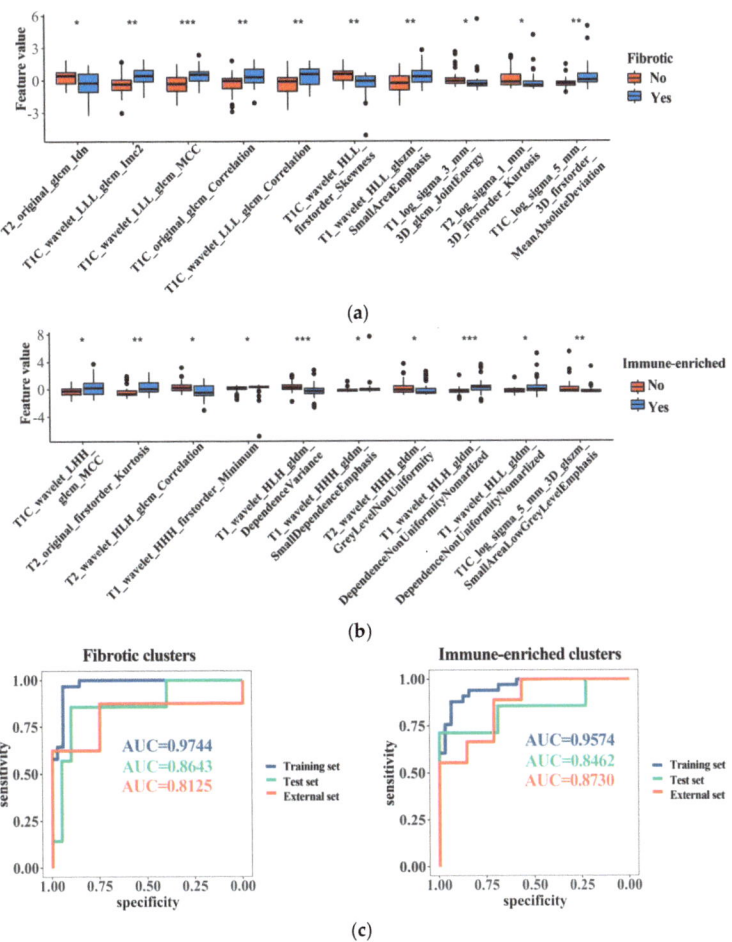

Figure 6. Radiomics features related to the TME clusters. (**a**) The top 10 most important radiomics features selected with random forest algorithm for identifying the "fibrotic" clusters; (**b**) the top 10 most important radiomics features selected with random forest algorithm for identifying the "immune-enriched" clusters; (**c**) discrimination ability of generated radiomics models for identifying the "fibrotic" or "immune-enriched" clusters. * $p < 0.05$; ** $p < 0.01$; *** $p < 0.001$.

4. Discussion

Mounting evidence has supported the fundamental role of TME in tumor genesis and progression [15,16], thus significantly impacting the tumor recurrence, prognosis, and therapeutic response [17]. Additionally, TME classification models have been reported for a variety of tumor types, which have been reported as valuable for predicting prognosis and selecting treatment [15,19,20]. Therefore, a comprehensive understanding of TME is essential for the precise diagnosis and thus better management of BSGs. BSGs are reported to be a group of tumors with significant heterogeneity [1,2,21], and we have found differences in tumor immune microenvironments between cases in previous studies [2]. However, there is still a lack of systematic research on the heterogeneity of BSGs in terms of TME, and TME classification for BSGs has not been systematically reported before this study.

Herein, we utilized a list of pan-cancer-conserved and TME-related GESs [15] to classify BSGs according to the TME status. Additionally, consistent with the findings on the other malignancies [15], BSGs are also grouped into four clusters, reflecting that the TME classification is conserved in BSGs. Interestingly, we observed the high inter-tumor heterogeneity of TME in BSGs, even in DIPGs, which are often unanimously recognized as immune-cold tumors [13]. These results suggest that the TME classification would be an important indicator for BSG subtyping. Also, we observed that the TME classification was associated with the tumor phenotype, had an independent influence on prognosis, and was correlated with the activities in malignancy-related pathways and radiation sensitivity. Further, a four-gene panel and a radiomics approach were developed to identify the TME clusters. This may be the first study to report a TME classification specifically for BSGs, which may be useful in deepening the understanding of BSGs and improving their precise diagnosis and treatments.

DIPGs comprise a group of BSGs that diffusely infiltrate pons and commonly harbor a K27M mutation in gene H3F3A [3,4]. It represents one of the deadliest pediatric brain malignancies, with a short medial survival of less than 12 months after diagnosis [3]. It is also universally concerned as an immune-cold tumor [4,13] that is innately resistant to immunotherapy such as an immune checkpoint blockade [2–4,41]. In this study, we also observed a higher proportion of the "fibrotic" cluster in DIPGs than the other BSGs (Figure 2b), and on the other hand, the immune-depleted clusters (the "fibrotic" cluster and the "depleted" cluster) constituted the majority of DIPGs (Figure S4A). However, we uncovered nearly 40% of DIPGs grouped into the immune-enriched clusters, suggesting a TME heterogeneity in DIPGs that would be transferred into their distinct clinical outcomes (Figure 3), differential response to radiation sensitivity (Figure 4), and immunotherapies as well. Therefore, the TME classification would impact outcomes in DIPG patients receiving experimental therapeutics and should thus be considered in the design for the according clinical trials. Additionally, the intrinsic mechanisms driving heterogeneity also pose an intriguing question that warrants further exploration.

Several studies have shown TME features as another dimension of prediction systems for prognosis, improving the predictive accuracy of current TNM staging systems [15,42,43]. We also revealed the TME classification as an independent predictor for BSG patients outcomes (Figure 3a,b). Accompanying the WHO grading system, DIPG, and radiotherapy, the TME classification provided additional valuable information, allowing for a more precise prediction for prognosis (Figure 3c) and highlighting its clinical significance as a new prognosis prediction system for BSG patients. Meanwhile, since the TME clusters have shown their independent prognostic value, it is suggested that novel treatments that can modify the TME status may have the potential to benefit BSG patients [16,44].

The determination of the GESs requires measuring hundreds of genes, which may restrict the clinical use of the TME classification. As a result, two simplified methods were developed to identify the TME subtypes. We developed a four-gene panel that demonstrated high accuracy in identifying TME clusters in both our cohort and external datasets. The four genes included in the panel were mechanistically reasonable, as CD3E is present in the majority of T cells, while COL3A1 and MMP1 are representative components and enzymes in the fibrotic extracellular matrix environment [15,45,46]. Moreover, since these genes have been validated through IHC to show significant differences between subtypes, it is suggested that the panel is not only reliable but also has the potential to be clinically determined using a common IHC method. Furthermore, an identification approach was developed using radiomics features and the SVM algorithm, which demonstrated satisfactory efficacy in identifying the TME clusters. This finding is consistent with similar research conducted on other types of tumors that show that the TME status can be predicted using radiomics approaches [47]. And future studies will include additional imaging features and more advanced algorithms in order to develop TME prediction models that are more effective and easier to interpret. These models will also be validated in larger sample sizes and across multiple centers.

However, there are some limitations in this study. Firstly, this is a post hoc study utilizing old data, most of which have been published [2], and would contain confounding factors restricting the extension of our result. For instance, the majority of DIPG tumor samples were collected from patients who received debulking surgery at our center [2,23]. Additionally, the DIPGs eligible for debulking surgery contained a higher proportion of MRI-contrast-enhanced appearances than the biopsy-eligible DIPGs that usually appear as homogenously non-contrast images. Therefore, the observation of high TME heterogeneity could be partly attributed to the DIPG type with contrasted MRI appearances. Secondly, due to the rarity of BSG and the difficulty in obtaining tumor tissues using neurosurgical approaches, the sample size in this study is relatively small, which might also introduce biases in the conclusion. A larger multi-center cohort established through international collaboration is thus warranted [6] to better understand the significance of this TME classification. Thirdly, due to the limited number and small scale of BSG trials, a study on the value of TME classification in therapeutic responses is lacking.

5. Conclusions

BSGs exhibited a high inter-tumor TME heterogeneity, such that they were classified into four TME clusters with distinct clinical outcomes and tumor biological properties. The TME classification can be well identified using a four-gene panel and a non-invasive radiomics method, thus facilitating its clinical application.

Supplementary Materials: The following supporting information can be downloaded at https://www.mdpi.com/article/10.3390/cancers15174224/s1, Figure S1: workflow of this study; Figure S2: batch effects were removed using Combat_seq; Figure S3: determination of cluster number; Figure S4: proportions of TME clusters in DIPGs and PA-like tumors; Figure S5: results of consensus cluster of external datasets; Figure S6: procedures of determining key genes; Table S1: antibodies or DAPI and the conditions used for multidimensional fluorescence staining; Table S2: procedures for multidimensional fluorescence staining; Table S3: results of univariate Cox regression.

Author Contributions: Conceptualization, X.X., Y.Z. and L.Z.; methodology, X.X., Y.W., Y.Z. and L.Z.; software, X.X., X.L. and Y.W.; validation, X.X., Y.W. and Y.Z.; formal analysis, X.X., X.L., Y.W., C.P., P.Z., G.G., T.L., Z.J. and Y.Z.; investigation, X.X., X.L., Y.W., G.G. and Y.Z.; resources, X.L., C.P., P.Z., T.L., Z.J. and L.Z.; data curation, X.L., Y.W., C.P., P.Z., G.G. and T.L.; writing—original draft preparation, X.X., X.L., Y.W., C.P., P.Z., G.G., T.L., Z.J., Y.Z. and L.Z.; writing—review and editing, X.X., X.L., Y.W., C.P., P.Z., G.G., T.L., Z.J., Y.Z. and L.Z.; visualization, Y.W., G.G. and P.Z.; supervision, Y.Z. and L.Z.; project administration, Y.Z.; funding acquisition, L.Z. All authors have read and agreed to the published version of the manuscript.

Funding: This research was funded by the Beijing Municipal Special Funds for Medical Research, grant number JingYiYan 2018-7.

Institutional Review Board Statement: The study was conducted in accordance with the Declaration of Helsinki and approved by the Institutional Review Board of Beijing Tiantan Hospital. The approval number is KY-2020-087-02, and the date of approval is 20 October 2020.

Informed Consent Statement: Patient consent was waived due to the respective nature of this study and previously obtained written consent in the previous study.

Data Availability Statement: The data presented in this study are available on request from the corresponding author.

Acknowledgments: We acknowledge our colleagues who contributed to this work but did not meet the criteria for authorship.

Conflicts of Interest: The authors declare no conflict of interest.

References

1. Grimm, S.A.; Chamberlain, M.C. Brainstem glioma: A review. *Curr. Neurol. Neurosci. Rep.* **2013**, *13*, 346. [CrossRef]
2. Chen, L.H.; Pan, C.; Diplas, B.H.; Xu, C.; Hansen, L.J.; Wu, Y.; Chen, X.; Geng, Y.; Sun, T.; Sun, Y.; et al. The integrated genomic and epigenomic landscape of brainstem glioma. *Nat. Commun.* **2020**, *11*, 3077. [CrossRef] [PubMed]

3. Perrone, M.G.; Ruggiero, A.; Centonze, A.; Carrieri, A.; Ferorelli, S.; Scilimati, A. Diffuse Intrinsic Pontine Glioma (DIPG) Breakthrough and Clinical Perspective. *Curr. Med. Chem.* **2021**, *28*, 3287–3317. [CrossRef] [PubMed]
4. Cooney, T.M.; Lubanszky, E.; Prasad, R.; Hawkins, C.; Mueller, S. Diffuse midline glioma: Review of epigenetics. *J. Neurooncol* **2020**, *150*, 27–34. [CrossRef]
5. Cucu, A.I.; Turliuc, S.; Costea, C.F.; Perciaccante, A.; Bianucci, R.; Donell, S.; Scripcariu, D.V.; Turliuc, M.D. The brainstem and its neurosurgical history. *Neurosurg. Rev.* **2021**, *44*, 3001–3022. [CrossRef] [PubMed]
6. Hu, X.; Fang, Y.; Hui, X.; Jv, Y.; You, C. Radiotherapy for diffuse brainstem glioma in children and young adults. *Cochrane Database Syst. Rev.* **2016**, *2016*, CD010439. [CrossRef] [PubMed]
7. Kim, H.J.; Suh, C.O. Radiotherapy for Diffuse Intrinsic Pontine Glioma: Insufficient but Indispensable. *Brain Tumor Res. Treat* **2023**, *11*, 79–85. [CrossRef]
8. Heravi Shargh, V.; Luckett, J.; Bouzinab, K.; Paisey, S.; Turyanska, L.; Singleton, W.G.B.; Lowis, S.; Gershkovich, P.; Bradshaw, T.D.; Stevens, M.F.G.; et al. Chemosensitization of Temozolomide-Resistant Pediatric Diffuse Midline Glioma Using Potent Nanoencapsulated Forms of a N(3)-Propargyl Analogue. *ACS Appl. Mater. Interfaces* **2021**, *13*, 35266–35280. [CrossRef]
9. Majzner, R.G.; Ramakrishna, S.; Yeom, K.W.; Patel, S.; Chinnasamy, H.; Schultz, L.M.; Richards, R.M.; Jiang, L.; Barsan, V.; Mancusi, R.; et al. GD2-CAR T cell therapy for H3K27M-mutated diffuse midline gliomas. *Nature* **2022**, *603*, 934–941. [CrossRef]
10. Bernstock, J.D.; Hoffman, S.E.; Kappel, A.D.; Valdes, P.A.; Essayed, W.; Klinger, N.V.; Kang, K.D.; Totsch, S.K.; Olsen, H.E.; Schlappi, C.W.; et al. Immunotherapy approaches for the treatment of diffuse midline gliomas. *Oncoimmunology* **2022**, *11*, 2124058 [CrossRef]
11. Dunn-Pirio, A.M.; Vlahovic, G. Immunotherapy approaches in the treatment of malignant brain tumors. *Cancer* **2017**, *123*, 734–750. [CrossRef] [PubMed]
12. Chen, Y.; Zhao, C.; Li, S.; Wang, J.; Zhang, H. Immune Microenvironment and Immunotherapies for Diffuse Intrinsic Pontine Glioma. *Cancers* **2023**, *15*, 602. [CrossRef]
13. Lieberman, N.A.P.; DeGolier, K.; Kovar, H.M.; Davis, A.; Hoglund, V.; Stevens, J.; Winter, C.; Deutsch, G.; Furlan, S.N.; Vitanza, N.A.; et al. Characterization of the immune microenvironment of diffuse intrinsic pontine glioma: Implications for development of immunotherapy. *Neuro Oncol.* **2019**, *21*, 83–94. [CrossRef] [PubMed]
14. Quail, D.F.; Joyce, J.A. Microenvironmental regulation of tumor progression and metastasis. *Nat. Med.* **2013**, *19*, 1423–1437 [CrossRef]
15. Bagaev, A.; Kotlov, N.; Nomie, K.; Svekolkin, V.; Gafurov, A.; Isaeva, O.; Osokin, N.; Kozlov, I.; Frenkel, F.; Gancharova, O.; et al. Conserved pan-cancer microenvironment subtypes predict response to immunotherapy. *Cancer Cell* **2021**, *39*, 845–865.e7 [CrossRef] [PubMed]
16. Xu, L.; Zou, C.; Zhang, S.; Chu, T.S.M.; Zhang, Y.; Chen, W.; Zhao, C.; Yang, L.; Xu, Z.; Dong, S.; et al. Reshaping the systemic tumor immune environment (STIE) and tumor immune microenvironment (TIME) to enhance immunotherapy efficacy in solid tumors. *J. Hematol. Oncol.* **2022**, *15*, 87. [CrossRef]
17. Wu, T.; Dai, Y. Tumor microenvironment and therapeutic response. *Cancer Lett.* **2017**, *387*, 61–68. [CrossRef]
18. Job, S.; Rapoud, D.; Dos Santos, A.; Gonzalez, P.; Desterke, C.; Pascal, G.; Elarouci, N.; Ayadi, M.; Adam, R.; Azoulay, D.; et al. Identification of Four Immune Subtypes Characterized by Distinct Composition and Functions of Tumor Microenvironment in Intrahepatic Cholangiocarcinoma. *Hepatology* **2020**, *72*, 965–981. [CrossRef]
19. Ye, L.; Wang, L.; Yang, J.; Hu, P.; Zhang, C.; Tong, S.; Liu, Z.; Tian, D. Identification of tumor antigens and immune subtypes in lower grade gliomas for mRNA vaccine development. *J. Transl. Med.* **2021**, *19*, 352. [CrossRef]
20. Wang, F. Identification of tumor antigens and immune subtypes of acute myeloid leukemia for mRNA vaccine development. *Clin Transl. Oncol.* **2023**, *25*, 2204–2223. [CrossRef]
21. Recinos, P.F.; Sciubba, D.M.; Jallo, G.I. Brainstem tumors: Where are we today? *Pediatr. Neurosurg.* **2007**, *43*, 192–201. [CrossRef] [PubMed]
22. Price, G.; Bouras, A.; Hambardzumyan, D.; Hadjipanayis, C.G. Current knowledge on the immune microenvironment and emerging immunotherapies in diffuse midline glioma. *eBioMedicine* **2021**, *69*, 103453. [CrossRef] [PubMed]
23. Zhang, L.; Chen, L.H.; Wan, H.; Yang, R.; Wang, Z.; Feng, J.; Yang, S.; Jones, S.; Wang, S.; Zhou, W.; et al. Exome sequencing identifies somatic gain-of-function PPM1D mutations in brainstem gliomas. *Nat. Genet* **2014**, *46*, 726–730. [CrossRef] [PubMed]
24. Pan, C.; Zhang, M.; Xiao, X.; Kong, L.; Wu, Y.; Zhao, X.; Sun, T.; Zhang, P.; Geng, Y.; Zuo, P.; et al. A multimodal imaging-based classification for pediatric diffuse intrinsic pontine gliomas. *Neurosurg. Rev.* **2023**, *46*, 151. [CrossRef] [PubMed]
25. Zhang, Y.; Parmigiani, G.; Johnson, W.E. ComBat-seq: Batch effect adjustment for RNA-seq count data. *NAR Genom. Bioinform.* **2020**, *2*, lqaa078. [CrossRef]
26. Schubert, M.; Klinger, B.; Klunemann, M.; Sieber, A.; Uhlitz, F.; Sauer, S.; Garnett, M.J.; Bluthgen, N.; Saez-Rodriguez, J. Perturbation-response genes reveal signaling footprints in cancer gene expression. *Nat. Commun.* **2018**, *9*, 20. [CrossRef]
27. Grass, G.D.; Alfonso, J.C.L.; Welsh, E.; Ahmed, K.A.; Teer, J.K.; Pilon-Thomas, S.; Harrison, L.B.; Cleveland, J.L.; Mule, J.J.; Eschrich, S.A.; et al. The Radiosensitivity Index Gene Signature Identifies Distinct Tumor Immune Microenvironment Characteristics Associated with Susceptibility to Radiation Therapy. *Int. J. Radiat. Oncol. Biol. Phys.* **2022**, *113*, 635–647. [CrossRef]
28. Yan, D.; Zhao, Q.; Du, Z.; Li, H.; Geng, R.; Yang, W.; Zhang, X.; Cao, J.; Yi, N.; Zhou, J.; et al. Development and validation of an immune-related gene signature for predicting the radiosensitivity of lower-grade gliomas. *Sci. Rep.* **2022**, *12*, 6698. [CrossRef]

29. Pan, C.C.; Liu, J.; Tang, J.; Chen, X.; Chen, F.; Wu, Y.L.; Geng, Y.B.; Xu, C.; Zhang, X.; Wu, Z.; et al. A machine learning-based prediction model of H3K27M mutations in brainstem gliomas using conventional MRI and clinical features. *Radiother. Oncol.* **2019**, *130*, 172–179. [CrossRef]
30. van Griethuysen, J.J.M.; Fedorov, A.; Parmar, C.; Hosny, A.; Aucoin, N.; Narayan, V.; Beets-Tan, R.G.H.; Fillion-Robin, J.C.; Pieper, S.; Aerts, H. Computational Radiomics System to Decode the Radiographic Phenotype. *Cancer Res.* **2017**, *77*, e104–e107. [CrossRef]
31. Louis, D.N.; Perry, A.; Wesseling, P.; Brat, D.J.; Cree, I.A.; Figarella-Branger, D.; Hawkins, C.; Ng, H.K.; Pfister, S.M.; Reifenberger, G.; et al. The 2021 WHO Classification of Tumors of the Central Nervous System: A summary. *Neuro Oncol.* **2021**, *23*, 1231–1251. [CrossRef] [PubMed]
32. Li, Y.; Beeraka, N.M.; Guo, W.; Lei, Y.; Hu, Q.; Guo, L.; Fan, R.; Liu, J.; Sui, A. Prognosis of Patients with Brainstem Glioblastoma Based on "age, surgery and radiotherapy": A SEER Database Analysis. *Technol. Cancer Res. Treat* **2022**, *21*, 15330338221082760. [CrossRef] [PubMed]
33. Kaminska, B.; Kocyk, M.; Kijewska, M. TGF beta signaling and its role in glioma pathogenesis. *Adv. Exp. Med. Biol.* **2013**, *986*, 171–187. [CrossRef] [PubMed]
34. Ludwig, K.; Kornblum, H.I. Molecular markers in glioma. *J. Neurooncol.* **2017**, *134*, 505–512. [CrossRef]
35. He, L.; Zhou, H.; Zeng, Z.; Yao, H.; Jiang, W.; Qu, H. Wnt/beta-catenin signaling cascade: A promising target for glioma therapy. *J. Cell Physiol.* **2019**, *234*, 2217–2228. [CrossRef] [PubMed]
36. Barthel, L.; Hadamitzky, M.; Dammann, P.; Schedlowski, M.; Sure, U.; Thakur, B.K.; Hetze, S. Glioma: Molecular signature and crossroads with tumor microenvironment. *Cancer Metastasis Rev.* **2022**, *41*, 53–75. [CrossRef]
37. Vallee, A.; Guillevin, R.; Vallee, J.N. Vasculogenesis and angiogenesis initiation under normoxic conditions through Wnt/beta-catenin pathway in gliomas. *Rev. Neurosci.* **2018**, *29*, 71–91. [CrossRef]
38. Lang, F.F.; Yung, W.K.; Raju, U.; Libunao, F.; Terry, N.H.; Tofilon, P.J. Enhancement of radiosensitivity of wild-type p53 human glioma cells by adenovirus-mediated delivery of the p53 gene. *J. Neurosurg.* **1998**, *89*, 125–132. [CrossRef]
39. Chedeville, A.L.; Madureira, P.A. The Role of Hypoxia in Glioblastoma Radiotherapy Resistance. *Cancers* **2021**, *13*, 542. [CrossRef]
40. Zhang, X.; Dong, N.; Hu, X. Wnt/beta-catenin signaling inhibitors. *Curr. Top Med. Chem.* **2023**, *23*, 880–896.
41. Persson, M.L.; Douglas, A.M.; Alvaro, F.; Faridi, P.; Larsen, M.R.; Alonso, M.M.; Vitanza, N.A.; Dun, M.D. The intrinsic and microenvironmental features of diffuse midline glioma: Implications for the development of effective immunotherapeutic treatment strategies. *Neuro Oncol.* **2022**, *24*, 1408–1422. [CrossRef] [PubMed]
42. Nepal, C.; Zhu, B.; O'Rourke, C.J.; Bhatt, D.K.; Lee, D.; Song, L.; Wang, D.; Van Dyke, A.L.; Choo-Wosoba, H.; Liu, Z.; et al. Integrative molecular characterisation of gallbladder cancer reveals micro-environment-associated subtypes. *J. Hepatol.* **2021**, *74*, 1132–1144. [CrossRef] [PubMed]
43. Wang, Q.W.; Bao, Z.S.; Jiang, T.; Zhu, Y.J. Tumor microenvironment is associated with clinical and genetic properties of diffuse gliomas and predicts overall survival. *Cancer Immunol. Immunother.* **2022**, *71*, 953–966. [CrossRef] [PubMed]
44. Zhang, J.; Huang, D.; Saw, P.E.; Song, E. Turning cold tumors hot: From molecular mechanisms to clinical applications. *Trends Immunol.* **2022**, *43*, 523–545. [CrossRef] [PubMed]
45. Ho, I.A.; Chan, K.Y.; Ng, W.H.; Guo, C.M.; Hui, K.M.; Cheang, P.; Lam, P.Y. Matrix metalloproteinase 1 is necessary for the migration of human bone marrow-derived mesenchymal stem cells toward human glioma. *Stem Cells* **2009**, *27*, 1366–1375. [CrossRef]
46. Yin, W.; Zhu, H.; Tan, J.; Xin, Z.; Zhou, Q.; Cao, Y.; Wu, Z.; Wang, L.; Zhao, M.; Jiang, X.; et al. Identification of collagen genes related to immune infiltration and epithelial-mesenchymal transition in glioma. *Cancer Cell. Int.* **2021**, *21*, 276. [CrossRef]
47. Khalili, N.; Kazerooni, A.F.; Familiar, A.; Haldar, D.; Kraya, A.; Foster, J.; Koptyra, M.; Storm, P.B.; Resnick, A.C.; Nabavizadeh, A. Radiomics for characterization of the glioma immune microenvironment. *NPJ Precis. Oncol.* **2023**, *7*, 59. [CrossRef]

Disclaimer/Publisher's Note: The statements, opinions and data contained in all publications are solely those of the individual author(s) and contributor(s) and not of MDPI and/or the editor(s). MDPI and/or the editor(s) disclaim responsibility for any injury to people or property resulting from any ideas, methods, instructions or products referred to in the content.

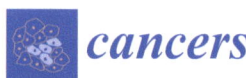

Review

Current Knowledge about the Peritumoral Microenvironment in Glioblastoma

Gianluca Trevisi [1,2,*] and Annunziato Mangiola [1]

[1] Department of Neurosciences, Imaging and Clinical Sciences, G. D'Annunzio University Chieti-Pescara, 66100 Chieti, Italy; annunziato.mangiola@unich.it
[2] Neurosurgical Unit, Ospedale Spirito Santo, 65122 Pescara, Italy
* Correspondence: gianluca.trevisi@unich.it

Simple Summary: In this manuscript, we review the most relevant biological findings on glioblastoma peritumoral tissue. This area, which is beyond frank tumoral tissue, presents a unique microenvironment with a peculiar cellular landscape and genomic and transcriptomic alterations that ultimately lead to glioblastoma progression or recurrence after treatment. Indeed, while some infiltrating tumor cells are found in about one third of cases, these alterations are seen even in non-infiltrated cases. This is of utmost translational interest, as the peritumoral brain zone (PBZ) is the real target of post-operative adjuvant treatment.

Abstract: Glioblastoma is a deadly disease, with a mean overall survival of less than 2 years from diagnosis. Recurrence after gross total surgical resection and adjuvant chemo-radiotherapy almost invariably occurs within the so-called peritumoral brain zone (PBZ). The aim of this narrative review is to summarize the most relevant findings about the biological characteristics of the PBZ currently available in the medical literature. The PBZ presents several peculiar biological characteristics. The cellular landscape of this area is different from that of healthy brain tissue and is characterized by a mixture of cell types, including tumor cells (seen in about 30% of cases), angiogenesis-related endothelial cells, reactive astrocytes, glioma-associated microglia/macrophages (GAMs) with anti-inflammatory polarization, tumor-infiltrating lymphocytes (TILs) with an "exhausted" phenotype and glioma-associated stromal cells (GASCs). From a genomic and transcriptomic point of view, compared with the tumor core and healthy brain tissue, the PBZ presents a "half-way" pattern with upregulation of genes related to angiogenesis, the extracellular matrix, and cellular senescence and with stemness features and downregulation in tumor suppressor genes. This review illustrates that the PBZ is a transition zone with a pre-malignant microenvironment that constitutes the base for GBM progression/recurrence. Understanding of the PBZ could be relevant to developing more effective treatments to prevent GBM development and recurrence.

Keywords: glioblastoma; glioma-associated microglia; glioma-associated stromal cells; immune infiltrate; microenvironment; peritumoral brain area; peritumor; tumor-infiltrating lymphocytes

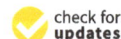

Citation: Trevisi, G.; Mangiola, A. Current Knowledge about the Peritumoral Microenvironment in Glioblastoma. *Cancers* 2023, 15, 5460. https://doi.org/10.3390/cancers15225460

Academic Editor: Frank A.E. Kruyt

Received: 23 September 2023
Revised: 31 October 2023
Accepted: 15 November 2023
Published: 17 November 2023

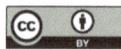

Copyright: © 2023 by the authors. Licensee MDPI, Basel, Switzerland. This article is an open access article distributed under the terms and conditions of the Creative Commons Attribution (CC BY) license (https://creativecommons.org/licenses/by/4.0/).

1. Introduction

Glioblastoma (GBM) is the most common and most deadly primary brain tumor in humans, being classified as the fourth and most malignant grade of central nervous system (CNS) tumors by the World Health Organization (WHO) classification system [1]. Before 2016, gliomas were divided into different types and grades (from 1, the most indolent, to 4, the most aggressive) according to their histological characteristics. Classical histological characteristics of GBM include a diffusely infiltrative growth pattern, nuclear atypia, mitotic activity, increased cellular density, pseudopalisades, microvascular proliferation and necrosis. The latter two were often considered as pathognomonic of GBM. However, in the last decade, molecular biology has figured strongly in the WHO CNS classification

Indeed, the new 2021 edition divided adult-type, diffuse gliomas into only three types: astrocytoma, IDH-mutant; oligodendroglioma, IDH-mutant and 1p/19q-codeleted; and glioblastoma, IDH-wildtype [2]. Therefore, all IDH-mutant diffuse astrocytic tumors are considered a single type (astrocytoma, IDH-mutant) and are then graded as CNS WHO grade 2, 3, or 4. Moreover, grading is no longer entirely histological, since the presence of CDKN2A/B homozygous deletion results in a CNS WHO grade of 4, even in the absence of microvascular proliferation or necrosis. Lastly, according to the 2021 classification, a diagnosis of glioblastoma should now be diagnosed in the setting of an IDH-wildtype diffuse and astrocytic glioma in adults if there is TERT promoter mutation or EGFR gene amplification or there are +7/−10 chromosome copy-number changes, regardless of histological features of a lower grading [2].

Gross total surgical resection (GTR) or maximal safe resection followed by radiochemotherapy is considered the treatment of choice for newly diagnosed glioblastoma [3–5]. The extent of resection has been extensively associated with prolonged survival in these tumors [6,7].

However, the above strategies have prolonged the overall survival of our patients by only a few months, averaging 20 months from diagnosis in recent series. It is a common clinical experience to observe tumor recurrence in the area surrounding the surgical margins, generally between 1 and 2 cm from the resection cavity, even in cases of GTR confirmed by post-operative MR scans performed with the most-advanced machines and techniques and followed by full adjuvant therapy [8].

This has long been known in the neurosurgical community, with discouraging early experiences of recurrences even after hemispherectomies in a small series of patients in the 1920s [9]. Histopathological and biomolecular evidence of tumor cells located at relevant distances from the tumor core, both in the same hemisphere and in the contralateral one, led to the diffuse opinion that glioblastoma should be considered a systematic brain disease and not a delineated tumor [10,11].

Our interest in the "periphery" of GBM, namely, the brain tissue around MR contrast enhancement and seen as apparently normal at surgical resection, started with the initial observation of longer survival in GBM patients with no tumor cell infiltration of apparently normal white matter compared to patients with white matter infiltration (21 vs. 12 months) [12].

As our research went on, we realized that the alterations in the "periphery" were not limited only to the presence of frank tumor cells but also included a different cellular and molecular microenvironment compared to healthy brain tissue. This was true also in cases where no tumor cell infiltration was detected. Whether this is related to intracerebral tumor cell migration [13], to tumor-initiating stem cells [14], or to "normal" brain cells undergoing a tumorigenic cascade cross-talking with and recruited by tumor cells [15] is a matter of debate.

Regardless of its origins, it is now accepted that the so-called peritumoral brain zone (PBZ) contributes to GBM heterogeneity and recurrence. Since the PBZ is what actually remains after surgical resection, being the real target of adjuvant therapies, it is evident that a deeper knowledge of its radiological, cellular, and molecular characteristics could be of paramount importance in GBM treatment.

Several strands of evidence have recently shown that the tumor microenvironment plays a crucial role in GBM progression and treatment resistance by promoting tumor growth and invasion while suppressing the immune response [16,17]. The immune microenvironment of GBM also contributes to treatment resistance by inhibiting the anti-tumor immune response [17]. Therefore, active research on therapies targeting the tumor microenvironment to enhance the immune response, disrupt tumor–stroma interactions, and make tumor cells more susceptible to treatment is ongoing [18–20].

The scope of this narrative review is to summarize the main findings on different aspects of the PBZ microenvironment in glioblastoma.

It is important to underline that, as mentioned above, grade 4 astrocytoma was introduced only in 2021 by the WHO CNS tumor classification [2]. This entity was defined as IDH-mutated glioblastoma in the 2016 WHO classification [21], and before 2016 it was known as "secondary" glioblastoma, that is, the result of an anaplastic transformation and malignant progression of a lower-grade glioma [22,23]. Therefore, the bulk of the literature currently available on the PBZ does not differentiate between glioblastoma and grade 4 astrocytoma.

However, it is a common experience that IDH-wildtype glioblastoma is by far the most common grade 4 glioma (90–95% of grade 4 gliomas); therefore, most of the data included in this review refer to the most common clinical entity.

Ethical Statement: The data included in Figures 1 and 2 were part of a prospective GBM biobanking study authorized by the Chieti-Pescara Local Ethics Committee (EC number: 08/21.05.2020). The patients gave written consent to the use of their radiological and surgical data in anonymous form.

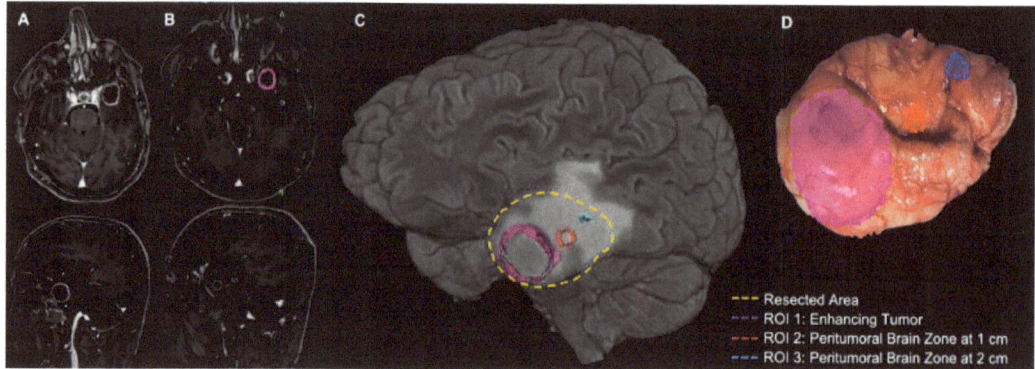

Figure 1. Exemplificative case of peritumoral brain zone (PBZ) sampling in left temporal pole glioblastoma. (**A**) Pre-operative contrast-enhanced T1w MR images. Note the tumor core composed of an inner necrotic area and an enhancing border. Peritumoral brain zone is beyond the enhancing border. (**B**) Pre-operative MR scans were imported into a neuronavigation workstation and several regions of interest (ROIs) were detected: enhancing tumor (pink ROI), two ROIs from PBZs at 1 cm from enhancing tumor (red and green ROIs), and one ROI from PBZ at 2 cm from enhancing tumor (blue ROI). (**C**) Three-dimensional surface rendering of the case with superimposed dotted lines showing the supratotal en-bloc resection (yellow dotted line) that includes enhancing tumor (pink dotted line) and the preselected ROIs of PBZ at 1 cm and 2 cm from enhancing tumor (red and blue dotted lines, respectively). Please note that FLAIR alteration goes far beyond enhancing tumors and that sampled PBZ ROIs are located within FLAIR alterations. A complete "FLAIRectomy" could not be performed in this case due to the risk of postoperative language deficits related to posterior superior temporal gyrus ("Wernicke area") involvement in FLAIR alteration. (**D**) Surgical sample with ROI overlay.

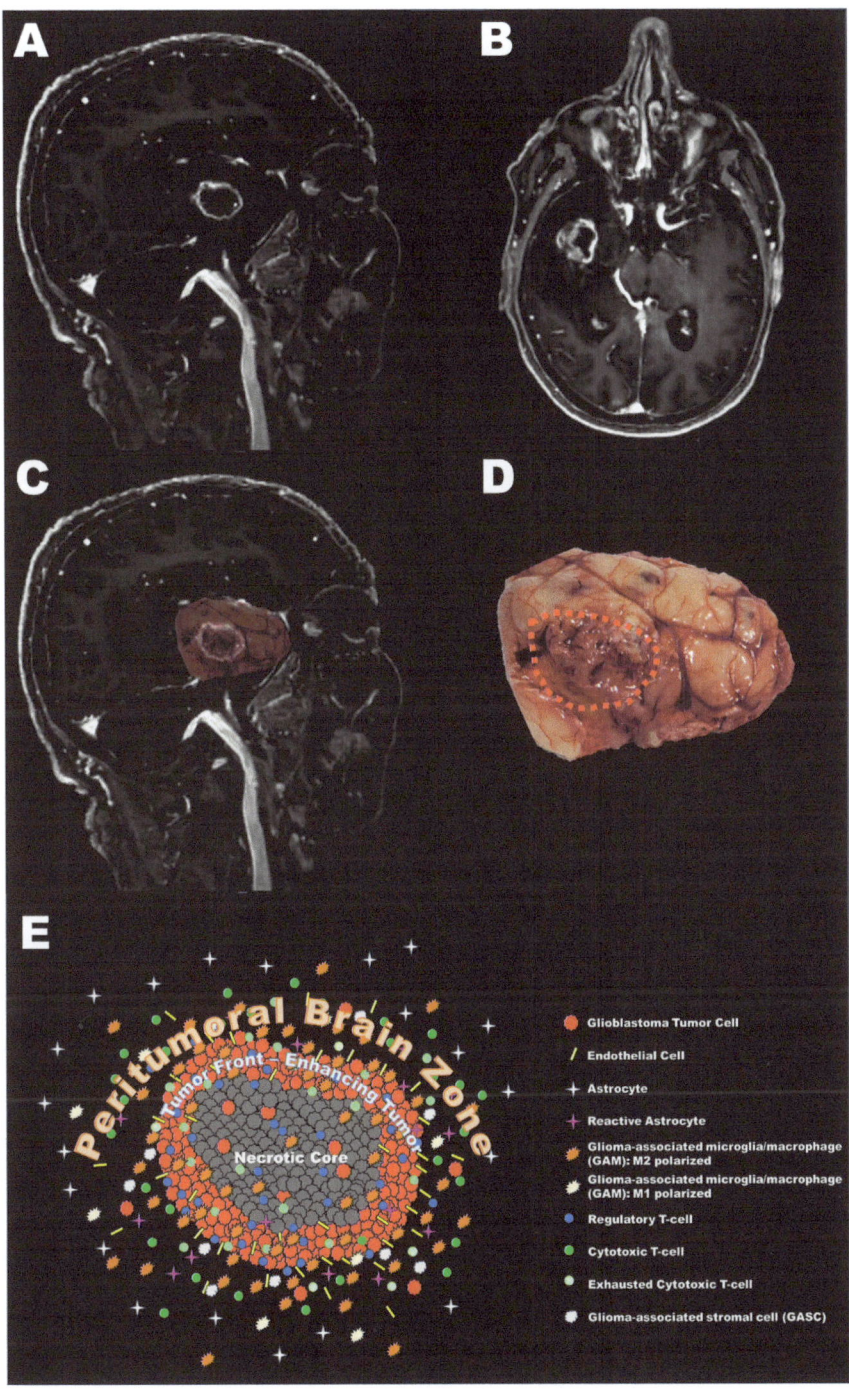

Figure 2. Right temporal glioblastoma. (**A**) T1w gadolinium enhanced MRI, sagittal view. (**B**) Axial plane. Note the necrotic core, the enhancing ring, and the peritumoral signal alteration (hypointense in T1-weighted scans). (**C**) Overlay of surgical sample on pre-operative scan. Please note the correspondence

of the tumor core, seen as altered brain parenchyma, even at gross visual inspection, with the enhancing area. (**D**) Surgical sample with an overlayed contouring of tumor core (red dotted line). (**E**) Graphical rendering of the cellular microenvironment seen when analyzing slices from a supratotal GBM resection. Cellular types are detailed on the right side. The distribution of cellular types between tumor core and peritumoral brain zone (PBZ) resembles evidence in the literature as per the main text of this manuscript.

2. Definition of the Peritumoral Brain Zone (PBZ)

When dealing with the PBZ (sometimes defined as the peripheral brain zone or as brain adjacent to tumor (BAT)), the first, difficult issue is its definition. The most-used definition of the PBZ is the area around the contrast-enhancing tumor seen in T1-weighted MR scans. This is quite a vague definition, since contrast enhancement is related to blood–brain barrier disruption and is not a fully reliable picture of tumor extension. Moreover, it is common to see a halo of hyperintensity in T2-weighted and FLAIR sequences around the enhancing tumor [24]. This signal abnormality is related to a mixture of increased cellularity/cellular infiltration and vasogenic edema, with tumor cell infiltration and even frank tumor tissue documented in up to 76% and 9% of samples, respectively, in a recent study [25]. On this basis, the surgical concept of "FLAIRectomy" has recently emerged [26,27]. More advanced radiological techniques based on diffusion-weighted sequences (ADC, FA, and DTI) appear to be more sensitive to changes in the peritumoral area and could be correlated with the degree of glioma infiltration [28,29]. The novel field of radiomics, which aims to extract large numbers of quantitative features from medical images using data-characterization algorithms, could help in the pre-operative analysis of the PBZ, and specific PBZ features could be predictive of survival [24–26,30–32].

In our neurosurgical practice, we defined, and whenever possible systematically sampled, preferentially via en-bloc supratotal resection, the PBZ as apparently normal brain tissue 1–2 cm around glioblastoma margins, defined through surgical magnification and with neuronavigation [14]. Believing in a small, but still significant, survival advantage of supratotal resection also in GBM [33], when regarded as functionally safe (e.g., in right fronto-polar GBMs), we extended our resection up to 3.5 cm from the enhancing tumor margin: tissue analysis from areas more distant from the tumor showed the same alterations found in areas located within 1 cm from the margin of the tumor [34]. Figure 1 shows an exemplificative case with our usual workflow in PBZ sampling.

3. Cellular Characteristics of the PBZ

3.1. Tumor Cells

An important concept is that the PBZ is not always infiltrated by frank tumor cells at pathological examination. However, even in these cases, cellular and molecular differences from healthy brain tissue can be detected.

GBM cell infiltration of the PBZ is generally seen in 35–45% of cases [15,24], with some authors reporting an even larger percentage of infiltration in their experience [25]. If present, the number of tumor cells detected in the PBZ is generally between 10 and 30% of the total number of cells in the specimen [35].

At surgical resection, tumor cells from the PBZ do not usually fluoresce when 5-aminolevulinic acid (5-ALA) is used [36]. These cells differ phenotypically from those obtained from the core of the tumor [37–39]. In particular, neoplastic cells from the PBZ show a lower stem-cell molecular signature than cells from the core of the tumor, differing in expression of CD133, Sox2, nestin, and musashi 1 [37–39]. Therefore, in vitro stemness characteristics, such as self-renewal, are reduced in peripheral tumor cells. However, conflicting results have been published about the in vivo tumorigenic potential of tumor cells from the PBZ. If cancer stem cells (CSCs) derived from the periphery of the tumor have shown little if no tumorigenic potential in animal models [40], a population of non-self-renewing tumorigenic cells has been demonstrated from the same area [39]. Tumor cells from the core and the periphery of a GBM also differ in their response to drugs and irradiation in vitro [38,41].

Nestin expression sharply decreases in peritumoral tissue compared to proper tumor areas. Despite being classically considered as a marker of neural stem cells, a mild nestin increase in apparently normal cells of the PBZ was shown [34]. This could be related to reactive changes in normal astrocytic cells, thus indicating an induced "pre-malignant" state. Expression of nestin and CD105 in endothelial cells of neo-formed microvessels of the PBZ morphologically quite similar to those present in the tumor [42] was also demonstrated.

Bastola and coworkers described uniquely elevated markers attributable to GBM core cells (CD44, MYC, HIF-1α, VIM, ANXA1, CDK6, and JAG1) and GBM edge cells (OLIG1, TC2, SRRM2, ERBB3, PHGDH, and RAP1GAP), showing that intercellular crosstalk from core GBM cells promotes aggressiveness of the edge counterparts, with HDAC1 as the initiator of the cross-talk and sCD109 acting as the mediator via HDAC1-C/EBPβ regulation [41].

Other genetic differences between tumor cells in the PBZ and tumor cells from the core of a GBM involve genes related to invasion (Galectin-1, Rac1, Rac3, RhoA GTPases, p27, and avb3 integrin), cell adhesion (CDH20 and PCDH19), migration (SNAI2, NANOG, USP6, and DISC1), and immune or inflammatory responses (TLR4) [43].

Among others, serine protease inhibitor clade A, member 3 (SERPINA3) protein is more expressed in the PBZ, and its expression correlates with poor prognosis. The in vitro knockdown of SERPINA decreases tumor cell proliferation, invasion, migration, transition to mesenchymal phenotype, stemness, and radioresistance [44].

3.2. Non-Neoplastic Cells

The majority of cells detected in the PBZ are peculiar non-neoplastic cells that can be found also when there is no evidence of tumor cell invasion [45]. Among these PBZ non-neoplastic cells, we will discuss the characteristics of angiogenesis-related endothelial cells and of the already mentioned reactive astrocytes, microglia, and other inflammatory and stromal cells. These cells are also detected in the core of the tumor and their vital role in controlling the course of pathology has been revealed in the last decade [46].

3.2.1. Endothelial Cells

Angiogenesis is a key feature of glioblastoma and several trials with anti-angiogenic drugs have been conducted in the last years, with limited impact in clinical practice [47]. However, this exuberant new vascularization is very inefficient, leading to highly hypoxic areas within the tumor and associated necrosis, with hypoxia-inducible factor-1 (HIF-1), the main transcription factor activated by hypoxia, upregulating several genes involved in angiogenesis, metabolic reprogramming, cell invasion, immunosuppression, and cancer stem-cell phenotypes [48]. Hypoxia has, therefore, a major role in GBM maintenance and progression [49].

Neo-angiogenic potential is shared by GBM cancer stem cells derived from both the core and the PBZ [50]. Moreover, neo-angiogenesis occurs in the peritumoral tissue even in the absence of cells with neoplastic morphology. This is suggested by the expression of HIF-1α, HIF2α, vascular endothelial growth factor (VEGF), and VEGF receptors (VEGFR1 and VEGFR2) in both GBM and peritumoral tissue, indicating that both areas contain, to some extent, cells that are either responsive to angiogenic stimuli or able to trigger angiogenic response. However, the vascular characteristics of the PBZ differ from those of the tumor core. Although nestin, CD105, and CD34 are clearly expressed in endothelial cells in the PBZ, HIF-1α and VEGFR-1/2 expression is either low or negative [51]. Also, VEGF-A expression in the PBZ is low compared with that in the core. VEGF-A expression is related to HIF-1α, and this axis plays a pivotal role in the development of the immunosuppressive microenvironment by inhibition of the maturation of dendritic cells, stimulation of the proliferation of regulatory T cells, and suppression of anti-tumor immunity [52,53].

3.2.2. Reactive Astrocytes

Reactive astrocytes are astrocytes that undergo morphological, molecular, and functional changes in response to pathological situations in surrounding tissue [54]. Useful markers for reactive astrocyte detection are GFAP, CD274, proliferation markers (such as Ki67, PCNA, and BrdU incorporation), aldehyde dehydrogenase-1 L1 (ALDH1L1), glutamine synthetase (GS), and aldolase-C (ALDOC) [54,55]. In gliomas, astrocytes display a reactive phenotype due to activated microglia induction and glioma cell contact, working synergistically to promote GBM proliferation and invasiveness [56,57]. Reactive astrocytes are also believed to offer chemoprotection to glioma cells via gap-junction communication and especially connexin 43 [58,59], and immunoprotection via paracrine secretion of several factors, including tenascin-C [60] and IL-10 [61]. A higher expression of factors related to reactive astrocytes is found in the PBZs of patients with shorter survival after surgical resection compared to longer-term-survival patients [62].

3.2.3. Glioma-Associated Microglia/Macrophages (GAMs)

Microglia, which are the brain-resident immune cells, and peripheral blood macrophages are the most common non-neoplastic cells detected in the GBM microenvironment [63]. As per reactive astrocytes, the pro-tumor role of microglia and macrophages in GBM growth and progression has been recently postulated [64]. In fact, these cells could contribute to immune evasion, growth, and invasion of GBM [65,66].

Three possible phenotypes have been described for microglia/macrophages [67–69]: the M0 phenotype, or resting microglia, contributing to the maintenance of a healthy environment for neuronal function; the activated M1 phenotype, or pro-inflammatory microglia, characterized by the ability to release pro-inflammatory cytokines/mediators such as IL-1β, IL-6, TNF-α, CCL2, reactive oxygen species (ROS), and nitric oxide (NO); and the activated M2 phenotype, or anti-inflammatory microglia, associated with the ability to produce anti-inflammatory and immune-suppressive factors, including ARG-1, Ym1 and CD36, as well as upregulate the cell surface markers CD163, CD204, and CD206 and anti-inflammatory cytokines, such as IL-10. M2 GAMs also secrete transforming growth factor beta (TGF-β), VEGF, and matrix metalloproteinase 9 (MMP9).

However, a rigid, dichotomic characterization (M1 vs. M2 phenotypes) is considered an oversimplification, and a new view based on the coexistence of multiple states is currently encouraged by experts in the field [70]. Glioma and microglia interaction result in a dynamic stimulus-dependent microglia phenotype expression [71–73]. In a condition mimicking the late stage of GBM in vitro, microglia present as a mixture of polarization phenotypes (M1 and M2a/b), while microglia exposed to factors resembling the early stage of pathology show a more specific pattern of activation, with increased M2b polarization status and upregulation of IL-10 only [71].

Ex vivo, glioma-associated microglia/macrophages (GAMs) show a heterogeneous M1/M2 polarization within the tumor and the PBZ. CD163+, M2-polarized GAMs, are highly expressed in the tumor core, with a core-to-PBZ decreasing gradient [74,75]. A correlation between high CD163 expression and reduced overall survival has been shown in GBM and grade 3 gliomas but not in grade 2 gliomas [74,76]. Nonetheless, iNOS + GAMs, that is, M1-polarized GAMs, also show a higher concentration in the tumor core compared with the PBZ [74], confirming that these cells are recruited by the tumor and that the notion of a stimulus-dependent microglia phenotype should replace the oversimplified M1/M2 polarization paradigm [72,73].

Regarding the role of GAMs in GBM progression, intense GAM–glioma cross-talk has been shown [77,78]. Most GAMs arise from circulating monocytes, whose recruitment and differentiation into GAMs is supported by CCL2 and CSF-1. Indeed, glioma cells release several other chemoattractive factors (e.g., MCP-1 and 3, HGF/SF, CX3CL1, GDNF, ATF, SDF-1, GM-CSF, etc.) to recruit GAMs to the tumor tissue. Moreover, tumor cells secrete inflammatory factors, chemokines, and signal molecules to promote the M2 polarization of GAMs, such as IL-4, CCL2, and TGF-β [79]. In turn, GAMs release several other factors to promote glioma cell invasion, such as TGF-β, STI1, EGF, IL-6, and IL-1β. In particular, TGF-β triggers the release of pro-MMP2 and versican from glioma cells and a cascade that ultimately leads GAM cells to produce active MMP2 and MMP9, which enhance degradation of the extracellular matrix and glioma invasion [77].

3.2.4. Tumor-Infiltrating Lymphocytes (TILs)

Other inflammatory cells found in the GBM microenvironment are T-cells and NK cells [80]. However, GBM is often described as a "cold tumor", due to the prevalence among tumor-infiltrating lymphocytes (TILs) of regulatory T-cells, a specialized subpopulation of T cells that act to suppress the immune response, thereby maintaining homeostasis and self-tolerance, and a relative lack of cytotoxic T-cells (CD8+). Moreover, it has been shown that TILs in GBM are more immunosuppressed than their peripheral counterparts, and dysfunction of these TILs, which often show an "exhausted" phenotype, is a hallmark of GBM [81].

T-cells, identified through CD3 positivity, are more prevalent in the tumor core than in the PBZ, with a similar gradient to CD163+, M2-like GAMs [75]. These M2-like immunosuppressive GAMs, as well as reactive astrocytes, release several immunosuppressive factors, such as IL-10 and TGF-β, both of which inhibit cytotoxic T-cell functions [82,83]; arginase, which inhibits T-cells through arginine depletion from the tumor microenvironment [84]; and indolamine 2,3-dioxygenase (IDO), which acts to recruit regulatory T-cells and inhibit cytotoxic T-cells through tryptophan depletion [85,86]. Our research group recently showed that IDO is expressed almost exclusively in the tumor core, with substantially no staining in the PBZ, and that IDO positively localizes with CD163+ cell clusters, confirming GAMs as the source of IDO secretion [75]. Also, a high HIF-1α concentration in the tumor core attracts regulatory T-cells and promotes the migration and differentiation of immunosuppressive GAMs, resulting in further suppression of cytotoxic T-cells.

In summary, when compared with the tumor core, the PBZ shows a higher density of CD8+ cytotoxic T-cells, a lower density of Foxp3+ regulatory T-cells, and a similar number of CD4+ T-cells, which include both regulatory and helper T-cells [87]. Interestingly, cytotoxic T-cells show a significantly lower expression of programmed cell death-1 (PD-1) in the PBZ compared with the tumor core [87]. Indeed, expression of PD-1, a T-cell surface protein serving as an immune checkpoint which downregulates the immune system to prevent auto-immunity [88,89], is upregulated by VEGF-A [90]. Of note, hypoxia in the tumor core induces VEGF expression via the HIF-1α pathway, which also induces the expression of the PD-1 ligand (PD-L1) [91].

3.2.5. Glioma-Associated Stromal Cells (GASCs)

It has been shown that in systemic carcinomas a significant component of the tumor stroma is constituted by cancer-associated fibroblasts (CAFs), also known as myofibroblasts [92]. Recently, GBM-associated stromal cells (GASCs) from histologically tumor-free PBZs with phenotypic and functional properties similar to CAFs have been isolated [93]. The nomenclature of these cells is still debated, as several names, including glioma-associated human MSCs (GA-hMSCs), glioma-associated or glioblastoma-derived MSCs (gbMSCs), glioma stroma MSCs (GS-MSCs), brain tumor-derived MSCs (BT-MSCs), mesenchymal stem-like cells (MSLCs), tumor MSCLs (tMSLCs), glioma stromal MSLCs (GS-MSLCs), CAF-like cells, and glioblastoma-associated stromal or glioma-associated stem cells (GASCs), have been used in the literature [94], inducing confusion and possible errors. Probably, the most problematic name used by some authors is glioma-associated stem cells, which could erroneously be interpreted as a synonym of glioma stem cells (GSCs). However, GASCs and GSCs are genetically different, as GASCs are typically diploid and do not harbor the genetic alterations commonly seen in GSCs, such as loss of chromosome 10 or gain of chromosome 7 [95,96].

Interest in GASCs is related to the evidence that their probable progenitor cells, namely, mesenchymal stem cells (MSC), also known as bone marrow-derived mesenchymal stem cells (bm-MSC), show anti-tumor behavior [97] and are regarded as carriers for cancer therapy [98]. Nonetheless, there is still an ongoing debate on the progenitor cells of GASCs which goes beyond the scope of this manuscript, and even their role in GBM behavior is debated [95,99–101].

However, several experimental data seem to confirm that tumor-resident GASCs have a pro-tumorigenic role. Indeed, GASCs have a complex cross-talk with GBM tumor cells [102]. Tumor cells recruit GASCs and enhance their angiogenic potential via platelet derived growth factor-BB (PDGF-BB), Matrix Metalloproteinase 1 (MMP1), IL-8, VEGF-A, and TGF-β1 secretion [103–106]. In turn, GASCs can facilitate tumor cell migration by remodeling the extracellular matrix [107], drive phenotypic changes in GBM cells, and stimulate GBM cells, leading to greater tumor infiltration [99,108]. The interaction of GASCs with GSCs could even produce fusion cells that were more angiogenic than the parental cells in animal models [109].

Two subtypes of GASCs differentiated by DNA methylation upon transcriptome analysis can be isolated: GASCs-A and GASCs-B [37]. The latter show pro-carcinogenic properties both in vitro and in vivo, promoting the development of tumor cells and endothelia. It has been shown that GASCs can stimulate glioma malignancy also through the M2 GAMs and are associated with the level of immune checkpoints in the glioma microenvironment [110].

3.3. Summary of Cellular Characteristics of the PBZ

Several cellular types play a role in GBM development and behavior. The PBZ shares most of these players with the tumor core. However, most of the involved cell types show different characteristics depending on their spatial distribution. Overall, an increasing malignant-behavior gradient is present from the PBZ to the tumor core, where GBM expresses the apex of its immunosuppressive properties. Hypoxia has a key role, orchestrating the molecular landscape of the tumor core. In turn, the tumor core influences angiogenesis in the PBZ, which still has some preserved immune properties that are progressively lost when approaching the tumor core.

Figure 2 shows a second exemplificative clinical case of a GBM undergoing supra total resection and sampling of the PBZ, with a graphical rendering of the main cellular populations in the tumor core and the PBZ.

Table 1 and Figure 3 summarize the main cellular properties of the peritumoral brain zone in glioblastoma and the cross-talk between different cellular populations to promote tumor growth, invasion, and immune-, chemo-, and radioresistance.

Table 1. Summary of main cellular characteristics of PBZ.

Cell Type	Peritumoral Brain Zone Cellular Characteristics	
	Details	Main References
Tumor-infiltrating cells	<ul><li>Seen in 35–45% of cases, representing 10–30% of cells in the specimen</li><li>No/low fluorescence at 5-ALA</li><li>Low stem-cell molecular signature</li><li>Show a different expression of tumor markers compared with tumor core neoplastic cells</li><li>Different in vitro response to drugs and radiation compared with tumor core neoplastic cells</li></ul>	<ul><li>Mangiola 2013 [15]; Lemée 2015 [24]</li><li>Idoate 2011 [36]</li><li>Clavreul 2015 [37]; Piccirillo 2012 [39]; Bastola 2020 [41]</li><li>Glas 2010 [38]; Nimbalkar 2021 [44]</li></ul>
Endothelial cells	<ul><li>Angiogenesis occurs in both tumor core and PBZ, also with no infiltrating tumor cells</li><li>HIFs are pivotal in GBM microenvironment</li><li>As in tumor core, in PBZ, endothelial cells express nestin, CD105, and CD34</li><li>Compared to tumor core, in PBZ, endothelial cells express low or null HIF-1α, VEGF-A, and VEGFR-1/2</li></ul>	<ul><li>D'Alessio 2016 [50]</li><li>Domènech 2021 [48]; Shi 2023 [49]</li><li>Tamura 2018 [51]</li></ul>

Table 1. Cont.

Cell Type	Peritumoral Brain Zone Cellular Characteristics	
	Details	Main References
Reactive astrocytes	• Promote GBM proliferation and invasiveness • Chemoprotection through gap junctions and connexin 43 • Immunoprotection through tenascin-C and IL-10 • Reduced survival in patients with higher density in PBZ	• Placone 2016 [56]; Liddelow 2017 [57] • Lin 2016 [58]; Munoz 2014 [59] • Huang 2010 [60]; Fujita 2008 [61] • Fazi 2015 [62]
Glioma-associated microglia and macrophages	• Recruited and polarized by tumor cells • Contribute to immune evasion, growth, and invasion of GBM • M2-polarized GAMs (anti-inflammatory phenotype) are prevalent, with a decreasing gradient from core to PBZ. They have a prominent pro-tumorigenic role • Also, M1-polarized GAMs (pro-inflammatory phenotype) are recruited by GBM, with a decreasing core-to-PBZ gradient, similar to M2 GAMs	• Annovazzi 2018 [76] • Hambardzumyan 2016 [77] • Hussain 2006 [65]; Watters 2005 [66] • Ge 2020 [79]; Lisi 2017 [74] • Rahimi Koshkaki 2020 [75]
Tumor-infiltrating lymphocytes	• PBZ shows higher number of PD-1-negative CD8+ cytotoxic T-cells • Cytotoxic T-cells in tumor core have an "exhausted" phenotype and the majority are PD-1+ (immunosuppressive) • Tumor core has higher density of regulatory T-cells (immunosuppressive) • Overall, more TILs in tumor core with same gradient of GAMs	• Tamura 2018 [87] • Woroniecka 2018 [81] • Rahimi Koshkaki 2020 [75]
Glioma-associated stromal cells	• Similar to cancer-associated fibroblasts seen in systemic cancers • Several names used in the literature • Unknown progenitor cells (mesenchymal stem cells?) • GASCs and GSCs are genetically different, as GASCs are typically diploid and do not harbor the genetic alterations commonly seen in GSCs, such as loss of chromosome 10 or gain of chromosome 7 • Tumor cells recruit GASCs and induce their angiogenic potential • GASCs facilitate tumor cell migration by remodeling the extracellular matrix and inducing phenotypic changes in GBM tumor cells • GASCs also interact with M2-polarized GAMs	• Clavreul 2012, 2014, 2020 [93–95] • Hossain 2015 [96] • Schichor 2006 [103] • Zhang 2021 [106] • Birnbaum 2011 [105] • Ho 2009 [104] • Lim 2018 [107] • Cai 2021 [110]

Abbreviations: 5-ALA: 5-aminolevulinic acid; GAMs: glioma-associated microglia and macrophages; GASCs: glioma-associated stromal cells; GBM: glioblastoma; GSCs: glioma stem cells; HIFs: hypoxia-inducible factors; PBZ: peritumoral brain zone; TILs: tumor-infiltrating lymphocytes; VEGF: vascular endothelial growth factor; VEGFR: vascular endothelial growth factor receptor; PD-1: programmed cell death protein 1.

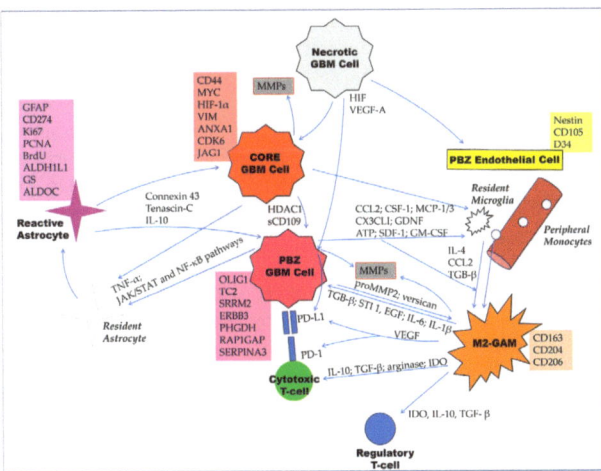

Figure 3. Main underlying mechanisms of the interplay of immune and other cells within the microenvironment of the peritumoral brain zone (PBZ) in GBM. Main cell markers are shown in rectangular

boxes at the side of any cell type. Core GBM cells promote aggressiveness of the PBZ counterparts with sCD109 acting as the mediator of HDAC1-C/EBPβ pathway. GBM cells induce reactive astrocytes via TNF-α secretion and through direct cell–cell contact by a variety of signaling pathways including the JAK/STAT and NF-κB pathways. In turn, reactive astrocytes offer chemoprotection to glioma cells via gap-junction communication (connexin 43) and immunoprotection via paracrine secretion of tenascin-C and IL-10. The necrotic core induces endothelial cell proliferation via the HIF-VEGF-A axis, which also induces MMP production and PD-L1 expression in GBM cells. Glioma cells attract resident microglia and peripheral monocytes and induce their transformation into M2 polarized glioma-associated microglia/macrophages (GAMs). The cross-talk between M2-GAMs and glioma cells leads to MMPs production and PD-L1 overexpression in GBM cells. M2-GAMs also suppress the immune system by secreting IDO, IL-10, and TGF-β, which activate regulatory T-cells and induce PD-1 expression by cytotoxic T-cells. These mechanisms are similar between the tumor core and the PBZ, with a decreasing gradient of immunosuppressive properties from the center to the periphery.

4. Molecular Characteristics of the PBZ

Here, we report the most relevant findings from immunohistochemistry analysis and the main genomic and transcriptomic characteristics of the PBZ in GBM. Some of these data have already been mentioned in the previous subsections as part of the narrative.

4.1. Immunohistochemistry

Glial fibrillary acidic protein (GFAP) immunolabeling in the PBZ is common and associated with reactive astrocytes.

Ki-67 immunoreactivity is dependent on the presence or not of infiltrating tumor cells

As already mentioned in the previous section, neo-vascularization markers, such as nestin and CD105, are expressed in the PBZ regardless of the presence of tumor cells [42]. Indeed, nestin is expressed also in reactive astrocytes and normal glia of the PBZ [34]. The presence and activation of mitogen-activated protein kinases both in tumors and the PBZ was also shown. These are signal transduction pathways activated by growth factors. In particular, the presence and activation of the extracellular signal-regulated kinase ERK1/2 and stress-activated protein kinases/c-Jun NH2-terminal kinases (JNKs) were detected [34,111]. As per nestin, this was shown independently of the presence of neoplastic cells and not only in reactive astrocytes, but also in apparently normal glial cells. ERKs play a crucial role in transducing growth factor signals to the nucleus and are involved in a wide range of biological responses, including cell proliferation, differentiation and motility; thus, this pathway might be involved in tumor progression. The role of JNK is more controversial. It is strongly expressed in the tumor core. Enhanced JNK activation has been found in brain tumor cell lines in response to epidermal growth factor, and the isoform JNK2a2 promotes phenotypes associated with tumorigenesis and proliferation [112,113]. However, JNK is also associated with apoptosis [114]. Prolonged OS has been shown in GBM patients who presented in their PBZs a higher expression of JNK in its activated form (pJNK), a higher ratio between pJNK and total JNK expression (pJNK/tJNK), and higher pJNK/nestin and (pJNK/tJNK)/nestin ratios [34].

Increased expression of HIF-1α as well as other hypoxia-regulated proteins, such as VEGF, in the PBZ have been correlated with reduced progression-free survival after surgery and adjuvant treatment [115].

The tumor border, sometimes called the infiltration zone, showed strong staining for the "signal transducer and activator of transcription" STAT-1, both in tumor elements and in reactive astrocytes and microglia of the non-invaded brain [116]. STAT proteins are intracellular transcription factors activated by the membrane cytokine receptor JAK (the JAJK/STAT pathway) that mediate many aspects of cellular immunity, proliferation, apoptosis, and differentiation. STAT-1 can be induced by interferon γ and growth factors such as the interleukins IL-6 and IL-10, growth hormone, thrombopoietin, and insulin-like growth-factor binding proteins (IGFBP-3). The role of STAT-1 expression in GBM and the PBZ is controversial. Its involvement in apoptosis could constitute a neuroprotective mechanism and could favor response to chemotherapy [116]. However, a correlation between increased STAT-1 expression and shorter overall survival has been documented [117]. This could be related to overexpression of STAT-1 in its inactivated form, as suggested by the restriction of the staining to the cytoplasm of tumor cells, indicating that in glioblastomas STAT-1 is not translocated to the nucleus [116].

Microglia of the PBZ also avidly stain for A1 adenosine receptor (A1AR), one of the receptors for the regulatory nucleoside adenosine expressed in response to cellular stress and damage, such as episodes of tissue hypoxia and inflammation. A1AR has anti-inflammatory properties and its expression seems to play an anti-tumorigenic role mediated by microglia cells [118].

Our research group recently showed that galectin-3-binding protein (LGALS3BP), a secreted, hyperglycosylated protein, is highly expressed, with a cytoplasmatic pattern, in the GBM tumor core, while it is barely detectable in the PBZ, where it is primarily confined to perineuronal glial cells [119]. This secreted protein has several proposed roles in contributing to a pro-tumorigenic microenvironment (for a review, consult Capone et al. [120]). While we could not show a correlation between this expression and any significant clinicpathological finding, we showed that tumor cells are the source of extracellular vesicle (EV)-associated LGALS3BP. Indeed, increased levels of EV-associated LGALS3BP were found in glioma patients compared with healthy donors, with increasing concentrations associated with increasing glioma grade [119,121]. These findings are relevant, since they show that GBM cells secrete LGALS3BP, probably to favor tumor progression in the PBZ, and circulating EV-associated LGALS3BP could have a role in "liquid biopsy" from plasma sampling in GBM diagnosis and monitoring. Moreover, LGALS3BP could be a target for non-internalizing antibody–drug conjugates [122], which are considered as a promising new frontier of personalized cancer medicine [123].

4.2. Genomic and Transcriptomic Characteristics

Studies from the French Grand Ouest Glioma Project could not find significant genomic alterations in non-infiltrated PBZs [24,35], while tumor-cell-infiltrated PBZs showed some genomic alterations in common with their tumor cores, in particular, chromosome 7 polysomy, EGFR amplification, and chromosome 10 deletion.

However, other research groups, including ours, could detect some abnormal gene expression in PBZs not invaded by tumor cells upon pathological analysis [15,124]. Indeed, when matching genomic alterations of a tumor core with the corresponding PBZ in a single patient, a variable amount of correlation was found [124,125]. Non-infiltrated PBZs and enhancing tumors were shown to share some genomic anomalies: del(1p36), del(2p21), MDM2 and CDK4 amplification, and amplification of 15q24.1, 219, and 222 [14]. CDK4 is a known cancer promoter gene involved in several systemic cancers, including breast carcinoma, that participates in the Cyclin D1 (CCND1)–CDK4/6–CDKN2A (p16INK4A)–Rb axis, which is often altered in the GBM [126]. Overexpression of CDK4 in the GBM PBZ is related to poor outcomes [125].

Indeed, gene expression shows only a partial overlap between the tumor core and the PBZ. Both tissues show upregulation of genes related to angiogenesis, the extracellular matrix, and cellular senescence and with stemness features, while downregulation is seen in tumor-suppressor genes, such as SLC17A7 and CHD5 [127]. Moreover, the PBZ shows upregulation of UBE2C, NUSAP1, IGFBP2, SERPINA3, and PBK genes when compared to the tumor core [127].

When summarizing transcriptomic data, it should be kept in mind that the possible infiltration of tumor-infiltrating cells or even of glioma stem cells could influence the reported data, as only a few manuscripts have tried to minimize this possible bias. We will therefore now focus on these studies.

When comparing tumor cores, non-invaded PBZs, and normal white matter from non-glioma patients, several differences in gene expression were found [15]. Briefly, tumor and PBZ samples showed significant changes in the expression of 1323 genes. Among genes with at least a 10-fold difference in expression level, 20 genes were overexpressed in GBM when compared to the PBZ, while 45 genes were downregulated. High overexpression was seen for genes involved in angiogenesis (VEGF and ANGPT2), genes associated with cell growth (IGFBP2 and GAP43) and with the cell-cycle activator CKS2, and genes encoding proteins associated with extracellular matrix formation, including COL4A1, COL4A2, COL1A1, COL3A1, and COL1A2. The majority of the 45 genes highly downregulated in GBM compared to the PBZ were involved in the development of the nervous system (MOG, RAPGEF5, GRM3, SH3GL3, NINJ2, UGT8, MOBP, and MBP).

PBZs with no tumor cell infiltration showed significant differences in the expression of 57 genes compared to white matter from control patients: 15 genes were overexpressed and 42 genes were downregulated in the PBZs. EGFR expression levels showed the largest difference between healthy white matter and PBZs, being highly expressed in the latter. Moreover, genes belonging to two main relevant biological processes were particularly deregulated in the PBZs. In detail, genes associated with growth and proliferation (CSRP2, TAZ, ID3, and DTNA) and cell motility/adhesion (HIST2H2AA, EGFR, IGFBP5, VCAM1, and CD99) were upregulated, while genes involved in neurogenesis (SYNJ1, NBEA, SERPINI1, CNTNAP2, and RELN) and several tumor-suppressor genes (BAI3, PEG3, PRDM2, and RB1CC1), along with the natural killer receptor KLRC1, were downregulated in the PBZs.

Interpretation of the above data is difficult, with the postulate of a "pre-cancerous" state of brain tissue surrounding the tumor under the influence of cross-talk between tumor cells and normal cells resulting in a recruitment of the latter cells in GBM proliferation and growth being an intriguing possibility.

In another work, GBM de novo tumor cores and PBZ transcriptomes were compared through a serial analysis of gene expression (SAGE) technique, and their miRNomes were compared through a subsequent microRNA deep sequencing [62]. The results were analyzed separately for short- (<36 months) and long-term ($\geq$36 months) survivors. In agreement with other groups' findings [35,45], the transcriptional features of the PBZ showed a predominance of the TCGA neural subtype [128], regardless of the presence or not of tumor cell infiltration and with no correlation with the tumor core features. The tumor center showed overexpression of several molecules belonging to the "mesenchymal signature" of glioblastoma, likely due to microglia and reactive astrocytes infiltration.

Chemokine (C-X-C motif) ligand 14 (CXCL14) RNA was found to be overexpressed in the tumor cores and PBZs of both long- and short-term survivors when compared to healthy white matter from non-glioma patients [62]. However, while in long-term survivors its expression resulted in comparable tumor centers and PBZs, in short-term survivors it was overexpressed in the majority of tumor center samples compared to paired PBZs [62]. CXCL14 is a small cytokine, mainly contributing to the regulation of immune cell migration [129], whose transcription is induced in microglia activated towards the pro-invasive, immunosuppressive (M2) phenotype by glioma cells in experimental conditions [130].

Transforming growth factor beta-induced (TGFBI) protein is considered a feature of the mesenchymal GBM subtype. TGFBI RNA was found to be overexpressed in both the tumor cores and PBZs of all patients compared to healthy white matter from controls, with significant overexpression in the tumor cores between long-term and short-term survivors [62]. TGFBI is a protein secreted in the extracellular matrix, the mediator of the non-SMAD-mediated TGFβ signaling pathway in GBM [131], that interacts with several other extracellular matrix components, such as collagens, in cell–cell or cell–substrate adhesion. TGFBI is preferentially secreted by M2-like GAMs and indicates poor prognosis in GBM patients [132].

Giambra and colleagues found some peculiar gains in some loci in the short arms of chromosomes 11 and 16 in PBZs, not shared by tumor cores, focusing on the possible role of the EXT2 gene, which is involved in the biosynthesis of the heparan sulfates—glycosaminoglycans distributed on the cell surfaces and in the extracellular matrices of most tissues which could be involved in angiogenesis and tumor proliferation [125].

mRNA analysis of tumor cores compared with their own PBZs showed several signs of a higher participation of reactive cell types, such as microglia and reactive astrocytes, which could be depicted as a generally more "mesenchymal" feature, in short-term survivors but not in long-term survivors [62]. Comparing the PBZs of short-term and long-term survivors, indications of a possible higher contribution of tumor "stromal" cells, such as IGFBP5 mRNA expressed by reactive astrocytes, in short-term cases were documented. In addition, a sound overexpression of the extracellular protein lumican in long-term survivors' PBZs as compared to short-term survivors' ones was detected. This stromal protein has recently been shown to positively correlate with prolonged survival after tumor resection in pancreatic ductal adenocarcinomas due to its limiting role in EGFR-expressing pancreatic cancer progression [133].

MicroRNA analysis showed overexpression of miRNAs involved in TGFβ active pathways and mediators of a general state of immune escape typically sustaining glioma growth in all tumor core and PBZ samples compared with heathy white matter. In particular, overexpression of miR-106b and miR-93, found to target a ligand of the activating receptor of natural killer (NK) cells (NKG2DL), and of the TGFβ-induced miR-183, reported to suppress tumor-associated NK cells, was detected. The latter "oncomiR" (miR-183-5p), together with the chromosome 7-located miR-182-5p and miR-96-5p, showed differential expression between PBZ samples with detectable tumor cell infiltration and non-infiltrated samples. These three miRNAs are recognized as mediators of TGFβ signaling in GBM [134].

Underexpression of miR-128a, miR-181a, miR-181b, and miR-181c in tumor centers compared to PBZs was shown [135]. These miRNAs show peak expression at the adult stage when compared to embryonic and early post-natal stages: this might indicate some non-random correlation with a de-differentiated state of tumor cells (having lost their "adult brain signatures").

Piwecka and collaborators showed that miR-625 was downregulated in the PBZ compared to normal tissue but not in the tumor core [136]. MiR-625 overexpression suppresses cell proliferation and colony formation, induces G0/G1 arrest, increases chemosensitivity to temozolomide by targeting AKT2 in glioma cell lines, and suppresses tumor growth and angiogenesis in animal models [137].

The target-mimetic, sponge/decoy function of long non-coding RNAs (lncRNAs) on microRNAs was recently uncovered: they can act as miRNA sponges, reducing their regulatory effect on mRNAs [138]. A higher expression of the highly expressed long non-coding RNA in glioblastoma (lncHERG), acting as an miR-940 sponge, was found to indicate a lower survival rate and poorer prognosis, being related to cell proliferation, migration, and invasion, both in vitro and in vivo. LncHERG expression was shown to be higher in glioblastoma than non-tumor tissues, while the tumor suppressor miR-940 was, on the contrary, shown to be downregulated in glioblastoma tissues compared to peritumoral tissues [139].

Very few data on PBZ proteomics are available [140], with some proteins being overexpressed in the PBZ, in particular, the histone H3F3A and the crystallin B α-chain (CRYAB), both recognized as oncogenes.

The main immunohistochemistry, genomic, and transcriptomic characteristics of the PBZ are summarized in Figure 4.

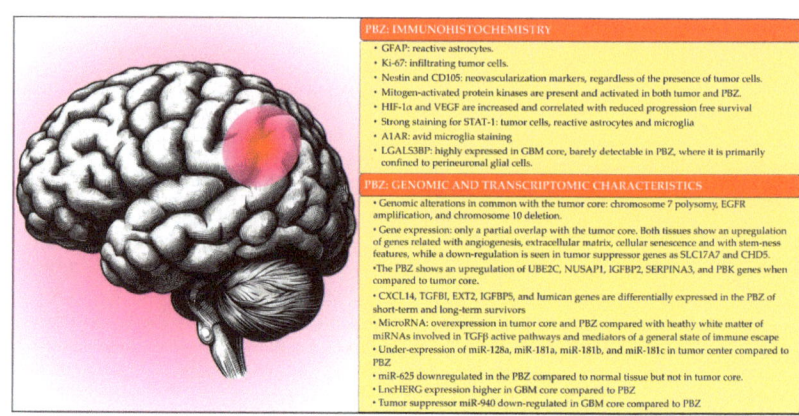

Figure 4. Main immunohistochemistry, genomic, and transcriptomic characteristics of peritumoral brain zone (PBZ).

5. Discussion

Analysis of the cellular and molecular characteristics of the PBZ is fundamental not only for understanding GBM pathophysiology but also to enhance therapeutic options since glioblastoma will almost inevitably recur from this tissue after extensive surgical resection and radio-chemotherapy. Indeed, several molecular mechanisms involved in the tumor core–PBZ cross-talk are currently regarded as potential therapeutic targets.

The key concepts of this review are:

- The PBZ is the real target of post-surgical therapies; therefore, understanding it is of paramount translational significance.
- Only in about one third of cases is it possible to detect tumor cells via microscopic analysis of the PBZ; nonetheless, we can observe distinct abnormal features also in cases of no infiltration.
- If some data on the PBZ can suggest the influence on the features of this area of tumor cells migrated well beyond the tumor border, diluted in brain parenchyma, and possibly having a "dormant" feature and therefore liable to be missed by pathological examination, others suggest the recruitment of surrounding cells reprogrammed towards a neoplastic phenotype.
- Angiogenesis and hypoxia play a pivotal role in influencing the tumor and PBZ microenvironment.
- An increasing immunocompromised gradient is seen from the PBZ to the tumor core
- The role of inflammatory cells has been illuminated in recent years, and several alterations in the PBZ can be related to an activation of microglia and astrocytes that could promote tumor growth and invasion.
- The transcriptomic profile of the PBZ is extremely complex, since this tissue differs from normal white matter, shares some tumor core characteristics, and possibly shows some peculiar alterations. Overall, the PBZ seems to be "half-way" on the road towards malignancy. However, the data are highly heterogeneous due to possible infiltration of glioma cells/glioma stem cells. Single-cell analysis could improve our understanding.

In summary, current data show that GBM actively induces transformation of the surrounding environment, inducing degradation of the extracellular matrix and recruiting astrocytes, microglia, macrophages, and regulatory T cells to promote an immunosuppressive environment. However, these mechanisms have a decreasing gradient at increasing distance from the tumor necrotic core, with the presence of still-competent immune cells in the PBZ, namely, a higher number of PD-1 negative CD8+ cytotoxic T-cells. Currently, sev eral ongoing trials are trying to enhance self-immunity [141,142]. Since the post-operative target of therapies is the PBZ, future research should focus on its molecular mechanisms, which only partially overlap with those of the tumor core.

Indeed, while a huge amount of data are available on the glioblastoma core, the PBZ is still relatively poorly investigated, with increasing interest in it having been shown only in the last few years in the medical literature. Moreover, it is difficult to reproduce the PBZ microenvironment in both in vitro and in vivo animal studies, as patient-derived cell lines can usually be obtained only from the most aggressive, tumor core-like GBM cells that infiltrate the PBZ. Therefore, most of the data on the PBZ can be derived by histopathologic and multi-omics analyses of appropriately selected surgical samples. Hence, it is fundamental for neurosurgeons to be directly involved in neuro-oncology research in order to opportunely select patients from whom PBZs can be safely sampled, pre-plan PBZ tissue resection with an adequate intraoperative methodology, and store the samples in an appropriate form for the planned biological analyses.

6. Conclusions

A better understanding of the PBZ would be of high translational potential. Indeed, the pathophysiology of the PBZ can be indicate early events of GBM tumorigenesis and help in detecting its initial alterations. From a surgical point of view, understanding of PBZ characteristics could help in the development of intraoperative techniques aiming to detect areas of alteration surrounding the macroscopically evident tumor. From a translational and therapeutic point of view, new molecular targets and possibly personalized adjuvant therapies could be developed with a better understanding of the PBZ, which is the real target of post-surgical therapies.

Author Contributions: G.T.: conceptualization; methodology; writing—original draft preparation. A.M.: writing—review and editing; supervision. All authors have read and agreed to the published version of the manuscript.

Funding: This research received no external funding.

Institutional Review Board Statement: The data included in Figures 1 and 2 were part of a prospective GBM biobanking study authorized by the Chieti-Pescara Local Ethics Committee (EC number: 08/21.05.2020).

Informed Consent Statement: The patients in Figures 1 and 2 gave written consent to the use of their radiological and surgical data in anonymous form.

Data Availability Statement: Data are contained within the article.

Conflicts of Interest: The authors declare no conflict of interest.

References

1. Ostrom, Q.T.; Cioffi, G.; Waite, K.; Kruchko, C.; Barnholtz-Sloan, J.S. CBTRUS Statistical Report: Primary Brain and Other Central Nervous System Tumors Diagnosed in the United States in 2014–2018. *Neuro-Oncology* **2021**, *23*, iii1–iii105. [CrossRef] [PubMed]
2. Louis, D.N.; Perry, A.; Wesseling, P.; Brat, D.J.; Cree, I.A.; Figarella-Branger, D.; Hawkins, C.; Ng, H.K.; Pfister, S.M.; Reifenberger, G.; et al. The 2021 WHO Classification of Tumors of the Central Nervous System: A summary. *Neuro-Oncology* **2021**, *23*, 1231–1251. [CrossRef]
3. Ziu, M.; Kim, B.Y.S.; Jiang, W.; Ryken, T.; Olson, J.J. The role of radiation therapy in treatment of adults with newly diagnosed glioblastoma multiforme: A systematic review and evidence-based clinical practice guideline update. *J. Neuro-Oncol.* **2020**, *150*, 215–267. [CrossRef]
4. Redjal, N.; Nahed, B.V.; Dietrich, J.; Kalkanis, S.N.; Olson, J.J. Congress of neurological surgeons systematic review and evidence-based guidelines update on the role of chemotherapeutic management and antiangiogenic treatment of newly diagnosed glioblastoma in adults. *J. Neuro-Oncol.* **2020**, *150*, 165–213. [CrossRef]
5. Domino, J.S.; Ormond, D.R.; Germano, I.M.; Sami, M.; Ryken, T.C.; Olson, J.J. Cytoreductive surgery in the management of newly diagnosed glioblastoma in adults: A systematic review and evidence-based clinical practice guideline update. *J. Neuro-Oncol.* **2020**, *150*, 121–142. [CrossRef]

6. Ius, T.; Sabatino, G.; Panciani, P.P.; Fontanella, M.M.; Rudà, R.; Castellano, A.; Barbagallo, G.M.V.; Belotti, F.; Boccaletti, R.; Catapano, G.; et al. Surgical management of Glioma Grade 4: Technical update from the neuro-oncology section of the Italian Society of Neurosurgery (SINch®): A systematic review. *J. Neuro-Oncol.* **2023**, *162*, 267–293. [CrossRef]
7. Mier-García, J.F.; Ospina-Santa, S.; Orozco-Mera, J.; Ma, R.; Plaha, P. Supramaximal versus gross total resection in Glioblastoma IDH wild-type and Astrocytoma, IDH-mutant, grade 4, effect on overall and progression free survival: Systematic review and meta-analysis. *J. Neuro-Oncol.* **2023**, *164*, 31–41. [CrossRef]
8. Petrecca, K.; Guiot, M.-C.; Panet-Raymond, V.; Souhami, L. Failure pattern following complete resection plus radiotherapy and temozolomide is at the resection margin in patients with glioblastoma. *J. Neuro-Oncol.* **2013**, *111*, 19–23. [CrossRef]
9. Dandy, W.E. Removal of Right Cerebral Hemisphere for Certain Tumors with Hemiplegia. *J. Am. Med. Assoc.* **1928**, *90*, 823–825. [CrossRef]
10. Capper, D.; Sahm, F.; Jeibmann, A.; Habel, A.; Paulus, W.; Troost, D.; von Deimling, A. Addressing Diffuse Glioma as a Systemic Brain Disease with Single-Cell Analysis. *Arch. Neurol.* **2012**, *69*, 523–526. [CrossRef]
11. Silbergeld, D.L.; Chicoine, M.R. Isolation and characterization of human malignant glioma cells from histologically normal brain. *J. Neurosurg.* **1997**, *86*, 525–531. [CrossRef] [PubMed]
12. Mangiola, A.; de Bonis, P.; Maira, G.; Balducci, M.; Sica, G.; Lama, G.; Lauriola, L.; Anile, C. Invasive tumor cells and prognosis in a selected population of patients with glioblastoma multiforme. *Cancer* **2008**, *113*, 841–846. [CrossRef]
13. The Cancer Genome Atlas Research Network. Comprehensive genomic characterization defines human glioblastoma genes and core pathways. *Nature* **2008**, *455*, 1061–1068. [CrossRef]
14. Fidoamore, A.; Cristiano, L.; Antonosante, A.; D'angelo, M.; Di Giacomo, E.; Astarita, C.; Giordano, A.; Ippoliti, R.; Benedetti, E.; Cimini, A. Glioblastoma Stem Cells Microenvironment: The Paracrine Roles of the Niche in Drug and Radioresistance. *Stem Cells Int.* **2016**, *2016*, 6809105. [CrossRef] [PubMed]
15. Mangiola, A.; Saulnier, N.; De Bonis, P.; Orteschi, D.; Sica, G.; Lama, G.; Pettorini, B.L.; Sabatino, G.; Zollino, M.; Lauriola, L.; et al. Gene Expression Profile of Glioblastoma Peritumoral Tissue: An Ex Vivo Study. *PLoS ONE* **2013**, *8*, e57145. [CrossRef]
16. Dapash, M.; Hou, D.; Castro, B.; Lee-Chang, C.; Lesniak, M.S. The Interplay between Glioblastoma and Its Microenvironment. *Cells* **2021**, *10*, 2257. [CrossRef] [PubMed]
17. DeCordova, S.; Shastri, A.; Tsolaki, A.G.; Yasmin, H.; Klein, L.; Singh, S.K.; Kishore, U. Molecular Heterogeneity and Immunosuppressive Microenvironment in Glioblastoma. *Front. Immunol.* **2020**, *11*, 1402. [CrossRef] [PubMed]
18. Simon, T.; Jackson, E.; Giamas, G. Breaking through the glioblastoma micro-environment via extracellular vesicles. *Oncogene* **2020**, *39*, 4477–4490. [CrossRef]
19. Ye, Z.; Ai, X.; Zhao, L.; Fei, F.; Wang, P.; Zhou, S. Phenotypic plasticity of myeloid cells in glioblastoma development, progression, and therapeutics. *Oncogene* **2021**, *40*, 6059–6070. [CrossRef]
20. Faisal, S.M.; Comba, A.; Varela, M.L.; Argento, A.E.; Brumley, E.; Abel, C.; Castro, M.G.; Lowenstein, P.R. The complex interactions between the cellular and non-cellular components of the brain tumor microenvironmental landscape and their therapeutic implications. *Front. Oncol.* **2022**, *12*, 1005069. [CrossRef]
21. Louis, D.N.; Perry, A.; Reifenberger, G.; Von Deimling, A.; Figarella-Branger, D.; Cavenee, W.K.; Ohgaki, H.; Wiestler, O.D.; Kleihues, P.; Ellison, D.W. The 2016 World Health Organization Classification of Tumors of the Central Nervous System: A summary. *Acta Neuropathol.* **2016**, *131*, 803–820. [CrossRef]
22. Ohgaki, H.; Kleihues, P. The Definition of Primary and Secondary Glioblastoma. *Clin. Cancer Res.* **2013**, *19*, 764–772. [CrossRef]
23. Ohgaki, H.; Kleihues, P. Genetic Pathways to Primary and Secondary Glioblastoma. *Am. J. Pathol.* **2007**, *170*, 1445–1453. [CrossRef] [PubMed]
24. Lemée, J.-M.; Clavreul, A.; Aubry, M.; Com, E.; De Tayrac, M.; Eliat, P.-A.; Henry, C.; Rousseau, A.; Mosser, J.; Menei, P. Characterizing the peritumoral brain zone in glioblastoma: A multidisciplinary analysis. *J. Neuro-Oncol.* **2015**, *122*, 53–61. [CrossRef] [PubMed]
25. Broggi, G.; Altieri, R.; Barresi, V.; Certo, F.; Barbagallo, G.M.V.; Zanelli, M.; Palicelli, A.; Magro, G.; Caltabiano, R. Histologic Definition of Enhancing Core and FLAIR Hyperintensity Region of Glioblastoma, IDH-Wild Type: A Clinico-Pathologic Study on a Single-Institution Series. *Brain Sci.* **2023**, *13*, 248. [CrossRef] [PubMed]
26. Altieri, R.; Barbagallo, D.; Certo, F.; Broggi, G.; Ragusa, M.; Di Pietro, C.; Caltabiano, R.; Magro, G.; Peschillo, S.; Purrello, M.; et al. Peritumoral Microenvironment in High-Grade Gliomas: From FLAIRectomy to Microglia–Glioma Cross-Talk. *Brain Sci.* **2021**, *11*, 200. [CrossRef] [PubMed]
27. Certo, F.; Altieri, R.; Maione, M.; Schonauer, C.; Sortino, G.; Fiumanò, G.; Tirrò, E.; Massimino, M.; Broggi, G.; Vigneri, P.; et al. FLAIRectomy in Supramarginal Resection of Glioblastoma Correlates with Clinical Outcome and Survival Analysis: A Prospective, Single Institution, Case Series. *Oper. Neurosurg.* **2021**, *20*, 151–163. [CrossRef]
28. Deng, Z.; Yan, Y.; Zhong, D.; Yang, G.; Tang, W.; Lü, F.; Xie, B.; Liu, B. Quantitative analysis of glioma cell invasion by diffusion tensor imaging. *J. Clin. Neurosci.* **2010**, *17*, 1530–1536. [CrossRef]
29. Lu, S.; Ahn, D.; Johnson, G.; Law, M.; Zagzag, D.; Grossman, R.I.; Bette, S.; Huber, T.; Gempt, J.; Boeckh-Behrens, T.; et al. Diffusion-Tensor MR Imaging of Intracranial Neoplasia and Associated Peritumoral Edema: Introduction of the Tumor Infiltration Index. *Radiology* **2004**, *232*, 221–228. [CrossRef]

30. Prasanna, P.; Patel, J.; Partovi, S.; Madabhushi, A.; Tiwari, P. Radiomic features from the peritumoral brain parenchyma on treatment-naïve multi-parametric MR imaging predict long versus short-term survival in glioblastoma multiforme: Preliminary findings. *Eur. Radiol.* **2017**, *27*, 4188–4197. [CrossRef]
31. Dasgupta, A.; Geraghty, B.; Maralani, P.J.; Malik, N.; Sandhu, M.; Detsky, J.; Tseng, C.-L.; Soliman, H.; Myrehaug, S.; Husain, Z.; et al. Quantitative mapping of individual voxels in the peritumoral region of IDH-wildtype glioblastoma to distinguish between tumor infiltration and edema. *J. Neuro-Oncol.* **2021**, *153*, 251–261. [CrossRef]
32. Malik, N.; Geraghty, B.; Dasgupta, A.; Maralani, P.J.; Sandhu, M.; Detsky, J.; Tseng, C.-L.; Soliman, H.; Myrehaug, S.; Husain, Z.; et al. MRI radiomics to differentiate between low grade glioma and glioblastoma peritumoral region. *J. Neuro-Oncol.* **2021**, *155*, 181–191. [CrossRef]
33. Guerrini, F.; Roca, E.; Spena, G. Supramarginal Resection for Glioblastoma: It Is Time to Set Boundaries! A Critical Review on a Hot Topic. *Brain Sci.* **2022**, *12*, 652. [CrossRef]
34. Mangiola, A.; Lama, G.; Giannitelli, C.; De Bonis, P.; Anile, C.; Lauriola, L.; La Torre, G.; Sabatino, G.; Maira, G.; Jhanwar-Uniyal, M.; et al. Stem Cell Marker Nestin and c-Jun NH2-Terminal Kinases in Tumor and Peritumor Areas of Glioblastoma Multiforme: Possible Prognostic Implications. *Clin. Cancer Res.* **2007**, *13*, 6970–6977. [CrossRef] [PubMed]
35. Aubry, M.; de Tayrac, M.; Etcheverry, A.; Clavreul, A.; Saikali, S.; Menei, P.; Mosser, J. From the core to beyond the margin: A genomic picture of glioblastoma intratumor heterogeneity. *Oncotarget* **2015**, *6*, 12094–12109. [CrossRef] [PubMed]
36. Idoate, M.A.; Díez Valle, R.; Echeveste, J.; Tejada, S. Pathological characterization of the glioblastoma border as shown during surgery using 5-aminolevulinic acid-induced fluorescence. *Neuropathology* **2011**, *31*, 575–582. [CrossRef] [PubMed]
37. Clavreul, A.; Etcheverry, A.; Tétaud, C.; Rousseau, A.; Avril, T.; Henry, C.; Mosser, J.; Menei, P. Identification of two glioblastoma-associated stromal cell subtypes with different carcinogenic properties in histologically normal surgical margins. *J. Neuro-Oncol.* **2015**, *122*, 1–10. [CrossRef] [PubMed]
38. Glas, M.; Rath, B.H.; Simon, M.; Reinartz, R.; Schramme, A.; Trageser, D.; Eisenreich, R.; Leinhaas, A.; Keller, M.; Schildhaus, H.; et al. Residual tumor cells are unique cellular targets in glioblastoma. *Ann. Neurol.* **2010**, *68*, 264–269. [CrossRef]
39. Piccirillo, S.G.M.; Dietz, S.; Madhu, B.; Griffiths, J.; Price, S.J.; Collins, V.P.; Watts, C. Fluorescence-guided surgical sampling of glioblastoma identifies phenotypically distinct tumour-initiating cell populations in the tumour mass and margin. *Br. J. Cancer* **2012**, *107*, 462–468. [CrossRef]
40. Piccirillo, S.G.M.; Combi, R.; Cajola, L.; Patrizi, A.; Redaelli, S.; Bentivegna, A.; Baronchelli, S.; Maira, G.; Pollo, B.; Mangiola, A.; et al. Distinct pools of cancer stem-like cells coexist within human glioblastomas and display different tumorigenicity and independent genomic evolution. *Oncogene* **2009**, *28*, 1807–1811. [CrossRef]
41. Bastola, S.; Pavlyukov, M.S.; Yamashita, D.; Ghosh, S.; Cho, H.; Kagaya, N.; Zhang, Z.; Minata, M.; Lee, Y.; Sadahiro, H.; et al. Glioma-initiating cells at tumor edge gain signals from tumor core cells to promote their malignancy. *Nat. Commun.* **2020**, *11*, 4660. [CrossRef]
42. Sica; Sica, G.; Lama, G.; Anile, C.; Geloso, M.C.; La Torre, G.; De Bonis, P.; Maira, G.; Lauriola, L.; Jhanwar-Uniyal, M.; et al. Assessment of angiogenesis by CD105 and nestin expression in peritumor tissue of glioblastoma. *Int. J. Oncol.* **2011**, *38*, 41–49. [CrossRef] [PubMed]
43. Lemée, J.-M.; Clavreul, A.; Menei, P. Intratumoral heterogeneity in glioblastoma: Don't forget the peritumoral brain zone. *Neuro-Oncology* **2015**, *17*, 1322–1332. [CrossRef]
44. Nimbalkar, V.P.; Kruthika, B.S.; Sravya, P.; Rao, S.; Sugur, H.S.; Verma, B.K.; Chickabasaviah, Y.T.; Arivazhagan, A.; Kondaiah, P.; Santosh, V. Differential gene expression in peritumoral brain zone of glioblastoma: Role of SERPINA3 in promoting invasion, stemness and radioresistance of glioma cells and association with poor patient prognosis and recurrence. *J. Neuro-Oncol.* **2021**, *152*, 55–65. [CrossRef]
45. Gill, B.J.; Pisapia, D.J.; Malone, H.R.; Goldstein, H.; Lei, L.; Sonabend, A.; Yun, J.; Samanamud, J.; Sims, J.S.; Banu, M.; et al. MRI-localized biopsies reveal subtype-specific differences in molecular and cellular composition at the margins of glioblastoma. *Proc. Natl. Acad. Sci. USA* **2014**, *111*, 12550–12555. [CrossRef]
46. Charles, N.A.; Holland, E.C.; Gilbertson, R.; Glass, R.; Kettenmann, H. The brain tumor microenvironment. *Glia* **2011**, *59*, 1169–1180. [CrossRef]
47. Ahir, B.K.; Engelhard, H.H.; Lakka, S.S. Tumor Development and Angiogenesis in Adult Brain Tumor: Glioblastoma. *Mol. Neurobiol.* **2020**, *57*, 2461–2478. [CrossRef] [PubMed]
48. Domènech, M.; Hernández, A.; Plaja, A.; Martínez-Balibrea, E.; Balañà, C. Hypoxia: The Cornerstone of Glioblastoma. *Int. J. Mol. Sci.* **2021**, *22*, 12608. [CrossRef] [PubMed]
49. Shi, T.; Zhu, J.; Zhang, X.; Mao, X. The Role of Hypoxia and Cancer Stem Cells in Development of Glioblastoma. *Cancers* **2023**, *15*, 2613. [CrossRef]
50. D'alessio, A.; Proietti, G.; Lama, G.; Biamonte, F.; Lauriola, L.; Moscato, U.; Vescovi, A.; Mangiola, A.; Angelucci, C.; Sica, G. Analysis of angiogenesis related factors in glioblastoma, peritumoral tissue and their derived cancer stem cells. *Oncotarget* **2016**, *7*, 78541–78556. [CrossRef]
51. Tamura, R.; Ohara, K.; Sasaki, H.; Morimoto, Y.; Yoshida, K.; Toda, M. Histopathological vascular investigation of the peritumoral brain zone of glioblastomas. *J. Neuro-Oncol.* **2018**, *136*, 233–241. [CrossRef]

52. Gabrilovich, D.I.; Chen, H.L.; Girgis, K.R.; Cunningham, H.T.; Meny, G.M.; Nadaf, S.; Kavanaugh, D.; Carbone, D.P. Production of vascular endothelial growth factor by human tumors inhibits the functional maturation of dendritic cells. *Nat. Med.* **1996**, *2*, 1096–1103. [CrossRef]
53. Ohm, J.E.; Gabrilovich, D.I.; Sempowski, G.D.; Kisseleva, E.; Parman, K.S.; Nadaf, S.; Carbone, D.P. VEGF inhibits T-cell development and may contribute to tumor-induced immune suppression. *Blood* **2003**, *101*, 4878–4886. [CrossRef] [PubMed]
54. Escartin, C.; Galea, E.; Lakatos, A.; O'callaghan, J.P.; Petzold, G.C.; Serrano-Pozo, A.; Steinhäuser, C.; Volterra, A.; Carmignoto, G.; Agarwal, A.; et al. Reactive astrocyte nomenclature, definitions, and future directions. *Nat. Neurosci.* **2021**, *24*, 312–325. [CrossRef] [PubMed]
55. Heiland, D.H.; Ravi, V.M.; Behringer, S.P.; Frenking, J.H.; Wurm, J.; Joseph, K.; Garrelfs, N.W.C.; Strähle, J.; Heynckes, S. Grauvogel, J.; et al. Tumor-associated reactive astrocytes aid the evolution of immunosuppressive environment in glioblastoma. *Nat. Commun.* **2019**, *10*, 2541. [CrossRef] [PubMed]
56. Placone, A.L.; Quiñones-Hinojosa, A.; Searson, P.C. The role of astrocytes in the progression of brain cancer: Complicating the picture of the tumor microenvironment. *Tumor Biol.* **2016**, *37*, 61–69. [CrossRef]
57. Liddelow, S.A.; Guttenplan, K.A.; Clarke, L.E.; Bennett, F.C.; Bohlen, C.J.; Schirmer, L.; Bennett, M.L.; Münch, A.E.; Chung, W.-S. Peterson, T.C.; et al. Neurotoxic reactive astrocytes are induced by activated microglia. *Nature* **2017**, *541*, 481–487. [CrossRef]
58. Lin, Q.; Liu, Z.; Ling, F.; Xu, G. Astrocytes protect glioma cells from chemotherapy and upregulate survival genes via gap junctional communication. *Mol. Med. Rep.* **2016**, *13*, 1329–1335. [CrossRef]
59. Munoz, J.L.; Rodriguez-Cruz, V.; Greco, S.J.; Ramkissoon, S.H.; Ligon, K.L.; Rameshwar, P. Temozolomide resistance in glioblastoma cells occurs partly through epidermal growth factor receptor-mediated induction of connexin. *Cell Death Dis.* **2014**, *5*, e1145. [CrossRef]
60. Huang, J.-Y.; Cheng, Y.-J.; Lin, Y.-P.; Lin, H.-C.; Su, C.-C.; Juliano, R.; Yang, B.-C. Extracellular Matrix of Glioblastoma Inhibits Polarization and Transmigration of T Cells: The Role of Tenascin-C in Immune Suppression. *J. Immunol.* **2010**, *185*, 1450–1459. [CrossRef]
61. Fujita, M.; Zhu, X.; Sasaki, K.; Ueda, R.; Low, K.L.; Pollack, I.F.; Okada, H. Inhibition of STAT3 Promotes the Efficacy of Adoptive Transfer Therapy Using Type-1 CTLs by Modulation of the Immunological Microenvironment in a Murine Intracranial Glioma. *J. Immunol.* **2008**, *180*, 2089–2098. [CrossRef]
62. Fazi, B.; Felsani, A.; Grassi, L.; Moles, A.; D'andrea, D.; Toschi, N.; Sicari, D.; De Bonis, P.; Anile, C.; Guerrisi, M.G.; et al. The transcriptome and miRNome profiling of glioblastoma tissues and peritumoral regions highlights molecular pathways shared by tumors and surrounding areas and reveals differences between short-term and long-term survivors. *Oncotarget* **2015**, *6*, 22526–22552. [CrossRef] [PubMed]
63. Roggendorf, W.; Strupp, S.; Paulus, W. Distribution and characterization of microglia/macrophages in human brain tumors. *Acta Neuropathol.* **1996**, *92*, 288–293. [CrossRef] [PubMed]
64. da Fonseca, A.C.C.; Badie, B. Microglia and Macrophages in Malignant Gliomas: Recent Discoveries and Implications for Promising Therapies. *J. Immunol. Res.* **2013**, *2013*, 264124. [CrossRef]
65. Hussain, S.F.; Yang, D.; Suki, D.; Aldape, K.; Grimm, E.; Heimberger, A.B. The role of human glioma-infiltrating microglia/macrophages in mediating antitumor immune responses. *Neuro-Oncology* **2006**, *8*, 261–279. [CrossRef]
66. Watters, J.J.; Schartner, J.M.; Badie, B. Microglia function in brain tumors. *J. Neurosci. Res.* **2005**, *81*, 447–455. [CrossRef] [PubMed]
67. Butovsky, O.; Jedrychowski, M.P.; Moore, C.S.; Cialic, R.; Lanser, A.J.; Gabriely, G.; Koeglsperger, T.; Dake, B.; Wu, P.M.; E Doykan, C.; et al. Identification of a unique TGF-β–dependent molecular and functional signature in microglia. *Nat. Neurosci.* **2014**, *17*, 131–143. [CrossRef]
68. Michelucci, A.; Heurtaux, T.; Grandbarbe, L.; Morga, E.; Heuschling, P. Characterization of the microglial phenotype under specific pro-inflammatory and anti-inflammatory conditions: Effects of oligomeric and fibrillar amyloid-β. *J. Neuroimmunol.* **2009**, *210*, 3–12. [CrossRef]
69. Tamura, R.; Tamura, R.; Tanaka, T.; Tanaka, T.; Yamamoto, Y.; Yamamoto, Y.; Akasaki, Y.; Akasaki, Y.; Sasaki, H.; Sasaki, H.; et al. Dual role of macrophage in tumor immunity. *Immunotherapy* **2018**, *10*, 899–909. [CrossRef]
70. Paolicelli, R.C.; Sierra, A.; Stevens, B.; Tremblay, M.-E.; Aguzzi, A.; Ajami, B.; Amit, I.; Audinat, E.; Bechmann, I.; Bennett, M.; et al. Microglia states and nomenclature: A field at its crossroads. *Neuron* **2022**, *110*, 3458–3483. [CrossRef]
71. Lisi, L.; Stigliano, E.; Lauriola, L.; Navarra, P.; Russo, C.D. Proinflammatory-Activated Glioma Cells Induce a Switch in Microglial Polarization and Activation Status, from a Predominant M2b Phenotype to a Mixture of M1 and M2a/B Polarized Cells. *ASN Neuro* **2014**, *6*, 171–183. [CrossRef] [PubMed]
72. Ransohoff, R.M. A polarizing question: Do M1 and M2 microglia exist? *Nat. Neurosci.* **2016**, *19*, 987–991. [CrossRef] [PubMed]
73. Xue, J.; Schmidt, S.V.; Sander, J.; Draffehn, A.; Krebs, W.; Quester, I.; De Nardo, D.; Gohel, T.D.; Emde, M.; Schmidleithner, L.; et al. Transcriptome-based network analysis reveals a spectrum model of human macrophage activation. *Immunity* **2014**, *40*, 274–288. [CrossRef]
74. Lisi, L.; Ciotti, G.M.P.; Braun, D.; Kalinin, S.; Currò, D.; Dello Russo, C.; Coli, A.; Mangiola, A.; Anile, C.; Feinstein, D.L.; et al. Expression of iNOS, CD163 and ARG-1 taken as M1 and M2 markers of microglial polarization in human glioblastoma and the surrounding normal parenchyma. *Neurosci. Lett.* **2017**, *645*, 106–112. [CrossRef] [PubMed]

75. Rahimi Koshkaki, H.; Minasi, S.; Ugolini, A.; Trevisi, G.; Napoletano, C.; Zizzari, I.G.; Gessi, M.; Giangaspero, F.; Mangiola, A.; Nuti, M.; et al. Immunohistochemical Characterization of Immune Infiltrate in Tumor Microenvironment of Glioblastoma. *J. Pers. Med.* **2020**, *10*, 112. [CrossRef]
76. Annovazzi, L.; Mellai, M.; Bovio, E.; Mazzetti, S.; Pollo, B.; Schiffer, D. Microglia immunophenotyping in gliomas. *Oncol. Lett.* **2018**, *15*, 998–1006. [CrossRef]
77. Hambardzumyan, D.; Gutmann, D.H.; Kettenmann, H. The role of microglia and macrophages in glioma maintenance and progression. *Nat. Neurosci.* **2016**, *19*, 20–27. [CrossRef]
78. Sampson, J.H.; Gunn, M.D.; Fecci, P.E.; Ashley, D.M. Brain immunology and immunotherapy in brain tumours. *Nat. Rev. Cancer* **2020**, *20*, 12–25. [CrossRef] [PubMed]
79. Ge, Z.; Ding, S. The Crosstalk between Tumor-Associated Macrophages (TAMs) and Tumor Cells and the Corresponding Targeted Therapy. *Front. Oncol.* **2020**, *10*, 590941. [CrossRef]
80. Kim, Y.-H.; Jung, T.-Y.; Jung, S.; Jang, W.-Y.; Moon, K.-S.; Kim, I.-Y.; Lee, M.-C.; Lee, J.-J. Tumour-infiltrating T-cell subpopulations in glioblastomas. *Br. J. Neurosurg.* **2012**, *26*, 21–27. [CrossRef]
81. Woroniecka, K.; Chongsathidkiet, P.; Rhodin, K.; Kemeny, H.; Dechant, C.; Farber, S.H.; Elsamadicy, A.A.; Cui, X.; Koyama, S.; Jackson, C.; et al. T-Cell Exhaustion Signatures Vary with Tumor Type and Are Severe in Glioblastoma. *Clin. Cancer Res.* **2018**, *24*, 4175–4186. [CrossRef]
82. Gong, D.; Shi, W.; Yi, S.-J.; Chen, H.; Groffen, J.; Heisterkamp, N. TGFβ signaling plays a critical role in promoting alternative macrophage activation. *BMC Immunol.* **2012**, *13*, 31. [CrossRef]
83. Vitkovic, L.; Maeda, S.; Sternberg, E. Anti-Inflammatory Cytokines: Expression and Action in the Brain. *Neuroimmunomodulation* **2001**, *9*, 295–312. [CrossRef] [PubMed]
84. Zhang, I.; Alizadeh, D.; Liang, J.; Zhang, L.; Gao, H.; Song, Y.; Ren, H.; Ouyang, M.; Wu, X.; D'apuzzo, M.; et al. Characterization of Arginase Expression in Glioma-Associated Microglia and Macrophages. *PLoS ONE* **2016**, *11*, e0165118. [CrossRef] [PubMed]
85. Wainwright, D.A.; Balyasnikova, I.V.; Chang, A.L.; Ahmed, A.U.; Moon, K.-S.; Auffinger, B.; Tobias, A.L.; Han, Y.; Lesniak, M.S. IDO Expression in Brain Tumors Increases the Recruitment of Regulatory T Cells and Negatively Impacts Survival. *Clin. Cancer Res.* **2012**, *18*, 6110–6121. [CrossRef] [PubMed]
86. Uyttenhove, C.; Pilotte, L.; Théate, I.; Stroobant, V.; Colau, D.; Parmentier, N.; Boon, T.; van den Eynde, B.J. Evidence for a tumoral immune resistance mechanism based on tryptophan degradation by indoleamine 2,3-dioxygenase. *Nat. Med.* **2003**, *9*, 1269–1274. [CrossRef]
87. Tamura, R.; Ohara, K.; Sasaki, H.; Morimoto, Y.; Kosugi, K.; Yoshida, K.; Toda, M. Difference in Immunosuppressive Cells Between Peritumoral Area and Tumor Core in Glioblastoma. *World Neurosurg.* **2018**, *120*, e601–e610. [CrossRef]
88. Ishida, Y.; Agata, Y.; Shibahara, K.; Honjo, T. Induced expression of PD-1, a novel member of the immunoglobulin gene superfamily, upon programmed cell death. *EMBO J.* **1992**, *11*, 3887–3895. [CrossRef]
89. Sharpe, A.H.; Pauken, K.E. The diverse functions of the PD1 inhibitory pathway. *Nat. Rev. Immunol.* **2017**, *18*, 153–167. [CrossRef]
90. Voron, T.; Colussi, O.; Marcheteau, E.; Pernot, S.; Nizard, M.; Pointet, A.-L.; Latreche, S.; Bergaya, S.; Benhamouda, N.; Tanchot, C.; et al. VEGF-A modulates expression of inhibitory checkpoints on CD8+ T cells in tumors. *J. Exp. Med.* **2015**, *212*, 139–148. [CrossRef]
91. Masoud, G.N.; Li, W. HIF-1α pathway: Role, regulation and intervention for cancer therapy. *Acta Pharm. Sin. B* **2015**, *5*, 378–389. [CrossRef] [PubMed]
92. Polanska, U.M.; Orimo, A. Carcinoma-associated fibroblasts: Non-neoplastic tumour-promoting mesenchymal cells. *J. Cell. Physiol.* **2013**, *228*, 1651–1657. [CrossRef] [PubMed]
93. Clavreul, A.; Guette, C.; Faguer, R.; Tétaud, C.; Boissard, A.; Lemaire, L.; Rousseau, A.; Avril, T.; Henry, C.; Coqueret, O.; et al. Glioblastoma-associated stromal cells (GASCs) from histologically normal surgical margins have a myofibroblast phenotype and angiogenic properties. *J. Pathol.* **2014**, *233*, 74–88. [CrossRef]
94. Clavreul, A.; Menei, P. Mesenchymal Stromal-Like Cells in the Glioma Microenvironment: What Are These Cells? *Cancers* **2020**, *12*, 2628. [CrossRef] [PubMed]
95. Clavreul, A.; Network, T.G.O.G.P.; Etcheverry, A.; Chassevent, A.; Quillien, V.; Avril, T.; Jourdan, M.-L.; Michalak, S.; François, P.; Carré, J.-L.; et al. Isolation of a new cell population in the glioblastoma microenvironment. *J. Neuro-Oncol.* **2012**, *106*, 493–504. [CrossRef]
96. Hossain, A.; Gumin, J.; Gao, F.; Figueroa, J.; Shinojima, N.; Takezaki, T.; Priebe, W.; Villarreal, D.; Kang, S.-G.; Joyce, C.; et al. Mesenchymal Stem Cells Isolated from Human Gliomas Increase Proliferation and Maintain Stemness of Glioma Stem Cells Through the IL-6/gp130/STAT3 Pathway. *Stem Cells* **2015**, *33*, 2400–2415. [CrossRef]
97. Ho, I.A.; Toh, H.C.; Ng, W.H.; Teo, Y.L.; Guo, C.M.; Hui, K.M.; Lam, P.Y. Human Bone Marrow-Derived Mesenchymal Stem Cells Suppress Human Glioma Growth through Inhibition of Angiogenesis. *Stem Cells* **2013**, *31*, 146–155. [CrossRef]
98. Hmadcha, A.; Martin-Montalvo, A.; Gauthier, B.R.; Soria, B.; Capilla-Gonzalez, V. Therapeutic Potential of Mesen-chymal Stem Cells for Cancer Therapy. *Front. Bioeng. Biotechnol.* **2020**, *8*, 43. [CrossRef]
99. Lim, E.-J.; Kim, S.; Oh, Y.; Suh, Y.; Kaushik, N.; Lee, J.-H.; Lee, H.-J.; Kim, M.-J.; Park, M.-J.; Kim, R.-K.; et al. Crosstalk between GBM cells and mesenchymal stemlike cells promotes the invasiveness of GBM through the C5a/p38/ZEB1 axis. *Neuro-Oncology* **2020**, *22*, 1452–1462. [CrossRef]

100. D'alessandris, Q.G.; Della Pepa, G.M.; Noya, C.; Olivi, A.; Pallini, R. Mesenchymal stem cells: Are they the good or the bad? *Neuro-Oncology* **2021**, *23*, 1203–1204. [CrossRef]
101. Kang, S.-G.; Lee, S.-J. Reply to D'Alessandris et al.: Clear evidence of differences between tumor-resident mesenchymal stemlike cells and bone marrow-derived mesenchymal stem cells. *Neuro-Oncology* **2021**, *23*, 1205–1206. [CrossRef]
102. Bajetto, A.; Thellung, S.; Dellacasagrande, I.; Pagano, A.; Barbieri, F.; Florio, T. Cross talk between mesenchymal and glioblastoma stem cells: Communication beyond controversies. *Stem Cells Transl. Med.* **2020**, *9*, 1310–1330. [CrossRef]
103. Schichor, C.; Birnbaum, T.; Etminan, N.; Schnell, O.; Grau, S.; Miebach, S.; Aboody, K.; Padovan, C.; Straube, A.; Tonn, J.-C.; et al. Vascular endothelial growth factor A contributes to glioma-induced migration of human marrow stromal cells (hMSC). *Exp. Neurol.* **2006**, *199*, 301–310. [CrossRef]
104. Ho, I.A.W.; Chan, K.Y.W.; Ng, W.-H.; Guo, C.M.; Hui, K.M.; Cheang, P.; Lam, P.Y.P. Matrix Metalloproteinase 1 Is Necessary for the Migration of Human Bone Marrow-Derived Mesenchymal Stem Cells Toward Human Glioma. *Stem Cells* **2009**, *27*, 1366–1375. [CrossRef] [PubMed]
105. Birnbaum, T.; Hildebrandt, J.; Nuebling, G.; Sostak, P.; Straube, A. Glioblastoma-dependent differentiation and angiogenic potential of human mesenchymal stem cells in vitro. *J. Neuro-Oncol.* **2011**, *105*, 57–65. [CrossRef] [PubMed]
106. Zhang, Q.; Xiang, W.; Xue, B.-Z.; Yi, D.-Y.; Zhao, H.-Y.; Fu, P. Growth factors contribute to the mediation of angiogenic capacity of glioma-associated mesenchymal stem cells. *Oncol. Lett.* **2021**, *21*, 215. [CrossRef] [PubMed]
107. Lim, E.-J.; Suh, Y.; Kim, S.; Kang, S.-G.; Lee, S.-J. Force-mediated proinvasive matrix remodeling driven by tumor-associated mesenchymal stem-like cells in glioblastoma. *BMB Rep.* **2018**, *51*, 182–187. [CrossRef]
108. Oliveira, M.N.; Pillat, M.M.; Motaln, H.; Ulrich, H.; Lah, T.T. Kinin-B1 Receptor Stimulation Promotes Invasion and is Involved in Cell-Cell Interaction of Co-Cultured Glioblastoma and Mesenchymal Stem Cells. *Sci. Rep.* **2018**, *8*, 1299. [CrossRef]
109. Sun, C.; Dai, X.; Zhao, D.; Wang, H.; Rong, X.; Huang, Q.; Lan, Q. Mesenchymal stem cells promote glioma neovascularization in vivo by fusing with cancer stem cells. *BMC Cancer* **2019**, *19*, 1240. [CrossRef] [PubMed]
110. Cai, X.; Yuan, F.; Zhu, J.; Yang, J.; Tang, C.; Cong, Z.; Ma, C. Glioma-Associated Stromal Cells Stimulate Glioma Malignancy by Regulating the Tumor Immune Microenvironment. *Front. Oncol.* **2021**, *11*, 672928. [CrossRef]
111. Lama, G.; Mangiola, A.; Anile, C.; Sabatino, G.; De Bonis, P.; Lauriola, L.; Giannitelli, C.; La Torre, G.; Jhanwar-Uniyal, M.; Sica, G.; et al. Activated ERK1/2 Expression in Glioblastoma Multiforme and in Peritumor Tissue. *Int. J. Oncol.* **2007**, *30*, 1333–1342. [CrossRef]
112. Antonyak, A.M.; Kenyon, L.C.; Godwin, A.K.; James, D.C.; Emlet, D.R.; Okamoto, I.; Tnani, M.; Holgado-Madruga, M.; Moscatello D.K.; Wong, A.J. Elevated JNK activation contributes to the pathogenesis of human brain tumors. *Oncogene* **2002**, *21*, 5038–5046. [CrossRef]
113. Cui, J.; Han, S.-Y.; Wang, C.; Su, W.; Harshyne, L.; Holgado-Madruga, M.; Wong, A.J. c-Jun NH2-Terminal Kinase 2α2 Promotes the Tumorigenicity of Human Glioblastoma Cells. *Cancer Res.* **2006**, *66*, 10024–10031. [CrossRef]
114. Sluss, H.K.; Barrett, T.; Dérijard, B.; Davis, R.J. Signal Transduction by Tumor Necrosis Factor Mediated by JNK Protein Kinases. *Mol. Cell Biol.* **1994**, *14*, 8376–8384. [PubMed]
115. Jensen, R.L.; Mumert, M.L.; Gillespie, D.L.; Kinney, A.Y.; Schabel, M.C.; Salzman, K.L. Preoperative dynamic contrast-enhanced MRI correlates with molecular markers of hypoxia and vascularity in specific areas of intratumoral microenvironment and is predictive of patient outcome. *Neuro-Oncology* **2014**, *16*, 280–291. [CrossRef] [PubMed]
116. Haybaeck, J.; Obrist, P.; Schindler, C.U.; Spizzo, G.; Doppler, W. STAT-1 Expression in Human Glioblastoma and Peritumoral Tissue. *Anticancer Res.* **2007**, *27*, 3829–3835.
117. Thota, B.; Arimappamagan, A.; Kandavel, T.; Shastry, A.H.; Pandey, P.; Chandramouli, B.A.; Hegde, A.S.; Kondaiah, P.; Santosh, V. STAT-1 expression is regulated by IGFBP-3 in malignant glioma cells and is a strong predictor of poor survival in patients with glioblastoma. *J. Neurosurg.* **2014**, *121*, 374–383. [CrossRef] [PubMed]
118. Synowitz, M.; Glass, R.; Fäber, K.; Markovic, D.; Kronenberg, G.; Herrmann, K.; Schnermann, J.; Nolte, C.; van Rooijen, N.; Kiwit J.; et al. A1 Adenosine Receptors in Microglia Control Glioblastoma-Host Interaction. *Cancer Res.* **2006**, *66*, 8550–8557. [CrossRef] [PubMed]
119. Dufrusine, B.; Capone, E.; Ponziani, S.; Lattanzio, R.; Lanuti, P.; Giansanti, F.; De Laurenzi, V.; Iacobelli, S.; Ippoliti, R.; Mangiola, A.; et al. Extracellular LGALS3BP: A potential disease marker and actionable target for antibody–drug conjugate therapy in glioblastoma. *Mol. Oncol.* **2023**, *17*, 1460–1473. [CrossRef]
120. Capone, E.; Iacobelli, S.; Sala, G. Role of galectin 3 binding protein in cancer progression: A potential novel therapeutic target. *J. Transl. Med.* **2021**, *19*, 405. [CrossRef]
121. Rana, R.; Chauhan, K.; Gautam, P.; Kulkarni, M.; Banarjee, R.; Chugh, P.; Chhabra, S.S.; Acharya, R.; Kalra, S.K.; Gupta, A.; et al. Plasma-Derived Extracellular Vesicles Reveal Galectin-3 Binding Protein as Potential Biomarker for Early Detection of Glioma. *Front. Oncol.* **2021**, *11*, 778754. [CrossRef]
122. Giansanti, F.; Capone, E.; Ponziani, S.; Piccolo, E.; Gentile, R.; Lamolinara, A.; Di Campli, A.; Sallese, M.; Iacobelli, V.; Cimini A.; et al. Secreted Gal-3BP is a novel promising target for non-internalizing Antibody–Drug Conjugates. *J. Control. Release* **2019**, *294*, 176–184. [CrossRef] [PubMed]
123. Ponziani, S.; Di Vittorio, G.; Pitari, G.; Cimini, A.M.; Ardini, M.; Gentile, R.; Iacobelli, S.; Sala, G.; Capone, E.; Flavell, D.J.; et al. Antibody-Drug Conjugates: The New Frontier of Chemotherapy. *Int. J. Mol. Sci.* **2020**, *21*, 5510. [CrossRef]

24. Giambra, M.; Messuti, E.; Di Cristofori, A.; Cavandoli, C.; Bruno, R.; Buonanno, R.; Marzorati, M.; Zambuto, M.; Rodriguez-Menendez, V.; Redaelli, S.; et al. Characterizing the Genomic Profile in High-Grade Gliomas: From Tumor Core to Peritumoral Brain Zone, Passing through Glioma-Derived Tumorspheres. *Biology* **2021**, *10*, 1157. [CrossRef] [PubMed]
25. Giambra, M.; Di Cristofori, A.; Conconi, D.; Marzorati, M.; Redaelli, S.; Zambuto, M.; Rocca, A.; Roumy, L.; Carrabba, G.; Lavitrano, M.; et al. Insights into the Peritumoural Brain Zone of Glioblastoma: CDK4 and EXT2 May Be Potential Drivers of Malignancy. *Int. J. Mol. Sci.* **2023**, *24*, 2835. [CrossRef]
26. Cen, L.; Carlson, B.L.; Schroeder, M.A.; Ostrem, J.L.; Kitange, G.J.; Mladek, A.C.; Fink, S.R.; Decker, P.A.; Wu, W.; Kim, J.-S.; et al. p16-Cdk4-Rb axis controls sensitivity to a cyclin-dependent kinase inhibitor PD0332991 in glioblastoma xenograft cells. *Neuro-Oncology* **2012**, *14*, 870–881. [CrossRef] [PubMed]
27. Giambra, M.; Di Cristofori, A.; Valtorta, S.; Manfrellotti, R.; Bigiogera, V.; Basso, G.; Moresco, R.M.; Giussani, C.; Bentivegna, A. The peritumoral brain zone in glioblastoma: Where we are and where we are going. *J. Neurosci. Res.* **2023**, *101*, 199–216. [CrossRef] [PubMed]
28. Verhaak, R.G.W.; Hoadley, K.A.; Purdom, E.; Wang, V.; Wilkerson, M.D.; Miller, C.R.; Ding, L.; Golub, T.; Jill, P.; Alexe, G.; et al. Integrated Genomic Analysis Identifies Clinically Relevant Subtypes of Glioblastoma Characterized by Abnormalities in PDGFRA, IDH1, EGFR, and NF1. *Cancer Cell* **2010**, *17*, 98–110. [CrossRef] [PubMed]
29. Lu, J.; Chatterjee, M.; Schmid, H.; Beck, S.; Gawaz, M. CXCL14 as an emerging immune and inflammatory modulator. *J. Inflamm.* **2016**, *13*, 1. [CrossRef] [PubMed]
30. Ellert-Miklaszewska, A.; Dabrowski, M.; Lipko, M.; Sliwa, M.; Maleszewska, M.; Kaminska, B. Molecular definition of the pro-tumorigenic phenotype of glioma-activated microglia. *Glia* **2013**, *61*, 1178–1190. [CrossRef]
31. Lin, B.; Madan, A.; Yoon, J.-G.; Fang, X.; Yan, X.; Kim, T.-K.; Hwang, D.; Hood, L.; Foltz, G. Massively Parallel Signature Sequencing and Bioinformatics Analysis Identifies Up-Regulation of TGFBI and SOX4 in Human Glioblastoma. *PLoS ONE* **2010**, *5*, e10210. [CrossRef]
32. Peng, P.; Zhu, H.; Liu, D.; Chen, Z.; Zhang, X.; Guo, Z.; Dong, M.; Wan, L.; Zhang, P.; Liu, G.; et al. TGFBI secreted by tumor-associated macrophages promotes glioblastoma stem cell-driven tumor growth via integrin $\alpha v \beta 5$-Src-Stat3 signaling. *Theranostics* **2022**, *12*, 4221–4236. [CrossRef] [PubMed]
33. Li, X.; Truty, M.A.; Kang, Y.; Chopin-Laly, X.; Zhang, R.; Roife, D.; Chatterjee, D.; Lin, E.; Thomas, R.M.; Wang, H.; et al. Extracellular Lumican Inhibits Pancreatic Cancer Cell Growth and Is Associated with Prolonged Survival after Surgery. *Clin. Cancer Res.* **2014**, *20*, 6529–6540. [CrossRef] [PubMed]
34. Song, L.; Liu, L.; Wu, Z.; Li, Y.; Ying, Z.; Lin, C.; Wu, J.; Hu, B.; Cheng, S.-Y.; Li, M.; et al. TGF-β induces miR-182 to sustain NF-κB activation in glioma subsets. *J. Clin. Investig.* **2012**, *122*, 3563–3578. [CrossRef] [PubMed]
35. Ciafrè, S.; Galardi, S.; Mangiola, A.; Ferracin, M.; Liu, C.-G.; Sabatino, G.; Negrini, M.; Maira, G.; Croce, C.; Farace, M. Extensive modulation of a set of microRNAs in primary glioblastoma. *Biochem. Biophys. Res. Commun.* **2005**, *334*, 1351–1358. [CrossRef] [PubMed]
36. Piwecka, M.; Rolle, K.; Belter, A.; Barciszewska, A.M.; Żywicki, M.; Michalak, M.; Nowak, S.; Naskręt-Barciszewska, M.Z.; Barciszewski, J. Comprehensive analysis of microRNA expression profile in malignant glioma tissues. *Mol. Oncol.* **2015**, *9*, 1324–1340. [CrossRef] [PubMed]
37. Zhang, J.; Zhang, J.; Zhang, J.; Qiu, W.; Xu, S.; Yu, Q.; Liu, C.; Wang, Y.; Lu, A.; Zhang, J.; et al. MicroRNA-625 inhibits the proliferation and increases the chemosensitivity of glioma by directly targeting AKTAm. *J. Cancer Res.* **2017**, *7*, 1835–1849.
38. Paraskevopoulou, M.D.; Hatzigeorgiou, A.G. Analyzing MiRNA-LncRNA Interactions. *Methods Mol. Biol.* **2016**, *1402*, 271–286. [CrossRef]
39. Shi, J.; Wang, Y.-J.; Sun, C.-R.; Qin, B.; Zhang, Y.; Chen, G. Long noncoding RNA lncHERG promotes cell proliferation, migration and invasion in glioblastoma. *Oncotarget* **2017**, *8*, 108031–108041. [CrossRef]
40. Lemée, J.-M.; Com, E.; Clavreul, A.; Avril, T.; Quillien, V.; de Tayrac, M.; Pineau, C.; Menei, P. Proteomic analysis of glioblastomas: What is the best brain control sample? *J. Proteom.* **2013**, *85*, 165–173. [CrossRef]
41. Zhang, N.; Wei, L.; Ye, M.; Kang, C.; You, H. Treatment Progress of Immune Checkpoint Blockade Therapy for Glioblastoma. *Front. Immunol.* **2020**, *11*, 592612. [CrossRef] [PubMed]
42. Huang, B.; Li, X.; Li, Y.; Zhang, J.; Zong, Z.; Zhang, H. Current Immunotherapies for Glioblastoma Multiforme. *Front. Immunol.* **2020**, *11*, 603911. [CrossRef] [PubMed]

Disclaimer/Publisher's Note: The statements, opinions and data contained in all publications are solely those of the individual author(s) and contributor(s) and not of MDPI and/or the editor(s). MDPI and/or the editor(s) disclaim responsibility for any injury to people or property resulting from any ideas, methods, instructions or products referred to in the content.

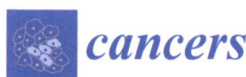

Review

Therapeutic Targeting of Glioblastoma and the Interactions with Its Microenvironment

Vassilis Genoud [1,2,3,4], Ben Kinnersley [1,2], Nicholas F. Brown [1,5], Diego Ottaviani [1,2] and Paul Mulholland [1,2,*]

1. Glioblastoma Research Group, University College London, London WC1E 6DD, UK; b.kinnersley@ucl.ac.uk (B.K.)
2. Department of Oncology, University College London Hospitals, London NW1 2PB, UK
3. Department of Oncology, University Hospitals of Geneva, 1205 Geneva, Switzerland
4. Centre for Translational Research in Onco-Haematology, University of Geneva, 1205 Geneva, Switzerland
5. Guy's Cancer, Guy's & St Thomas' NHS Foundation Trust, London SE1 3SS, UK
* Correspondence: paul.mulholland@nhs.net

Simple Summary: Glioblastoma (GBM) is the most aggressive brain tumour. Patients with GBM have a dismal survival and there is a distinct lack of curative treatments. We are increasingly understanding that the GBM tumour is composed not only of tumour cells but a complex tumour microenvironment (TME) of neuronal, glial and immune cells. Research into this area is important because the diversity of tumour cells and interactions with the TME contribute to the aggressiveness and treatment resistance of GBM. In this work, we review the multiple types of cells forming GBM and their interactions and provide examples of how our improved understanding can suggest potential new treatment strategies for this devastating disease.

Abstract: Glioblastoma (GBM) is the most common primary malignant brain tumour, and it confers a dismal prognosis despite intensive multimodal treatments. Whilst historically, research has focussed on the evolution of GBM tumour cells themselves, there is growing recognition of the importance of studying the tumour microenvironment (TME). Improved characterisation of the interaction between GBM cells and the TME has led to a better understanding of therapeutic resistance and the identification of potential targets to block these escape mechanisms. This review describes the network of cells within the TME and proposes treatment strategies for simultaneously targeting GBM cells, the surrounding immune cells, and the crosstalk between them.

Keywords: glioblastoma (GBM); heterogeneity; tumour microenvironment (TME); myeloid cells; microglia; tumour associated macrophages (TAMs); therapeutic targeting

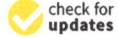

Citation: Genoud, V.; Kinnersley, B.; Brown, N.F.; Ottaviani, D.; Mulholland, P. Therapeutic Targeting of Glioblastoma and the Interactions with Its Microenvironment. *Cancers* 2023, *15*, 5790. https://doi.org/10.3390/cancers15245790

Academic Editor: David Wong

Received: 17 October 2023
Revised: 1 December 2023
Accepted: 7 December 2023
Published: 10 December 2023

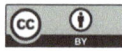

Copyright: © 2023 by the authors. Licensee MDPI, Basel, Switzerland. This article is an open access article distributed under the terms and conditions of the Creative Commons Attribution (CC BY) license (https://creativecommons.org/licenses/by/4.0/).

1. Introduction

Glioblastoma (GBM) is a disease of significant unmet need with a median overall survival of only nine months [1]. The standard treatment for GBM comprises maximal safe surgery, adjuvant radiotherapy (RT) with concurrent temozolomide (TMZ), and then adjuvant TMZ [2]. Despite there being many clinical trials over the last two decades, the management of the disease has not changed. Methylation of the O6-methylguanine-DNA methyltransferase (MGMT) promoter is the most impactful prognostic biomarker, and it confers a better prognosis and predicts response to treatment [3].

Although novel treatments have not demonstrated substantial improvement in overall survival (OS) in phase III clinical trials, subsets of patients with GBM appear to benefit. Bevacizumab, an anti-vascular endothelial growth factor (VEGF) monoclonal antibody (Ab), was shown to improve progression-free survival (PFS) but not OS [4]. Tumour treating fields (TTFs), an approach that uses alternating electrical fields, were reported to confer a modest OS benefit in newly diagnosed patients with GBM [5] but has not been widely adopted. Recently, the therapeutic vaccine DC-VaxL, which adds dendritic cell (DC) therapy to standard therapy in newly diagnosed patients, demonstrated a median OS of 19.3 months compared to 16.5 months in matched historical controls [6]. Immune checkpoint inhibitors (ICIs) with anti-PD-1 and anti-CTLA4 have radically changed the treatment of many other tumour types but have not demonstrated a survival advantage in GBM thus far [7,8]; however, further evaluation is ongoing, with neoadjuvant ICI showing promising initial results [9,10]. Finally, the remarkable success of chimeric antigen receptor (CAR) T-cell therapy in haematological cancers drives the exploration of this therapy in solid tumours, including GBM [11].

Clinical trials have demonstrated that GBM is largely resistant to immunotherapeutic approaches as it is an immunologically "cold" tumour [12]. The low immunogenicity of GBM is characterised by low T cell infiltration and absence of DC, a low tumour mutational burden, limited MHC-I expression, a highly immunosuppressive tumour microenvironment (TME), and a lack of conventional draining lymph nodes [13–15]. More detailed analyses of how treatments impact GBM and its TME are needed to identify potential therapeutic limitations and resistance pathways. Additionally, studies focusing on the origin of GBM and the complex crosstalk between a tumour and the surrounding cells will further improve our understanding of tumour development and the dynamic response to treatment. Additionally, detailed molecular analyses have aided the understanding of the cellular interactions and transcriptional pathways underlying GBM tumour composition. Identifying shared features between injuries and tumorigenesis has helped us understand the impact of inflammation on brain parenchyma and its potential link to the origins of GBM [16].

In this review, we will first describe our current understanding of the origins and genetic evolution of GBM. We will then focus on the interplay among tumour cells, astrocytes, and neurons as a cell network. The role of infiltrating immune cells in GBM will be described, and we will conclude with the therapeutic opportunities offered by targeting these cells and their interactions.

2. Molecular Subtype and GBM Stem Cells

In 2010, as part of the TCGA project, a pivotal paper by Verhaak et al. described four distinct molecular subtypes of GBM: proneural, neural, classical and mesenchymal [17]. Key genetic driver alterations are associated with each subtype: *PDGFRA* amplification for proneural, *EGFR* overexpression or amplification for neural, *EGFR* mutation, amplification, or overexpression for classical, and *NF1* mutation or deletion for mesenchymal [18]. Subsequently, as molecular techniques evolved from bulk to single-cell tumour profiling, similarities with the normal neural lineage were identified [19]. These lineages are referred to as oligodendrocyte-progenitor-cell-like (OPC-like), neural-progenitor-cell-like (NPC-like), and astrocyte-like (AC-like). Additionally, mesenchymal-like (MES-like) cells found in GBM are not observed in normal neural development but are induced in response to injury [19].

The cell of origin of GBM is still debatable. Evidence points towards either neural progenitor cells (NPCs) or oligodendrocyte progenitor cells (OPCs), as experimentally inducing somatic mutations in stem cells from either NPCs or OPCs can lead to tumour development [20]. Additionally, the subventricular zone (SVZ) has been identified as a potential stem-cell niche and the possible site of origin of GBM [21]. While the cell-state composition of the tumour mass is likely to be impacted by the cell of origin, its evolution is also influenced by various parameters, including mutations acquired during tumour development and interactions with the TME [22–24]. Specifically, *TP53* or *NF1* mutations in neural stem cells (NSCs) lead to the development of OPC progeny [21]. There is also high intra-tumoural heterogeneity, with the coexistence of up to five spatially resolved gene signatures, including NPC-like, OPC-like reactive astrocytes, MES-like, and MES-hypoxia, in the majority of GBM tumour samples analysed in a recent study [25].

As a tumour grows, it induces injury-associated inflammation, disrupting the physiological organisation of the brain parenchyma via mechanical, chemical, and even surgical or treatment-related impacts [26]. Injury-associated inflammation and wound response gene expression signatures have been described, and they can account for a significant proportion of the transcriptional heterogeneity of GBM [27]. Furthermore, the presence of GBM stem cells (GSCs) in the tumour bulk is positively correlated with tumour invasion, and OPCs can migrate to injury sites and proliferate to differentiate and promote remyelination [28].

Specific GBM molecular subtypes can impact prognosis, with the MES-like signature and the clustering pattern of AC-like tumour cells being associated with poor patient outcomes [29]. However, the prognosis is improved if the AC-like tumour cells are dispersed and in contact with other subtypes [30]. The MES-like subtype displays features of reactive astrocytes and is induced by the presence of tumour-associated macrophages (TAMs), which are enriched in regions of the tumour with the MES-like signature [31]. RNA velocity analysis suggests that MES-like cells are derived from an AC-like state in most tumours [30], but direct evolution from NPCs to MESs has also been described, drawing into question the necessity of the development of a transient astrocyte state [32].

Overall, the described molecular signatures illustrate the complexity of cellular interactions and dynamics within GBM tumours, with GSC plasticity driving evolution to escape treatment effects and leading to resistance to therapy and tumour recurrence [33,34]. Understanding the evolution and dynamics of these molecular subtypes will improve our understanding of the impact of treatment.

3. Blood–Brain Barrier Disruption in GBM

The physiological blood–brain barrier (BBB) is composed of astrocyte endfeet and tight junctions between endothelial cells and pericytes, which limit the accessibility of pathogens and many molecules, including chemotherapy, to the central nervous system (CNS) [35]. GBM growth induces physical distortion of the BBB, and the associated inflammation with neo-angiogenesis leads to the formation of leaky blood vessels, further disrupting its integrity [36,37]. Consequently, tumours are more permeable and show an increase in blood perfusion. VEGF is the major cytokine driving neo-angiogenesis; it decreases the expression of intercellular adhesion molecule (ICAM-1) and vascular cell adhesion molecule 1 (VCAM-1), thus limiting the adhesion and infiltration of immune cells to and into the tumour [38]. The aberrant and disorganised vascular morphology within the GBM tumour also limits the distribution of oxygen or nutrient supplies, leading to hypoxia and treatment resistance [39–41]. Through the induction of the transcription factor HIF1α, hypoxia regulates many genes implicated in diverse features, such as angiogenesis, survival, treatment resistance, genomic instability, and invasion [42–44]. Expression of HIF1α is associated with an increase in MDR1, which can drive chemoresistance. In vitro experiments in GBM cells have demonstrated hypoxia-induced resistance to cisplatin, TMZ and etoposide, as well as the overexpression of CD133, a marker associated with stemness [42,45,46]. As hypoxia limits the generation of reactive oxygen species (ROS), it can dampen the effectiveness of RT [46,47], and the limited perfusion of the tumour core causes necrotic areas and hypoxic regions that attract macrophages with immunosuppressive functions to develop [48].

4. The Complex Glioblastoma Microenvironment

The CNS parenchyma comprises neurons, astrocytes, oligodendrocytes, and microglial cells with complementary functions. Improved understanding of the complex crosstalk between the highly heterogeneous GBM cells and diversity of cell types in the surrounding TME will hopefully elucidate novel antitumour therapeutic strategies.

4.1. Astrocytes

Astrocytes maintain the structure and balance of the brain's parenchyma as they buffer the metabolic environment and provide an energy substrate (glucose and lactate) for neurons [49]. In the presence of GBM tumour cells, astrocytes detect damage-associated molecular patterns through pattern recognition receptors and sense mechanical stress and injury. These triggers activate a specific molecular signalling network through the JAK/STAT pathway, leading to reactive astrocytes in a process known as astrogliosis [50]. Along with JAK/STAT activation, reactive astrocytes overexpress GFAP and can express the immunosuppressive molecule PD-L1 [51,52]. Reactive astrocytes produce high levels of immunosuppressive chemokines in the TME, including IL-10 and TGF-β [51]. As a feedback loop, IL-10 and IFNγ induce the reactive state of astrocytes through JAK/STAT activation [51,53]. Increased extracellular ATP from parenchymal damage leads to ATP secretion from astrocytes and the recruitment of microglia. Moreover, pro-inflammatory reactive astrocytes are less efficient at maintaining the integrity of the BBB and further contribute to local inflammation [51,54,55]. Thus, given their role in inducing the immunosuppressive state of the GBM TME, limiting the formation of reactive astrocytes could favour therapeutic interventions.

4.2. Neurons

GBM tumours comprise a complex neuronal and axonal architecture [56], and they can directly form synapses with glioma cells to drive their proliferation via glutamatergic signalling [57]. GBM cells also interact with neurons through paracrine signalling with neuroligin-3, brain-derived neurotrophic factor, and AMPAR-mediated excitatory electrochemical synapses from neurons, promoting tumour growth [58–61]. Similarly, GBM cells can influence neurons through the secretion of non-synaptic glutamate [62,63] and can reduce the activation of inhibitory interneurons [64]. Gliomas may also increase the risk of epilepsy by influencing glutamatergic and GABAergic signalling in neurons [65], with studies in awake patients observing more neuronal excitability in the GBM-infiltrated cortex [59]. Short-range electrocorticography on the tumour-infiltrated cortex revealed functional remodelling of language circuits as some tumour regions with TSP-1$^+$ tumour cells maintained functional connectivity with neurons. This molecularly distinct GBM subpopulation is responsive to neuronal signals and has a synaptogenic, proliferative, invasive, and integrative profile, ultimately conveying a poor prognosis [16]. Moreover, it has been proposed that gliomas originating from functionally connected cortical regions are more connected to neurons and will promote the invasion of specific GBM subpopulations [16].

4.3. Glioblastoma Connectome

Large subpopulations of GBM cells are connected via tumour microtubes (TMs), which are the mechanical base for a tumour cell network, through gap junctions [66,67]. TMs can support the exchange of cell nuclei, microvesicles, mitochondria, Ca^{2+}, and chemotherapy molecules and are ultimately associated with treatment resistance [66,67]. Glutamatergic synapses in these networks can activate tumour cells and are associated with increased tumour cell proliferation and invasion [58–61]. These connections between tumour cells have been linked to invasiveness in other malignancies, such as breast, colon, and prostate cancer [68], and more recently to GBM [69]. Historically, it was believed that GBM invades the surrounding brain parenchyma by following anatomic structures, such as blood vessels, nerves, and astrocytic tracts [70]. However, a recent study identified GBM tumour cells with a neuronal molecular state that lacked connections with other tumour cells or astrocytes and that were the main drivers of diffuse brain invasion [16,71]. The molecular state of unconnected tumour cells was more enriched for neuronal and NPC-like cells and less enriched for MES-like cells [16]. GBM cell invasion resembles neuronal migration during development, with glutamatergic stimulation of synapses increasing the invasiveness of GBM cells, leading to TM formation. After invading surrounding tissue, invading unconnected tumour cells connect with the tumour mass and surrounding astrocytes to form what has been described as the "GBM connectome" [16]. Connected tumour cells are enriched for astrocytic, mesenchymal, and non-neuronal cell states that are consistent with injury response states. Confirming these findings, the upregulation of neuronal signalling programs is associated with invasiveness at recurrence of GBM [72].

4.4. Myeloid Cells

Myeloid cells in GBM comprise bone-marrow-derived macrophages and microglia which are brain-resident cells originating embryologically from the yolk sac. These two populations represent more than 95% of the immune infiltrate in GBM [73]. In the healthy brain microglia secrete neurotrophic factors and promote synaptic pruning to maintain CNS homeostasis [74,75]. Gliomas with an increased number of tumour-associated macrophages (TAMs) are associated with a higher grade and poor survival at diagnosis and at recurrence [76–78].

In GBM, TAMs are predominantly pro-inflammatory and secrete various cytokines including TNFα, IL-1a, IL-6, and IL-12, but they also have immuno-suppressive properties which are mainly through IL-10 and TGF-β secretion [79,80]. TAMs recruit polymorphonuclear neutrophils (PMNs) that generate ROS and nitric oxide (NO), further contributing to the inflamed and immunosuppressive TME. Single-cell RNA sequencing (scRNA-Seq) studies have described an enriched TAM population in the core of the tumour, which harbours a pro-inflammatory phenotype, whereas, at the tumour periphery, microglia with anti-inflammatory properties are more prominent [81–84]. Differences in the myeloid component of GBM were also noted between the tumour at diagnosis and at recurrence, as proportionally more microglia cells were present in GBM at diagnosis and proportionally more TAMs were present in recurrent GBM [85]. TAMs promote the differentiation of GBM towards the MES-like signature mainly through TNFα, C1q, IL-1a, and IFNγ [32] and the loss of *NF1* and *PTEN* in MES-like GBM cells is associated with greater TAM infiltration [86].

TAMs are highly plastic and dynamic, with their different states being defined by multiple gene signatures [85]. M1 and M2 phenotypes were proposed to distinguish classically and alternatively activated macrophages, respectively [87]. In vitro, M1 macrophages are induced after exposure to pro-inflammatory cytokines (such as TNFα or IFNγ) and produce pro-inflammatory factors [88]. M2 differentiation is triggered by anti-inflammatory cytokines (such as IL-4, IL-10, and IL-13), and these macrophages are less cytotoxic and produce immunosuppressive cytokines, such as IL-10 and TGF-β [89]. In GBM, most TAMs are described as being polarised to M2 and will limit T cell activity, secrete extracellular matrix components, and stimulate angiogenesis [43]. Arguably, this dichotomy is mainly observed in vitro, as in GBM patients, scRNA-Seq could not confirm the presence of these two polarised M1/M2 stages [90,91]. Although CD163 and CD206 have been proposed to help discriminate between the two extremes [91], many macrophages co-express M1 and M2 markers, and instead, a continuum with many states between the M1 and M2 spectrum exists [92,93]. Moreover, dynamic changes in the tumour and the TME that are driven by tumour growth and therapeutic interaction impact the TAM phenotype [88]. With single-cell resolution enabling the detection of smaller populations that can be diluted in bulk analysis, new TAM subtypes in the GBM TME have recently been described. The MARCO^{hi} macrophages and CD163$^+$-HMOX1$^+$ microglia are present only in mesenchymal GBM [94,95], with MARCO^{hi} macrophages inducing the mesenchymal transition and with HMOX1$^+$ microglia driving T cell exhaustion. High-grade glioma-associated microglia are proliferative and proinflammatory, and they promote GBM progression through the induction of the inflammasome [96]. CD73^{hi} macrophages are immunosuppressive, and their signature persists after anti-PD-1 treatment [97]. This population does not directly impact prognosis, but knocking out CD73 in mice led to increased iNOS$^+$ myeloid cells and enhanced antitumor efficacy of an ICI treatment [97], indicating that CD73^{hi} macrophages drive some immunosuppressive TME features.

Myeloid-derived suppressor cells (MDSCs) represent another myeloid population in the TME and are divided into monocytic and granulocytic MDSCs [98]. MDSCs harbour immunosuppressive features as they increase the catabolism of L-arginine by using arginase-1, depleting an essential amino acid for T cell proliferation. MDSCs can also generate ROS, impacting T cell efficacy [99], and they contribute to IL-10 and TGF-β secretion in the TME.

Neutrophil infiltration is associated with poor prognosis and treatment resistance in GBM [100]. A recent study identified a substantial neutrophil infiltration in the GBM TME [101], with CXCL8 and IL-8 being the main chemokines attracting neutrophils to the centre of the tumour [102]. Neutrophils secrete elastase, promoting tumour proliferation and angiogenesis [103], and they contribute to the immunosuppressive TME through the secretion of arginase-1, GM-CSF, and S100A4 [100,104].

4.5. Dendritic Cells

DCs are key to bridging innate and adaptive immunity by presenting antigens (Ag) to T and B cells [105]. They are not seen in the physiological brain parenchyma but, rather, during chronic inflammation. CCL5 and XCL1 can recruit DCs to the GBM TME, as observed in mouse models [106]. Based on the scRNA-Seq profiling of GBM tumours, it was estimated that about 4.5% of cells in the GBM TME have a molecular DC signature [73]. If present, DCs can secrete IL-12, which recruits $CD8^+$ T cells and reinvigorates anergic T cells [105]. Regulatory DCs have also been described and can promote regulatory T cells (Tregs) [107] while limiting $CD8^+$ T cell recruitment [108].

4.6. Lymphoid Cells

Natural killer (NK) cells exert contact-dependent cytotoxic activity through the secretion of granzyme B and perforins [109]. NK cells are found in the GBM TME [110], but radio-chemotherapy can decrease their presence [111]. NK cells are inhibited by the expression of MHC-I, which is often downregulated in GBM [112], and NK cell functionality is enhanced when NKp30 binds to B7-H6 on tumour cells [113].

T cells are the hallmark effectors of anti-tumour immunity. Their cytotoxic activity can lead to tumour eradication in other cancers and in mouse models of GBM, especially with ICI treatment [114]. However, generally, only a small number of T cells are present in the GBM TME, and when present, they exhibit an exhausted phenotype due to chronic exposure to Ag, which is associated with a lack of stimulation that leads to ineffective anti-tumour activity [115]. Many studies have explored the potential of ICI to enhance T cell activity in patients with GBM, but these have mostly failed to demonstrate significant clinical improvement [7]. Two companion studies have, however, observed that the neoadjuvant administration of anti-PD-1 Ab showed a signal towards improved OS, which will need to be validated in larger cohorts [9,10].

Tregs are immunosuppressive T cells, and their presence in GBM is associated with poor prognosis [116,117]. In contrast to CD4+/CD8+ T cells, Tregs highly express the transcription factor FOXP3, which downregulates the expression of pro-inflammatory cytokines such as IL-2 through the induction of two other transcription factors, NFAT and NFkB [118]. Innate immune cells secrete CXCL9, -10, -11, CXCR3, and CCL5-CCR5, which attract Tregs in the GBM TME [119]. As an autocrine loop, Tregs also secrete IL-10 and TGF-β, which further promotes the transition of T cells into Tregs and supports local immunosuppression [120,121]. Tregs also express high levels of the immunosuppressive molecules CTLA-4, PD-1, and GITR, thus providing inhibitory signals for all infiltrating immune cells.

5. Therapeutic Perspectives

Understanding the complex interactions between the multiple cell types underlying the GBM TME and their respective states or molecular profiles can help in the design of treatment strategies. Figure 1 illustrates these different cell types, and Table 1 highlights potential therapeutic approaches targeting the different components of GBM, as well as potential anticipated limitations.

No new systemic anti-cancer therapies have been approved for GBM for nearly twenty years, and whilst many cancers have benefited from ICI, GBM has been left trailing behind. Clinical trials evaluating ICIs have had little or no impact on the overall clinical outcomes of patients with GBM. However, case reports have demonstrated the potential for clinical benefit in an as-yet unidentified subpopulation of GBM, and early trials of neo-adjuvant PD-1 therapy appear promising, as do other forms of immunotherapy, such as CAR-T cell therapies and the recent results from DC Vax-L [6,122–125]. Improved outcomes from these immunotherapies were mainly observed in patients with methylated MGMT promoter tumours. This raises the question of these tumours having a potentially more immunotherapy-permissive TME and warrants further investigation.

Table 1. Examples of therapeutic strategies for targeting GBM and TME interactions. ICI, immune checkpoint inhibitor; TMB, tumour mutational burden; Ab, antibody; TAMs, tumour-associated macrophages; DCs, dendritic cells; NK, natural killer; BBB, blood–brain barrier; TME, tumour microenvironment; GBM, glioblastoma; GSCs, glioblastoma stem cells; DCs, dendritic cells.

Cell Targeted	Mechanism Targeted	Potential Strategy	Potential Limitations
GBM			
Tumour cells	Enhancing immunogenicity	Increasing MHC-I expression Increasing TMB and, therefore, neoantigen presentation with RT/TMZ treatment	Dampened NK cell response Sub-clonal TMB is associated with poor response to ICIs Effect may be restricted to MGMT-methylated GBM
Tumour cells, immune cells	Blocking negative regulators of antitumour immune response	ICIs	Lack of T cell infiltration, highly immunosuppressive TME
GSCs	Targeting specific markers Promoting GSC differentiation	Inhibition of CD133/ GPD1/ L1CAM Graphene oxide, Sulindac	Lack of truly specific targets, intrinsic treatment resistance
Tumour cells	Limiting the impact of hypoxia	HIF1α inhibition	Limited efficacy thus far
TME—normal brain			
Astrocytes	Limiting astrogliosis to suppress reactive astrocyte formation	JAK/STAT inhibition	Limited data available
Neurons	Targeting AMPAR signal	Perempanel treatment	Limited data available
Connectome	Targeting gap junctions	Connexin 43 targeting	Limited data available
TME—immune component			
TAMs	Limiting infiltration	CCL2 inhibition	Limited data available
	Limiting M2 polarization	CSF-1R inhibition	Induced resistance
	Enhancing phagocytosis	CD47 inhibition	Haematological side effects
	Depleting specific populations	CD73$^+$ or MARCO^{high} depletion	Limited data available
DCs	Enhancing immune activation	Therapeutic vaccines	Efficacy dependent on T cell homing to the tumour
Neutrophils	Limiting infiltration	Blocking chemokines	
Tregs	Depleting cells	IL-25 depleting Ab	Limited data available
T cells	Enhancing targeting and activation	CAR-T cell therapy	Antigen loss, on-target off-tumour effect
NK cells	Enhancing activation	Activating cytokines	Limited data available
CNS—integrity			
BBB	Increasing permeability	Focused ultrasound	Transient effect

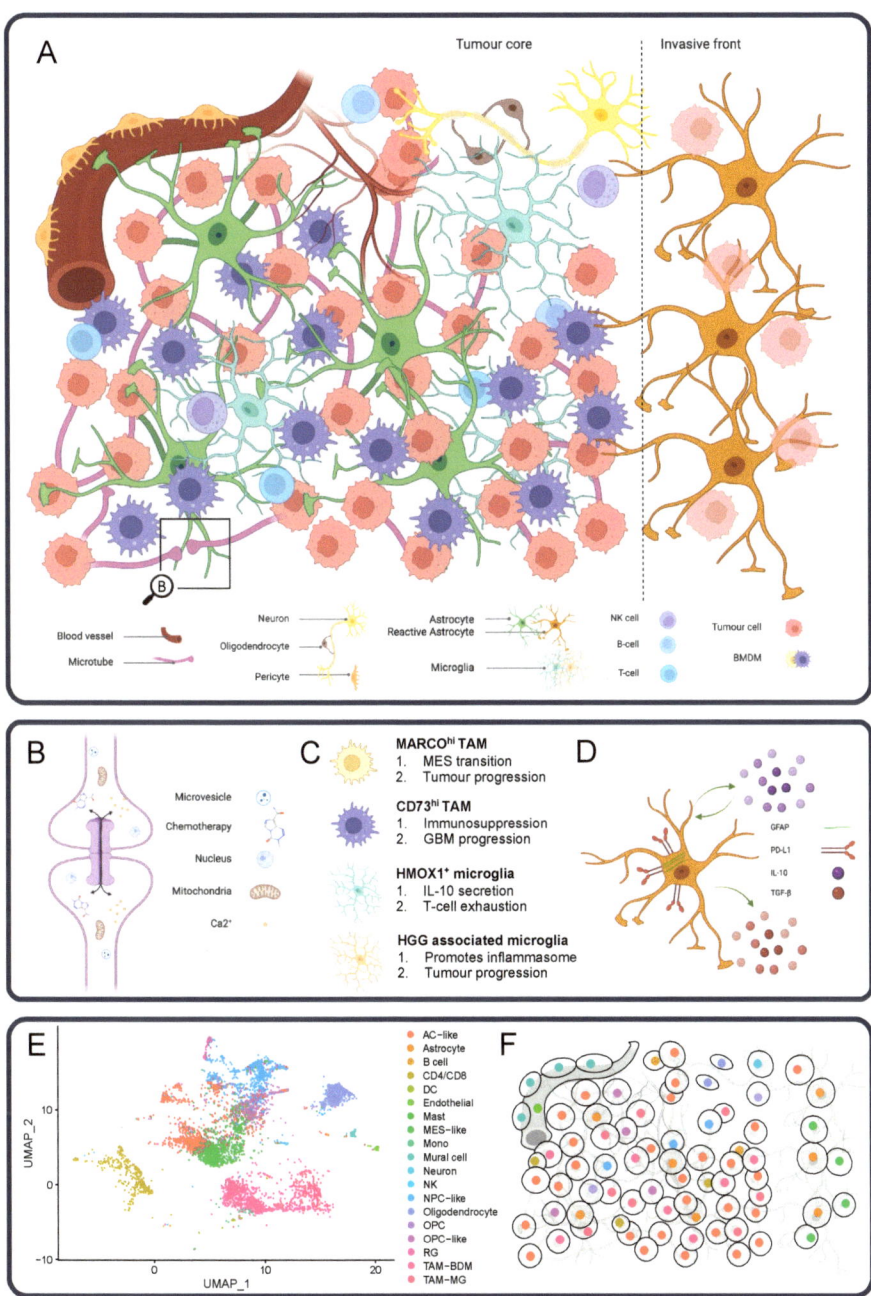

Figure 1. The complexity of the glioblastoma tumour microenvironment and the differences in techniques used to analyse it. (**A**) Schematic representation of the multiple cells composing the microenvironment of GBM. (**B**) Detailed representation of tumour microtubes and the different elements exchanged through this system. (**C**) Illustration of recently identified subpopulations of myeloid cells (MARCO^{hi} tumour-associated macrophages (TAM), CD73^{hi} TAM, HMOX1$^+$ microglia,

and high-grade glioma (HGG)-associated microglia) and their associated primary biological functions (**D**) Representation of reactive astrocytes expressing GFAP and PD-L1 and secreting the immunosuppressive cytokines IL-10 and TGF-β. (**E**) UMAP plot indicating the diversity of cell populations in GBM. Single-nucleus RNA-Seq data were obtained from GBM-CPTAC [126], processed using Seurat [127], and mapped to GBmap reference cell types [128] using Azimuth [129]. (**F**) Illustrative representation of spatial transcriptomics with single-cell resolution offered by new technological advances. This allows the identification of the complexity of the GBM TME by using gene expression to identify the different cells while keeping the biological architecture. The figure was created with BioRender.com, accessed on 16 October 2023.

Specific glioblastoma cell populations play prominent roles in tumour resistance or invasion. However, targeting these populations may not be sufficient as many other players support tumour growth in the TME. While the genomic profiling of GBM has identified several key dysregulated signalling pathways [130], targeted therapies have been ineffective in GBM, with intra-tumoural heterogeneity being a likely key factor driving this treatment resistance. The interaction between GBM cells and the TME drives immunosuppression and tumour progression. Consequently, an effective approach to therapy in glioblastoma is likely to involve simultaneously targeting GBM cells, the surrounding immune cells, and the crosstalk between them.

Multipotent GSCs drive tumour initiation and self-renewal, which supports tumour progression and therapy resistance. Therapeutic strategies targeting GSCs could increase treatment success [42,43,47,131,132]. In vitro studies showed that while TMZ initially inhibits GSC proliferation, MES-like tumour cells are resistant to this treatment, driving tumour recurrence [133,134]. The altered metabolic pathways of GSCs have been successfully targeted with epigallocatechin gallate, a bioactive polyphenol inhibiting transglutaminase which has been shown to restore the sensitivity of GSCs to TMZ and inhibit their proliferation in vitro [135]. However, it remains unclear if this strategy will translate to clinical trials. Additionally, targeting newer GSC-specific markers, such as the stem-like cell marker SOX2 that promotes tumour progression [136] or *SOCS3*, *USP8*, and *DOT1L*, which were recently linked to GSC growth, may be more efficient [137].

The molecular subtype of GBM cells is dynamic during treatment, as GBM cells with NPC- and OPC-like tumour signatures, which are more sensitive to RT, shift to an MES-like signature after RT. Consequently, RT enriches tumours for the MES-like subtype, which is more resistant to RT, which is possibly because of their proximity to RT-resistant reactive astrocytes. Additionally, RT leads to an acute accumulation of TAMs in the peritumoral area driving resistance to RT, as TAM depletion restores sensitivity to RT [138,139]. Altogether these changes in the TME after RT lead to an overall MES-like transformation, which is also the most stable subtype throughout various treatments [140].

Reactive astrocytes resist apoptosis through Fas or TRAIL pathways and have more DNA damage repair pathways than normal astrocytes [141]. Reactive astrocytes induced by activating injury pathways at the tumour margin can cause recurrence in that location [142]. This is not only due to tumour cells remaining after treatment but also because of their pro-tumoral profile [142]. Limiting the reactive injury response would, therefore, be a rational strategy for limiting tumour growth and resistance. The induction of reactive astrocytes mainly depends on the activation of the JAK/STAT pathway, which could be limited by specific inhibitors such as ruxolitinib [51]. Another strategy could be to target the tumour–astrocyte connectome, as this can drive treatment resistance. The inhibition of connexin 43 in TMs showed promising results in a pre-clinical model when combined with TMZ [143]. Additionally, in vitro experiments targeting AMPAR signalling with the anti-seizure medication perampanel limited the neuronal input to tumour cells and showed a synergistic effect with TMZ [144].

TAMs are critical for promoting tumour progression and immunosuppression in GBM and have likely contributed to the failure of immunotherapies in GBM thus far. Limiting TAMs' infiltration or modulating their pro-tumoural polarisation are promising therapeutic strategies. The CCL2/CCR2 chemokine axis is implicated in TAM infiltration, and the inhibition of CCL2 led to lower TAM recruitment and improved ICI efficacy in a mouse model of GBM [145,146]. However, the efficacy may have been blunted by the increased immunosuppressive microglia observed in CCR2 knockout mice [85]. TAMs express CSF-1R, which regulates survival and key TAM functions. The modulation of CSF-1R signalling can be used to reprogram TAMs and limit immunosuppressive polarisation. The small molecule BLZ945 inhibits CSF-1R. Although it does not deplete TAMs, it induces polarisation towards a more M1 phenotype, reducing tumour progression [138]. The concurrent inhibition of the IGFR/PI3K pathway should be explored, as GBM cells can acquire resistance to BLZ945 through this pathway [147]. BLZ945 also enhances the initial response to RT [139] and the efficacy of anti-PD-1 therapy [148]. However, CSF-1R inhibition with PLX3397 monotherapy in humans was ineffective [149]. The CD47/signal-regulatory protein alpha (SIRPα) pathway is a critical innate macrophage checkpoint, as CD47 expression on tumour cells limits the phagocytic function of TAMs. [150]. In mice, depleting CD47 increases the phagocytosis of macrophages and limits glioblastoma tumour progression [151]. Targeting specific TAM subpopulations, such as $CD73^+$ cells, extended the survival of mice with glioblastoma and showed synergistic effects when combined with anti-PD-1 and anti-CTLA-4 therapy [97]. In the same manner, Ab targeting of $MARCO^{hi}$ macrophages limited the transition of tumour cells to the MES-like subtype and the stemness features of GSCs [95].

Considering the failure of ICIs in GBM, accumulating evidence points towards the lack of efficient T cell priming by DCs [152]. A recent study compared the immune profiles of brain metastases with those of primary GBM tumours. As the primary tumours were not in the CNS, metastases exhibited more efficient T cell priming by peripheral DCs, generating a more effective T cell response against brain metastases compared to that of GBM [153]. FLT3L-mediated DC population expansion led to enhanced immune priming in a mouse model of GBM [154], and the recent encouraging results of DC-Vax-L [6] support the exploration of DC-targeted therapies.

CAR-T cell therapy for GBM could bypass the need for local T cell activation, as lymphocytes are activated ex vivo. CAR constructs targeting single tumour antigens have shown only occasional clinical improvements, but the field is now moving toward targeting multiple antigens with multivalent CARs, which is supported by a pre-clinical study where a trivalent CAR directed toward HER2, IL13Ra2, and EphA2 showed better cytotoxicity than that of monovalent CAR T cells [155].

Depleting Tregs by targeting CD25 initially faced limitations, as the anti-CD25 antibody also blocked bystander IL-2 receptor signalling, limiting T cell antitumour activity [156]. However, recent developments showed that improved antibody specificity could efficiently deplete Tregs without impacting IL-2 signalling, supporting further evaluation of this strategy [156].

Targeting other immune cells could help shape a more immuno-permissive TME. The administration of NK cells activated with IFNγ, IL-2, and anti-CD3 to enhance their cytotoxicity improved PFS in a phase III clinical trial, although the primary endpoint of improved OS was not met [157].

Finally, as the BBB and irregular neovessels limit the optimal delivery [158] and therapeutic concentrations of drugs [159], the recent development of transient BBB opening with focused ultrasound [160] could pave the way for new chemotherapeutic protocols or large molecules, such as antibody or antibody–drug conjugates, in patients with GBM.

6. Conclusions and Future Directions

Advances in genomic techniques have led to a better understanding of the intratumoural heterogeneity of GBM, although this has yet to make a therapeutic impact. With the development of spatial transcriptomics, our understanding of the interactions within the TME will be further improved and may be used to identify location-dependent cell interactions that are lost in single-cell data (Figure 1), and this technology is already improving with the development of sub-cellular resolution. For example, Figure 1E depicts the diversity of cells composing human GBM based on a single-cell RNA sequencing analysis. Cells are clustered based on the similarities in their gene expression profiles. Figure 1F illustrates a spatial transcriptomics readout in which the histological cell architecture is maintained, and single-cell identities are similarly determined according to their gene expression profiles.

Identifying the different components of the TME, their physical connections, and their interactions reveals new mechanisms of targeting glioblastoma. As illustrated by previous clinical studies, targeting only one subpopulation of GBM tumour cells or only one pathway, such as EGFRvIII$^+$ or PD-1, is not effective due to target loss and tumour resistance. Concurrent targeting of tumour cells and the TAM compartment or reactive astrocytes has therapeutic potential, as they form a connectome that contributes to invasion and treatment resistance. For example, reactive astrocytes that are induced by the JAK/STAT pathway could be targeted by a JAK inhibitor such as ruxolitinib, a drug that was initially developed for myelofibrosis.

The broader immune system can modify the therapeutic response in GBM. For example, the gut–brain axis has recently been associated with neurological disorders [161]. Studies of GBM have identified different compositions of the gut microbiome in both patients and GBM-bearing mice compared to healthy controls [162]. There is also an association between antibiotic treatment and GBM growth in mice [163], and a recent study showed that GBM can present bacterial epitopes that drive a specific T cell response [164]. As observed in other tumour types, the gut microbiome composition can alter ICI efficacy [165,166]. Therefore, further evaluation of the gut–brain axis is warranted to optimise therapeutic strategies using GBM immunotherapy.

In conclusion, recent studies and technological developments have advanced our understanding of the complex and intricate interactions between glioblastoma and the tumour microenvironment, providing insights into how glioblastoma evades current treatments and paving the way towards more effective therapies in the future.

Author Contributions: V.G., B.K., N.F.B., D.O. and P.M. all conceived, wrote, and reviewed the manuscript. All authors have read and agreed to the published version of the manuscript.

Funding: The work of V.G. was supported by the Swiss National Science Foundation (P500PM_210845). P.M. was supported by the University College London Hospitals/University College London Biomedical Research Centre and The National Brain Appeal.

Conflicts of Interest: The authors declare no conflict of interest.

References

1. Brown, N.F.; Ottaviani, D.; Tazare, J.; Gregson, J.; Kitchen, N.; Brandner, S.; Fersht, N.; Mulholland, P. Survival Outcomes and Prognostic Factors in Glioblastoma. *Cancers* **2022**, *14*, 3161. [CrossRef] [PubMed]
2. Stupp, R.; Mason, W.P.; van den Bent, M.J.; Weller, M.; Fisher, B.; Taphoorn, M.J.; Belanger, K.; Brandes, A.A.; Marosi, C.; Bogdahn U.; et al. Radiotherapy plus concomitant and adjuvant temozolomide for glioblastoma. *N. Engl. J. Med.* **2005**, *352*, 987–996. [CrossRef] [PubMed]
3. Hegi, M.E.; Diserens, A.C.; Gorlia, T.; Hamou, M.F.; de Tribolet, N.; Weller, M.; Kros, J.M.; Hainfellner, J.A.; Mason, W.; Mariani L.; et al. MGMT gene silencing and benefit from temozolomide in glioblastoma. *N. Engl. J. Med.* **2005**, *352*, 997–1003. [CrossRef] [PubMed]
4. Chinot, O.L.; Wick, W.; Mason, W.; Henriksson, R.; Saran, F.; Nishikawa, R.; Carpentier, A.F.; Hoang-Xuan, K.; Kavan, P.; Cernea D.; et al. Bevacizumab plus radiotherapy-temozolomide for newly diagnosed glioblastoma. *N. Engl. J. Med.* **2014**, *370*, 709–722. [CrossRef] [PubMed]
5. Stupp, R.; Taillibert, S.; Kanner, A.; Read, W.; Steinberg, D.M.; Lhermitte, B.; Toms, S.; Idbaih, A.; Ahluwalia, M.S.; Fink, K.; et al. Effect of Tumor-Treating Fields Plus Maintenance Temozolomide vs Maintenance Temozolomide Alone on Survival in Patients With Glioblastoma. *JAMA* **2017**, *318*, 2306. [CrossRef] [PubMed]
6. Liau, L.M.; Ashkan, K.; Brem, S.; Campian, J.L.; Trusheim, J.E.; Iwamoto, F.M.; Tran, D.D.; Ansstas, G.; Cobbs, C.S.; Heth, J.A. et al. Association of Autologous Tumor Lysate-Loaded Dendritic Cell Vaccination With Extension of Survival Among Patients With Newly Diagnosed and Recurrent Glioblastoma: A Phase 3 Prospective Externally Controlled Cohort Trial. *JAMA Oncol.* **2023**, *9*, 112–121. [CrossRef] [PubMed]

7. Reardon, D.A.; Brandes, A.A.; Omuro, A.; Mulholland, P.; Lim, M.; Wick, A.; Baehring, J.; Ahluwalia, M.S.; Roth, P.; Bahr, O.; et al. Effect of Nivolumab vs Bevacizumab in Patients With Recurrent Glioblastoma: The CheckMate 143 Phase 3 Randomized Clinical Trial. *JAMA Oncol.* **2020**, *6*, 1003–1010. [CrossRef]
8. Mulholland, P.J.; Brown, N.F.; McBain, C.; Brazil, L.; Peoples, S.; Jefferies, S.; Harris, F.; Plaha, P.; Vinayan, A.; Brooks, C.; et al. A randomised phase II multicentre study of ipilimumab with temozolomide vs temozolomide alone after surgery and chemoradiotherapy in patients with recently diagnosed glioblastoma: Ipi-Glio. *J. Clin. Oncol.* **2023**, *41*, LBA2023. [CrossRef]
9. Schalper, K.A.; Rodriguez-Ruiz, M.E.; Diez-Valle, R.; Lopez-Janeiro, A.; Porciuncula, A.; Idoate, M.A.; Inoges, S.; de Andrea, C.; Lopez-Diaz de Cerio, A.; Tejada, S.; et al. Neoadjuvant nivolumab modifies the tumor immune microenvironment in resectable glioblastoma. *Nat. Med.* **2019**, *25*, 470–476. [CrossRef]
10. Cloughesy, T.F.; Mochizuki, A.Y.; Orpilla, J.R.; Hugo, W.; Lee, A.H.; Davidson, T.B.; Wang, A.C.; Ellingson, B.M.; Rytlewski, J.A.; Sanders, C.M.; et al. Neoadjuvant anti-PD-1 immunotherapy promotes a survival benefit with intratumoral and systemic immune responses in recurrent glioblastoma. *Nat. Med.* **2019**, *25*, 477–486. [CrossRef]
11. Migliorini, D.; Dietrich, P.Y.; Stupp, R.; Linette, G.P.; Posey, A.D., Jr.; June, C.H. CAR T-Cell Therapies in Glioblastoma: A First Look. *Clin. Cancer Res.* **2018**, *24*, 535–540. [CrossRef] [PubMed]
12. Fridman, W.H.; Pages, F.; Sautes-Fridman, C.; Galon, J. The immune contexture in human tumours: Impact on clinical outcome. *Nat. Rev. Cancer* **2012**, *12*, 298–306. [CrossRef] [PubMed]
13. Berghoff, A.S.; Kiesel, B.; Widhalm, G.; Rajky, O.; Ricken, G.; Wohrer, A.; Dieckmann, K.; Filipits, M.; Brandstetter, A.; Weller, M.; et al. Programmed death ligand 1 expression and tumor-infiltrating lymphocytes in glioblastoma. *Neuro Oncol.* **2015**, *17*, 1064–1075. [CrossRef] [PubMed]
14. Wu, A.; Wiesner, S.; Xiao, J.; Ericson, K.; Chen, W.; Hall, W.A.; Low, W.C.; Ohlfest, J.R. Expression of MHC I and NK ligands on human CD133+ glioma cells: Possible targets of immunotherapy. *J. Neurooncol.* **2007**, *83*, 121–131. [CrossRef] [PubMed]
15. Schumacher, T.N.; Schreiber, R.D. Neoantigens in cancer immunotherapy. *Science* **2015**, *348*, 69–74. [CrossRef] [PubMed]
16. Venkataramani, V.; Yang, Y.; Schubert, M.C.; Reyhan, E.; Tetzlaff, S.K.; Wissmann, N.; Botz, M.; Soyka, S.J.; Beretta, C.A.; Pramatarov, R.L.; et al. Glioblastoma hijacks neuronal mechanisms for brain invasion. *Cell* **2022**, *185*, 2899–2917.e2831. [CrossRef] [PubMed]
17. DeCordova, S.; Shastri, A.; Tsolaki, A.G.; Yasmin, H.; Klein, L.; Singh, S.K.; Kishore, U. Molecular Heterogeneity and Immunosuppressive Microenvironment in Glioblastoma. *Front. Immunol.* **2020**, *11*, 1402. [CrossRef]
18. Verhaak, R.G.; Hoadley, K.A.; Purdom, E.; Wang, V.; Qi, Y.; Wilkerson, M.D.; Miller, C.R.; Ding, L.; Golub, T.; Mesirov, J.P.; et al. Integrated genomic analysis identifies clinically relevant subtypes of glioblastoma characterized by abnormalities in PDGFRA, IDH1, EGFR, and NF1. *Cancer Cell* **2010**, *17*, 98–110. [CrossRef]
19. Neftel, C.; Laffy, J.; Filbin, M.G.; Hara, T.; Shore, M.E.; Rahme, G.J.; Richman, A.R.; Silverbush, D.; Shaw, M.L.; Hebert, C.M.; et al. An Integrative Model of Cellular States, Plasticity, and Genetics for Glioblastoma. *Cell* **2019**, *178*, 835–849.e821. [CrossRef]
20. Alcantara Llaguno, S.R.; Wang, Z.; Sun, D.; Chen, J.; Xu, J.; Kim, E.; Hatanpaa, K.J.; Raisanen, J.M.; Burns, D.K.; Johnson, J.E.; et al. Adult Lineage-Restricted CNS Progenitors Specify Distinct Glioblastoma Subtypes. *Cancer Cell* **2015**, *28*, 429–440. [CrossRef]
21. Lee, J.H.; Lee, J.E.; Kahng, J.Y.; Kim, S.H.; Park, J.S.; Yoon, S.J.; Um, J.Y.; Kim, W.K.; Lee, J.K.; Park, J.; et al. Human glioblastoma arises from subventricular zone cells with low-level driver mutations. *Nature* **2018**, *560*, 243–247. [CrossRef] [PubMed]
22. Eramo, A.; Ricci-Vitiani, L.; Zeuner, A.; Pallini, R.; Lotti, F.; Sette, G.; Pilozzi, E.; Larocca, L.M.; Peschle, C.; De Maria, R. Chemotherapy resistance of glioblastoma stem cells. *Cell. Death Differ.* **2006**, *13*, 1238–1241. [CrossRef] [PubMed]
23. Auffinger, B.; Spencer, D.; Pytel, P.; Ahmed, A.U.; Lesniak, M.S. The role of glioma stem cells in chemotherapy resistance and glioblastoma multiforme recurrence. *Expert Rev. Neurother* **2015**, *15*, 741–752. [CrossRef] [PubMed]
24. Prager, B.C.; Bhargava, S.; Mahadev, V.; Hubert, C.G.; Rich, J.N. Glioblastoma Stem Cells: Driving Resilience through Chaos. *Trends Cancer* **2020**, *6*, 223–235. [CrossRef]
25. Zheng, Y.; Carrillo-Perez, F.; Pizurica, M.; Heiland, D.H.; Gevaert, O. Spatial cellular architecture predicts prognosis in glioblastoma. *Nat. Commun.* **2023**, *14*, 4122. [CrossRef]
26. Turnquist, C.; Harris, B.T.; Harris, C.C. Radiation-induced brain injury: Current concepts and therapeutic strategies targeting neuroinflammation. *Neuro-Oncol. Adv.* **2020**, *2*, vdaa057. [CrossRef] [PubMed]
27. Richards, L.M.; Whitley, O.K.N.; MacLeod, G.; Cavalli, F.M.G.; Coutinho, F.J.; Jaramillo, J.E.; Svergun, N.; Riverin, M.; Croucher, D.C.; Kushida, M.; et al. Gradient of Developmental and Injury Response transcriptional states defines functional vulnerabilities underpinning glioblastoma heterogeneity. *Nat. Cancer* **2021**, *2*, 157–173. [CrossRef]
28. Bien-Moller, S.; Balz, E.; Herzog, S.; Plantera, L.; Vogelgesang, S.; Weitmann, K.; Seifert, C.; Fink, M.A.; Marx, S.; Bialke, A.; et al. Association of Glioblastoma Multiforme Stem Cell Characteristics, Differentiation, and Microglia Marker Genes with Patient Survival. *Stem Cells Int.* **2018**, *2018*, 9628289. [CrossRef]
29. Torrisi, F.; Alberghina, C.; D'Aprile, S.; Pavone, A.M.; Longhitano, L.; Giallongo, S.; Tibullo, D.; Di Rosa, M.; Zappalà, A.; Cammarata, F.P. The hallmarks of glioblastoma: Heterogeneity, intercellular crosstalk and molecular signature of invasiveness and progression. *Biomedicines* **2022**, *10*, 806. [CrossRef]
30. Couturier, C.P.; Ayyadhury, S.; Le, P.U.; Nadaf, J.; Monlong, J.; Riva, G.; Allache, R.; Baig, S.; Yan, X.; Bourgey, M.; et al. Single-cell RNA-seq reveals that glioblastoma recapitulates a normal neurodevelopmental hierarchy. *Nat. Commun.* **2020**, *11*, 3406. [CrossRef]

31. Hara, T.; Chanoch-Myers, R.; Mathewson, N.D.; Myskiw, C.; Atta, L.; Bussema, L.; Eichhorn, S.W.; Greenwald, A.C.; Kinker, G.S.; Rodman, C. Interactions between cancer cells and immune cells drive transitions to mesenchymal-like states in glioblastoma. *Cancer Cell* 2021, *39*, 779–792.e711. [CrossRef] [PubMed]
32. Brooks, L.J.; Simpson Ragdale, H.; Hill, C.S.; Clements, M.; Parrinello, S. Injury programs shape glioblastoma. *Trends Neurosci.* 2022, *45*, 865–876. [CrossRef] [PubMed]
33. Dirkse, A.; Golebiewska, A.; Buder, T.; Nazarov, P.V.; Muller, A.; Poovathingal, S.; Brons, N.H.C.; Leite, S.; Sauvageot, N.; Sarkisjan, D.; et al. Stem cell-associated heterogeneity in Glioblastoma results from intrinsic tumor plasticity shaped by the microenvironment. *Nat. Commun.* 2019, *10*, 1787. [CrossRef]
34. Gangoso, E.; Southgate, B.; Bradley, L.; Rus, S.; Galvez-Cancino, F.; McGivern, N.; Guc, E.; Kapourani, C.A.; Byron, A.; Ferguson, K.M.; et al. Glioblastomas acquire myeloid-affiliated transcriptional programs via epigenetic immunoediting to elicit immune evasion. *Cell* 2021, *184*, 2454–2470. [CrossRef]
35. Wang, D.; Wang, C.; Wang, L.; Chen, Y. A comprehensive review in improving delivery of small-molecule chemotherapeutic agents overcoming the blood-brain/brain tumor barriers for glioblastoma treatment. *Drug Deliv.* 2019, *26*, 551–565. [CrossRef]
36. Wolburg, H.; Noell, S.; Fallier-Becker, P.; Mack, A.F.; Wolburg-Buchholz, K. The disturbed blood-brain barrier in human glioblastoma. *Mol. Aspects Med.* 2012, *33*, 579–589. [CrossRef]
37. Dubois, L.G.; Campanati, L.; Righy, C.; D'Andrea-Meira, I.; Spohr, T.C.; Porto-Carreiro, I.; Pereira, C.M.; Balca-Silva, J.; Kahn, S.A.; DosSantos, M.F.; et al. Gliomas and the vascular fragility of the blood brain barrier. *Front. Cell Neurosci.* 2014, *8*, 418. [CrossRef]
38. Yang, J.; Yan, J.; Liu, B. Targeting VEGF/VEGFR to Modulate Antitumor Immunity. *Front. Immunol.* 2018, *9*, 978. [CrossRef]
39. Liebelt, B.D.; Shingu, T.; Zhou, X.; Ren, J.; Shin, S.A.; Hu, J. Glioma Stem Cells: Signaling, Microenvironment, and Therapy. *Stem Cells Int.* 2016, *2016*, 7849890. [CrossRef]
40. Hardee, M.E.; Zagzag, D. Mechanisms of glioma-associated neovascularization. *Am. J. Pathol.* 2012, *181*, 1126–1141. [CrossRef]
41. Jhaveri, N.; Chen, T.C.; Hofman, F.M. Tumor vasculature and glioma stem cells: Contributions to glioma progression. *Cancer Lett.* 2016, *380*, 545–551. [CrossRef] [PubMed]
42. Uribe, D.; Torres, A.; Rocha, J.D.; Niechi, I.; Oyarzun, C.; Sobrevia, L.; San Martin, R.; Quezada, C. Multidrug resistance in glioblastoma stem-like cells: Role of the hypoxic microenvironment and adenosine signaling. *Mol. Aspects Med.* 2017, *55*, 140–151. [CrossRef] [PubMed]
43. Lau, E.Y.; Ho, N.P.; Lee, T.K. Cancer Stem Cells and Their Microenvironment: Biology and Therapeutic Implications. *Stem Cells Int.* 2017, *2017*, 3714190. [CrossRef] [PubMed]
44. Semenza, G.L. Defining the role of hypoxia-inducible factor 1 in cancer biology and therapeutics. *Oncogene* 2010, *29*, 625–634. [CrossRef] [PubMed]
45. Nardinocchi, L.; Pantisano, V.; Puca, R.; Porru, M.; Aiello, A.; Grasselli, A.; Leonetti, C.; Safran, M.; Rechavi, G.; Givol, D.; et al. Zinc downregulates HIF-1alpha and inhibits its activity in tumor cells in vitro and in vivo. *PLoS ONE* 2010, *5*, e15048. [CrossRef] [PubMed]
46. Ahmed, E.M.; Bandopadhyay, G.; Coyle, B.; Grabowska, A. A HIF-independent, CD133-mediated mechanism of cisplatin resistance in glioblastoma cells. *Cell Oncol.* 2018, *41*, 319–328. [CrossRef] [PubMed]
47. Dalerba, P.; Cho, R.W.; Clarke, M.F. Cancer stem cells: Models and concepts. *Annu. Rev. Med.* 2007, *58*, 267–284. [CrossRef]
48. Guo, X.; Xue, H.; Shao, Q.; Wang, J.; Guo, X.; Chen, X.; Zhang, J.; Xu, S.; Li, T.; Zhang, P.; et al. Hypoxia promotes glioma-associated macrophage infiltration via periostin and subsequent M2 polarization by upregulating TGF-beta and M-CSFR. *Oncotarget* 2016, *7*, 80521–80542. [CrossRef]
49. Matyash, V.; Kettenmann, H. Heterogeneity in astrocyte morphology and physiology. *Brain Res. Rev.* 2010, *63*, 2–10. [CrossRef]
50. Liddelow, S.A.; Barres, B.A. Reactive Astrocytes: Production, Function, and Therapeutic Potential. *Immunity* 2017, *46*, 957–967. [CrossRef]
51. Henrik Heiland, D.; Ravi, V.M.; Behringer, S.P.; Frenking, J.H.; Wurm, J.; Joseph, K.; Garrelfs, N.W.C.; Strahle, J.; Heynckes, S.; Grauvogel, J.; et al. Tumor-associated reactive astrocytes aid the evolution of immunosuppressive environment in glioblastoma. *Nat. Commun.* 2019, *10*, 2541. [CrossRef]
52. Pittet, C.L.; Newcombe, J.; Antel, J.P.; Arbour, N. The majority of infiltrating CD8 T lymphocytes in multiple sclerosis lesions is insensitive to enhanced PD-L1 levels on CNS cells. *Glia* 2011, *59*, 841–856. [CrossRef]
53. He, F.; Ge, W.; Martinowich, K.; Becker-Catania, S.; Coskun, V.; Zhu, W.; Wu, H.; Castro, D.; Guillemot, F.; Fan, G.; et al. A positive autoregulatory loop of Jak-STAT signaling controls the onset of astrogliogenesis. *Nat. Neurosci.* 2005, *8*, 616–625. [CrossRef]
54. Liddelow, S.A.; Guttenplan, K.A.; Clarke, L.E.; Bennett, F.C.; Bohlen, C.J.; Schirmer, L.; Bennett, M.L.; Munch, A.E.; Chung, W.S.; Peterson, T.C.; et al. Neurotoxic reactive astrocytes are induced by activated microglia. *Nature* 2017, *541*, 481–487. [CrossRef]
55. Zamanian, J.L.; Xu, L.; Foo, L.C.; Nouri, N.; Zhou, L.; Giffard, R.G.; Barres, B.A. Genomic analysis of reactive astrogliosis. *J. Neurosci.* 2012, *32*, 6391–6410. [CrossRef]
56. Krishna, S.; Choudhury, A.; Keough, M.B.; Seo, K.; Ni, L.; Kakaizada, S.; Lee, A.; Aabedi, A.; Popova, G.; Lipkin, B.; et al. Glioblastoma remodelling of human neural circuits decreases survival. *Nature* 2023, *617*, 599–607. [CrossRef]
57. Radin, D.P.; Tsirka, S.E. Interactions between Tumor Cells, Neurons, and Microglia in the Glioma Microenvironment. *Int. J. Mol. Sci.* 2020, *21*, 8476. [CrossRef]

58. Venkataramani, V.; Tanev, D.I.; Strahle, C.; Studier-Fischer, A.; Fankhauser, L.; Kessler, T.; Korber, C.; Kardorff, M.; Ratliff, M.; Xie, R.; et al. Glutamatergic synaptic input to glioma cells drives brain tumour progression. *Nature* **2019**, *573*, 532–538. [CrossRef] [PubMed]
59. Venkatesh, H.S.; Morishita, W.; Geraghty, A.C.; Silverbush, D.; Gillespie, S.M.; Arzt, M.; Tam, L.T.; Espenel, C.; Ponnuswami, A.; Ni, L.; et al. Electrical and synaptic integration of glioma into neural circuits. *Nature* **2019**, *573*, 539–545. [CrossRef] [PubMed]
60. Venkatesh, H.S.; Tam, L.T.; Woo, P.J.; Lennon, J.; Nagaraja, S.; Gillespie, S.M.; Ni, J.; Duveau, D.Y.; Morris, P.J.; Zhao, J.J.; et al. Targeting neuronal activity-regulated neuroligin-3 dependency in high-grade glioma. *Nature* **2017**, *549*, 533–537. [CrossRef] [PubMed]
61. Venkatesh, H.S.; Johung, T.B.; Caretti, V.; Noll, A.; Tang, Y.; Nagaraja, S.; Gibson, E.M.; Mount, C.W.; Polepalli, J.; Mitra, S.S.; et al. Neuronal Activity Promotes Glioma Growth through Neuroligin-3 Secretion. *Cell* **2015**, *161*, 803–816. [CrossRef]
62. Buckingham, S.C.; Campbell, S.L.; Haas, B.R.; Montana, V.; Robel, S.; Ogunrinu, T.; Sontheimer, H. Glutamate release by primary brain tumors induces epileptic activity. *Nat. Med.* **2011**, *17*, 1269–1274. [CrossRef] [PubMed]
63. Campbell, S.L.; Buckingham, S.C.; Sontheimer, H. Human glioma cells induce hyperexcitability in cortical networks. *Epilepsia* **2012**, *53*, 1360–1370. [CrossRef]
64. Campbell, S.L.; Robel, S.; Cuddapah, V.A.; Robert, S.; Buckingham, S.C.; Kahle, K.T.; Sontheimer, H. GABAergic disinhibition and impaired KCC2 cotransporter activity underlie tumor-associated epilepsy. *Glia* **2015**, *63*, 23–36. [CrossRef] [PubMed]
65. Hua, T.; Shi, H.; Zhu, M.; Chen, C.; Su, Y.; Wen, S.; Zhang, X.; Chen, J.; Huang, Q.; Wang, H. Glioma-neuronal interactions in tumor progression: Mechanism, therapeutic strategies and perspectives (Review). *Int. J. Oncol.* **2022**, *61*, 104. [CrossRef] [PubMed]
66. Osswald, M.; Jung, E.; Sahm, F.; Solecki, G.; Venkataramani, V.; Blaes, J.; Weil, S.; Horstmann, H.; Wiestler, B.; Syed, M.; et al. Brain tumour cells interconnect to a functional and resistant network. *Nature* **2015**, *528*, 93–98. [CrossRef] [PubMed]
67. Weil, S.; Osswald, M.; Solecki, G.; Grosch, J.; Jung, E.; Lemke, D.; Ratliff, M.; Hanggi, D.; Wick, W.; Winkler, F. Tumor microtubes convey resistance to surgical lesions and chemotherapy in gliomas. *Neuro Oncol.* **2017**, *19*, 1316–1326. [CrossRef] [PubMed]
68. Friedl, P.; Locker, J.; Sahai, E.; Segall, J.E. Classifying collective cancer cell invasion. *Nat. Cell Biol.* **2012**, *14*, 777–783. [CrossRef] [PubMed]
69. Gritsenko, P.G.; Atlasy, N.; Dieteren, C.E.J.; Navis, A.C.; Venhuizen, J.H.; Veelken, C.; Schubert, D.; Acker-Palmer, A.; Westerman, B.A.; Wurdinger, T.; et al. p120-catenin-dependent collective brain infiltration by glioma cell networks. *Nat. Cell Biol.* **2020**, *22*, 97–107. [CrossRef]
70. Cuddapah, V.A.; Robel, S.; Watkins, S.; Sontheimer, H. A neurocentric perspective on glioma invasion. *Nat. Rev. Neurosci.* **2014**, *15*, 455–465. [CrossRef]
71. Garofano, L.; Migliozzi, S.; Oh, Y.T.; D'Angelo, F.; Najac, R.D.; Ko, A.; Frangaj, B.; Caruso, F.P.; Yu, K.; Yuan, J.; et al. Pathway-based classification of glioblastoma uncovers a mitochondrial subtype with therapeutic vulnerabilities. *Nat. Cancer* **2021**, *2*, 141–156. [CrossRef] [PubMed]
72. Varn, F.S.; Johnson, K.C.; Martinek, J.; Huse, J.T.; Nasrallah, M.P.; Wesseling, P.; Cooper, L.A.D.; Malta, T.M.; Wade, T.E.; Sabedot, T.S.; et al. Glioma progression is shaped by genetic evolution and microenvironment interactions. *Cell* **2022**, *185*, 2184–2199.e2116. [CrossRef] [PubMed]
73. Darmanis, S.; Sloan, S.A.; Croote, D.; Mignardi, M.; Chernikova, S.; Samghababi, P.; Zhang, Y.; Neff, N.; Kowarsky, M.; Caneda, C.; et al. Single-Cell RNA-Seq Analysis of Infiltrating Neoplastic Cells at the Migrating Front of Human Glioblastoma. *Cell Rep.* **2017**, *21*, 1399–1410. [CrossRef]
74. Parkhurst, C.N.; Yang, G.; Ninan, I.; Savas, J.N.; Yates, J.R., 3rd; Lafaille, J.J.; Hempstead, B.L.; Littman, D.R.; Gan, W.B. Microglia promote learning-dependent synapse formation through brain-derived neurotrophic factor. *Cell* **2013**, *155*, 1596–1609. [CrossRef]
75. Hong, S.; Dissing-Olesen, L.; Stevens, B. New insights on the role of microglia in synaptic pruning in health and disease. *Curr. Opin. Neurobiol.* **2016**, *36*, 128–134. [CrossRef] [PubMed]
76. Gielen, P.R.; Schulte, B.M.; Kers-Rebel, E.D.; Verrijp, K.; Bossman, S.A.; Ter Laan, M.; Wesseling, P.; Adema, G.J. Elevated levels of polymorphonuclear myeloid-derived suppressor cells in patients with glioblastoma highly express S100A8/9 and arginase and suppress T cell function. *Neuro Oncol.* **2016**, *18*, 1253–1264. [CrossRef] [PubMed]
77. Richard, S.A. Explicating the Pivotal Pathogenic, Diagnostic, and Therapeutic Biomarker Potentials of Myeloid-Derived Suppressor Cells in Glioblastoma. *Dis. Markers* **2020**, *2020*, 8844313. [CrossRef]
78. Alban, T.J.; Alvarado, A.G.; Sorensen, M.D.; Bayik, D.; Volovetz, J.; Serbinowski, E.; Mulkearns-Hubert, E.E.; Sinyuk, M.; Hale, J.S.; Onzi, G.R.; et al. Global immune fingerprinting in glioblastoma patient peripheral blood reveals immune-suppression signatures associated with prognosis. *JCI Insight* **2018**, *3*, e122264. [CrossRef]
79. Jurga, A.M.; Paleczna, M.; Kuter, K.Z. Overview of General and Discriminating Markers of Differential Microglia Phenotypes. *Front. Cell Neurosci.* **2020**, *14*, 198. [CrossRef]
80. Colonna, M.; Butovsky, O. Microglia Function in the Central Nervous System During Health and Neurodegeneration. *Annu. Rev. Immunol.* **2017**, *35*, 441–468. [CrossRef]
81. Chen, Z.; Feng, X.; Herting, C.J.; Garcia, V.A.; Nie, K.; Pong, W.W.; Rasmussen, R.; Dwivedi, B.; Seby, S.; Wolf, S.A.; et al. Cellular and Molecular Identity of Tumor-Associated Macrophages in Glioblastoma. *Cancer Res.* **2017**, *77*, 2266–2278. [CrossRef] [PubMed]
82. Muller, A.; Brandenburg, S.; Turkowski, K.; Muller, S.; Vajkoczy, P. Resident microglia, and not peripheral macrophages, are the main source of brain tumor mononuclear cells. *Int. J. Cancer* **2015**, *137*, 278–288. [CrossRef] [PubMed]

83. Landry, A.P.; Balas, M.; Alli, S.; Spears, J.; Zador, Z. Distinct regional ontogeny and activation of tumor associated macrophages in human glioblastoma. *Sci. Rep.* **2020**, *10*, 19542. [CrossRef] [PubMed]
84. Ochocka, N.; Segit, P.; Walentynowicz, K.A.; Wojnicki, K.; Cyranowski, S.; Swatler, J.; Mieczkowski, J.; Kaminska, B. Single-cell RNA sequencing reveals functional heterogeneity of glioma-associated brain macrophages. *Nat. Commun.* **2021**, *12*, 1151. [CrossRef] [PubMed]
85. Pombo Antunes, A.R.; Scheyltjens, I.; Lodi, F.; Messiaen, J.; Antoranz, A.; Duerinck, J.; Kancheva, D.; Martens, L.; De Vlaminck, K.; Van Hove, H.; et al. Single-cell profiling of myeloid cells in glioblastoma across species and disease stage reveals macrophage competition and specialization. *Nat. Neurosci.* **2021**, *24*, 595–610. [CrossRef]
86. Chen, P.; Zhao, D.; Li, J.; Liang, X.; Li, J.; Chang, A.; Henry, V.K.; Lan, Z.; Spring, D.J.; Rao, G.; et al. Symbiotic Macrophage-Glioma Cell Interactions Reveal Synthetic Lethality in PTEN-Null Glioma. *Cancer Cell* **2019**, *35*, 868–884.e866. [CrossRef] [PubMed]
87. Martinez, F.O.; Gordon, S. The M1 and M2 paradigm of macrophage activation: Time for reassessment. *F1000Prime Rep.* **2014**, *6*, 13. [CrossRef]
88. Xuan, W.; Lesniak, M.S.; James, C.D.; Heimberger, A.B.; Chen, P. Context-Dependent Glioblastoma-Macrophage/Microglia Symbiosis and Associated Mechanisms. *Trends Immunol.* **2021**, *42*, 280–292. [CrossRef]
89. Mantovani, A.; Sica, A.; Sozzani, S.; Allavena, P.; Vecchi, A.; Locati, M. The chemokine system in diverse forms of macrophage activation and polarization. *Trends Immunol.* **2004**, *25*, 677–686. [CrossRef]
90. Abdelfattah, N.; Kumar, P.; Wang, C.; Leu, J.S.; Flynn, W.F.; Gao, R.; Baskin, D.S.; Pichumani, K.; Ijare, O.B.; Wood, S.L.; et al. Single-cell analysis of human glioma and immune cells identifies S100A4 as an immunotherapy target. *Nat. Commun.* **2022**, *13*, 767. [CrossRef]
91. Muller, S.; Kohanbash, G.; Liu, S.J.; Alvarado, B.; Carrera, D.; Bhaduri, A.; Watchmaker, P.B.; Yagnik, G.; Di Lullo, E.; Malatesta, M.; et al. Single-cell profiling of human gliomas reveals macrophage ontogeny as a basis for regional differences in macrophage activation in the tumor microenvironment. *Genome Biol.* **2017**, *18*, 234. [CrossRef] [PubMed]
92. Martinez-Lage, M.; Lynch, T.M.; Bi, Y.; Cocito, C.; Way, G.P.; Pal, S.; Haller, J.; Yan, R.E.; Ziober, A.; Nguyen, A.; et al. Immune landscapes associated with different glioblastoma molecular subtypes. *Acta Neuropathol. Commun.* **2019**, *7*, 203. [CrossRef] [PubMed]
93. Miyazaki, T.; Ishikawa, E.; Matsuda, M.; Sugii, N.; Kohzuki, H.; Akutsu, H.; Sakamoto, N.; Takano, S.; Matsumura, A. Infiltration of CD163-positive macrophages in glioma tissues after treatment with anti-PD-L1 antibody and role of PI3Kgamma inhibitor as a combination therapy with anti-PD-L1 antibody in in vivo model using temozolomide-resistant murine glioma-initiating cells. *Brain Tumor Pathol.* **2020**, *37*, 41–49. [CrossRef] [PubMed]
94. Ravi, V.M.; Will, P.; Kueckelhaus, J.; Sun, N.; Joseph, K.; Salie, H.; Vollmer, L.; Kuliesiute, U.; von Ehr, J.; Benotmane, J.K.; et al. Spatially resolved multi-omics deciphers bidirectional tumor-host interdependence in glioblastoma. *Cancer Cell* **2022**, *40*, 639–655.e613. [CrossRef] [PubMed]
95. Sa, J.K.; Chang, N.; Lee, H.W.; Cho, H.J.; Ceccarelli, M.; Cerulo, L.; Yin, J.; Kim, S.S.; Caruso, F.P.; Lee, M.; et al. Transcriptional regulatory networks of tumor-associated macrophages that drive malignancy in mesenchymal glioblastoma. *Genome Biol.* **2020**, *21*, 216. [CrossRef] [PubMed]
96. Liu, H.; Sun, Y.; Zhang, Q.; Jin, W.; Gordon, R.E.; Zhang, Y.; Wang, J.; Sun, C.; Wang, Z.J.; Qi, X.; et al. Pro-inflammatory and proliferative microglia drive progression of glioblastoma. *Cell Rep.* **2021**, *36*, 109718. [CrossRef]
97. Goswami, S.; Walle, T.; Cornish, A.E.; Basu, S.; Anandhan, S.; Fernandez, I.; Vence, L.; Blando, J.; Zhao, H.; Yadav, S.S.; et al. Immune profiling of human tumors identifies CD73 as a combinatorial target in glioblastoma. *Nat. Med.* **2020**, *26*, 39–46. [CrossRef]
98. Mi, Y.; Guo, N.; Luan, J.; Cheng, J.; Hu, Z.; Jiang, P.; Jin, W.; Gao, X. The Emerging Role of Myeloid-Derived Suppressor Cells in the Glioma Immune Suppressive Microenvironment. *Front. Immunol.* **2020**, *11*, 737. [CrossRef]
99. Groth, C.; Hu, X.; Weber, R.; Fleming, V.; Altevogt, P.; Utikal, J.; Umansky, V. Immunosuppression mediated by myeloid-derived suppressor cells (MDSCs) during tumour progression. *Br. J. Cancer* **2019**, *120*, 16–25. [CrossRef]
100. Massara, M.; Persico, P.; Bonavita, O.; Mollica Poeta, V.; Locati, M.; Simonelli, M.; Bonecchi, R. Neutrophils in Gliomas. *Front. Immunol.* **2017**, *8*, 1349. [CrossRef]
101. Maas, R.R.; Soukup, K.; Fournier, N.; Massara, M.; Galland, S.; Kornete, M.; Wischnewski, V.; Lourenco, J.; Croci, D.; Alvarez Prado, A.F.; et al. The local microenvironment drives activation of neutrophils in human brain tumors. *Cell* **2023**, *186*, 4546–4566. [CrossRef]
102. Masucci, M.T.; Minopoli, M.; Carriero, M.V. Tumor Associated Neutrophils. Their Role in Tumorigenesis, Metastasis, Prognosis and Therapy. *Front. Oncol.* **2019**, *9*, 1146. [CrossRef]
103. Wu, L.; Zhang, X.H. Tumor-Associated Neutrophils and Macrophages-Heterogenous but Not Chaotic. *Front. Immunol.* **2020**, *11*, 553967. [CrossRef]
104. Khan, S.; Mittal, S.; McGee, K.; Alfaro-Munoz, K.D.; Majd, N.; Balasubramaniyan, V.; de Groot, J.F. Role of Neutrophils and Myeloid-Derived Suppressor Cells in Glioma Progression and Treatment Resistance. *Int. J. Mol. Sci.* **2020**, *21*, 1954. [CrossRef]
105. Mildner, A.; Jung, S. Development and function of dendritic cell subsets. *Immunity* **2014**, *40*, 642–656. [CrossRef] [PubMed]
106. Bottcher, J.P.; Reis e Sousa, C. The Role of Type 1 Conventional Dendritic Cells in Cancer Immunity. *Trends Cancer* **2018**, *4*, 784–792. [CrossRef] [PubMed]

107. Henry, C.J.; Ornelles, D.A.; Mitchell, L.M.; Brzoza-Lewis, K.L.; Hiltbold, E.M. IL-12 produced by dendritic cells augments CD8+ T cell activation through the production of the chemokines CCL1 and CCL17. *J. Immunol.* **2008**, *181*, 8576–8584. [CrossRef] [PubMed]
108. Srivastava, S.; Jackson, C.; Kim, T.; Choi, J.; Lim, M. A Characterization of Dendritic Cells and Their Role in Immunotherapy in Glioblastoma: From Preclinical Studies to Clinical Trials. *Cancers* **2019**, *11*, 537. [CrossRef]
109. Paul, S.; Lal, G. The Molecular Mechanism of Natural Killer Cells Function and Its Importance in Cancer Immunotherapy. *Front. Immunol.* **2017**, *8*, 1124. [CrossRef] [PubMed]
110. Yang, I.; Han, S.J.; Sughrue, M.E.; Tihan, T.; Parsa, A.T. Immune cell infiltrate differences in pilocytic astrocytoma and glioblastoma: Evidence of distinct immunological microenvironments that reflect tumor biology. *J. Neurosurg.* **2011**, *115*, 505–511. [CrossRef]
111. Fadul, C.E.; Fisher, J.L.; Gui, J.; Hampton, T.H.; Cote, A.L.; Ernstoff, M.S. Immune modulation effects of concomitant temozolomide and radiation therapy on peripheral blood mononuclear cells in patients with glioblastoma multiforme. *Neuro Oncol.* **2011**, *13*, 393–400. [CrossRef] [PubMed]
112. Facoetti, A.; Nano, R.; Zelini, P.; Morbini, P.; Benericetti, E.; Ceroni, M.; Campoli, M.; Ferrone, S. Human leukocyte antigen and antigen processing machinery component defects in astrocytic tumors. *Clin. Cancer Res.* **2005**, *11*, 8304–8311. [CrossRef] [PubMed]
113. Jiang, T.; Wu, W.; Zhang, H.; Zhang, X.; Zhang, D.; Wang, Q.; Huang, L.; Wang, Y.; Hang, C. High expression of B7-H6 in human glioma tissues promotes tumor progression. *Oncotarget* **2017**, *8*, 37435–37447. [CrossRef] [PubMed]
114. Speranza, M.C.; Passaro, C.; Ricklefs, F.; Kasai, K.; Klein, S.R.; Nakashima, H.; Kaufmann, J.K.; Ahmed, A.K.; Nowicki, M.O.; Obi, P.; et al. Preclinical investigation of combined gene-mediated cytotoxic immunotherapy and immune checkpoint blockade in glioblastoma. *Neuro Oncol.* **2018**, *20*, 225–235. [CrossRef] [PubMed]
115. Ott, M.; Tomaszowski, K.H.; Marisetty, A.; Kong, L.Y.; Wei, J.; Duna, M.; Blumberg, K.; Ji, X.; Jacobs, C.; Fuller, G.N.; et al. Profiling of patients with glioma reveals the dominant immunosuppressive axis is refractory to immune function restoration. *JCI Insight* **2020**, *5*, e134386. [CrossRef]
116. Sayour, E.J.; McLendon, P.; McLendon, R.; De Leon, G.; Reynolds, R.; Kresak, J.; Sampson, J.H.; Mitchell, D.A. Increased proportion of FoxP3+ regulatory T cells in tumor infiltrating lymphocytes is associated with tumor recurrence and reduced survival in patients with glioblastoma. *Cancer Immunol. Immunother* **2015**, *64*, 419–427. [CrossRef] [PubMed]
117. Heimberger, A.B.; Abou-Ghazal, M.; Reina-Ortiz, C.; Yang, D.S.; Sun, W.; Qiao, W.; Hiraoka, N.; Fuller, G.N. Incidence and prognostic impact of FoxP3+ regulatory T cells in human gliomas. *Clin. Cancer Res.* **2008**, *14*, 5166–5172. [CrossRef] [PubMed]
118. Lu, L.; Barbi, J.; Pan, F. The regulation of immune tolerance by FOXP3. *Nat. Rev. Immunol.* **2017**, *17*, 703–717. [CrossRef]
119. Vilgelm, A.E.; Richmond, A. Chemokines Modulate Immune Surveillance in Tumorigenesis, Metastasis, and Response to Immunotherapy. *Front. Immunol.* **2019**, *10*, 333. [CrossRef]
120. Jarnicki, A.G.; Lysaght, J.; Todryk, S.; Mills, K.H. Suppression of antitumor immunity by IL-10 and TGF-beta-producing T cells infiltrating the growing tumor: Influence of tumor environment on the induction of CD4+ and CD8+ regulatory T cells. *J. Immunol.* **2006**, *177*, 896–904. [CrossRef]
121. Li, C.; Jiang, P.; Wei, S.; Xu, X.; Wang, J. Regulatory T cells in tumor microenvironment: New mechanisms, potential therapeutic strategies and future prospects. *Mol. Cancer* **2020**, *19*, 116. [CrossRef]
122. Johnson, L.A.; Scholler, J.; Ohkuri, T.; Kosaka, A.; Patel, P.R.; McGettigan, S.E.; Nace, A.K.; Dentchev, T.; Thekkat, P.; Loew, A.; et al. Rational development and characterization of humanized anti-EGFR variant III chimeric antigen receptor T cells for glioblastoma. *Sci. Transl. Med.* **2015**, *7*, 275ra222. [CrossRef]
123. O'Rourke, D.M.; Nasrallah, M.P.; Desai, A.; Melenhorst, J.J.; Mansfield, K.; Morrissette, J.J.D.; Martinez-Lage, M.; Brem, S.; Maloney, E.; Shen, A.; et al. A single dose of peripherally infused EGFRvIII-directed CAR T cells mediates antigen loss and induces adaptive resistance in patients with recurrent glioblastoma. *Sci. Transl. Med.* **2017**, *9*, eaaa0984. [CrossRef] [PubMed]
124. Sengupta, S.; Thaci, B.; Crawford, A.C.; Sampath, P. Interleukin-13 receptor alpha 2-targeted glioblastoma immunotherapy. *Biomed Res. Int.* **2014**, *2014*, 952128. [CrossRef] [PubMed]
125. Ahmed, N.; Brawley, V.; Hegde, M.; Bielamowicz, K.; Kalra, M.; Landi, D.; Robertson, C.; Gray, T.L.; Diouf, O.; Wakefield, A.; et al. HER2-Specific Chimeric Antigen Receptor-Modified Virus-Specific T Cells for Progressive Glioblastoma: A Phase 1 Dose-Escalation Trial. *JAMA Oncol.* **2017**, *3*, 1094–1101. [CrossRef] [PubMed]
126. Wang, L.-B.; Karpova, A.; Gritsenko, M.A.; Kyle, J.E.; Cao, S.; Li, Y.; Rykunov, D.; Colaprico, A.; Rothstein, J.H.; Hong, R. Proteogenomic and metabolomic characterization of human glioblastoma. *Cancer Cell* **2021**, *39*, 509–528.e520. [CrossRef] [PubMed]
127. Hao, Y.; Stuart, T.; Kowalski, M.H.; Choudhary, S.; Hoffman, P.; Hartman, A.; Srivastava, A.; Molla, G.; Madad, S.; Fernandez-Granda, C.; et al. Dictionary learning for integrative, multimodal and scalable single-cell analysis. *Nat. Biotechnol.* **2023**, 1–12. [CrossRef] [PubMed]
128. Ruiz-Moreno, C.; Salas, S.M.; Samuelsson, E.; Brandner, S.; Kranendonk, M.E.; Nilsson, M.; Stunnenberg, H.G. Harmonized single-cell landscape, intercellular crosstalk and tumor architecture of glioblastoma. *BioRxiv* **2022**.
129. Hao, Y.; Hao, S.; Andersen-Nissen, E.; Mauck, W.M., 3rd; Zheng, S.; Butler, A.; Lee, M.J.; Wilk, A.J.; Darby, C.; Zager, M.; et al. Integrated analysis of multimodal single-cell data. *Cell* **2021**, *184*, 3573–3587.e3529. [CrossRef]
130. Khan, F.; Pang, L.; Dunterman, M.; Lesniak, M.S.; Heimberger, A.B.; Chen, P. Macrophages and microglia in glioblastoma: Heterogeneity, plasticity, and therapy. *J. Clin. Invest.* **2023**, *133*, e163446. [CrossRef]
131. Seano, G. Targeting the perivascular niche in brain tumors. *Curr. Opin. Oncol.* **2018**, *30*, 54–60. [CrossRef] [PubMed]

132. Persano, L.; Rampazzo, E.; Basso, G.; Viola, G. Glioblastoma cancer stem cells: Role of the microenvironment and therapeutic targeting. *Biochem. Pharmacol.* **2013**, *85*, 612–622. [CrossRef] [PubMed]
133. Beier, D.; Rohrl, S.; Pillai, D.R.; Schwarz, S.; Kunz-Schughart, L.A.; Leukel, P.; Proescholdt, M.; Brawanski, A.; Bogdahn, U.; Trampe-Kieslich, A.; et al. Temozolomide preferentially depletes cancer stem cells in glioblastoma. *Cancer Res.* **2008**, *68*, 5706–5715 [CrossRef] [PubMed]
134. Garnier, D.; Meehan, B.; Kislinger, T.; Daniel, P.; Sinha, A.; Abdulkarim, B.; Nakano, I.; Rak, J. Divergent evolution of temozolomide resistance in glioblastoma stem cells is reflected in extracellular vesicles and coupled with radiosensitization. *Neuro Oncol.* **2018**, *20*, 236–248. [CrossRef]
135. Zhang, Y.; Wang, S.X.; Ma, J.W.; Li, H.Y.; Ye, J.C.; Xie, S.M.; Du, B.; Zhong, X.Y. EGCG inhibits properties of glioma stem-like cells and synergizes with temozolomide through downregulation of P-glycoprotein inhibition. *J. Neurooncol.* **2015**, *121*, 41–52 [CrossRef] [PubMed]
136. Zhang, S.; Xiong, X.; Sun, Y. Functional characterization of SOX2 as an anticancer target. *Signal Transduct. Target Ther.* **2020**, *5*, 135 [CrossRef] [PubMed]
137. MacLeod, G.; Bozek, D.A.; Rajakulendran, N.; Monteiro, V.; Ahmadi, M.; Steinhart, Z.; Kushida, M.M.; Yu, H.; Coutinho, F.J.; Cavalli, F.M.G.; et al. Genome-Wide CRISPR-Cas9 Screens Expose Genetic Vulnerabilities and Mechanisms of Temozolomide Sensitivity in Glioblastoma Stem Cells. *Cell Rep.* **2019**, *27*, 971–986.e979. [CrossRef]
138. Pyonteck, S.M.; Akkari, L.; Schuhmacher, A.J.; Bowman, R.L.; Sevenich, L.; Quail, D.F.; Olson, O.C.; Quick, M.L.; Huse, J.T.; Teijeiro, V.; et al. CSF-1R inhibition alters macrophage polarization and blocks glioma progression. *Nat. Med.* **2013**, *19*, 1264–1272 [CrossRef] [PubMed]
139. Akkari, L.; Bowman, R.L.; Tessier, J.; Klemm, F.; Handgraaf, S.M.; de Groot, M.; Quail, D.F.; Tillard, L.; Gadiot, J.; Huse, J.T.; et al. Dynamic changes in glioma macrophage populations after radiotherapy reveal CSF-1R inhibition as a strategy to overcome resistance. *Sci. Transl Med.* **2020**, *12*, eaaw7843. [CrossRef]
140. Wang, L.; Jung, J.; Babikir, H.; Shamardani, K.; Jain, S.; Feng, X.; Gupta, N.; Rosi, S.; Chang, S.; Raleigh, D.; et al. A single-cell atlas of glioblastoma evolution under therapy reveals cell-intrinsic and cell-extrinsic therapeutic targets. *Nat. Cancer* **2022**, *3*, 1534–1552 [CrossRef]
141. Song, J.H.; Bellail, A.; Tse, M.C.; Yong, V.W.; Hao, C. Human astrocytes are resistant to Fas ligand and tumor necrosis factor-related apoptosis-inducing ligand-induced apoptosis. *J. Neurosci.* **2006**, *26*, 3299–3308. [CrossRef] [PubMed]
142. Okolie, O.; Bago, J.R.; Schmid, R.S.; Irvin, D.M.; Bash, R.E.; Miller, C.R.; Hingtgen, S.D. Reactive astrocytes potentiate tumor aggressiveness in a murine glioma resection and recurrence model. *Neuro Oncol.* **2016**, *18*, 1622–1633. [CrossRef]
143. Schneider, M.; Vollmer, L.; Potthoff, A.L.; Ravi, V.M.; Evert, B.O.; Rahman, M.A.; Sarowar, S.; Kueckelhaus, J.; Will, P.; Zurhorst D.; et al. Meclofenamate causes loss of cellular tethering and decoupling of functional networks in glioblastoma. *Neuro Oncol* **2021**, *23*, 1885–1897. [CrossRef] [PubMed]
144. Salmaggi, A.; Corno, C.; Maschio, M.; Donzelli, S.; D'Urso, A.; Perego, P.; Ciusani, E. Synergistic Effect of Perampanel and Temozolomide in Human Glioma Cell Lines. *J. Pers. Med.* **2021**, *11*, 390. [CrossRef] [PubMed]
145. Flores-Toro, J.A.; Luo, D.; Gopinath, A.; Sarkisian, M.R.; Campbell, J.J.; Charo, I.F.; Singh, R.; Schall, T.J.; Datta, M.; Jain, R.K.; et al. CCR2 inhibition reduces tumor myeloid cells and unmasks a checkpoint inhibitor effect to slow progression of resistant murine gliomas. *Proc. Natl. Acad. Sci. USA* **2020**, *117*, 1129–1138. [CrossRef]
146. Shao, Z.; Tan, Y.; Shen, Q.; Hou, L.; Yao, B.; Qin, J.; Xu, P.; Mao, C.; Chen, L.N.; Zhang, H.; et al. Molecular insights into ligand recognition and activation of chemokine receptors CCR2 and CCR3. *Cell Discov.* **2022**, *8*, 44. [CrossRef]
147. Quail, D.F.; Bowman, R.L.; Akkari, L.; Quick, M.L.; Schuhmacher, A.J.; Huse, J.T.; Holland, E.C.; Sutton, J.C.; Joyce, J.A. The tumor microenvironment underlies acquired resistance to CSF-1R inhibition in gliomas. *Science* **2016**, *352*, aad3018. [CrossRef]
148. Cui, X.; Ma, C.; Vasudevaraja, V.; Serrano, J.; Tong, J.; Peng, Y.; Delorenzo, M.; Shen, G.; Frenster, J.; Morales, R.T.; et al. Dissecting the immunosuppressive tumor microenvironments in Glioblastoma-on-a-Chip for optimized PD-1 immunotherapy. *Elife* **2020**, *9* e52253. [CrossRef]
149. Butowski, N.; Colman, H.; De Groot, J.F.; Omuro, A.M.; Nayak, L.; Wen, P.Y.; Cloughesy, T.F.; Marimuthu, A.; Haidar, S.; Perry, A. et al. Orally administered colony stimulating factor 1 receptor inhibitor PLX3397 in recurrent glioblastoma: An Ivy Foundation Early Phase Clinical Trials Consortium phase II study. *Neuro Oncol.* **2016**, *18*, 557–564. [CrossRef]
150. Chen, P.; Hsu, W.H.; Han, J.; Xia, Y.; DePinho, R.A. Cancer Stemness Meets Immunity: From Mechanism to Therapy. *Cell Rep* **2021**, *34*, 108597. [CrossRef]
151. Ma, D.; Liu, S.; Lal, B.; Wei, S.; Wang, S.; Zhan, D.; Zhang, H.; Lee, R.S.; Gao, P.; Lopez-Bertoni, H.; et al. Extracellular Matrix Protein Tenascin C Increases Phagocytosis Mediated by CD47 Loss of Function in Glioblastoma. *Cancer Res.* **2019**, *79*, 2697–2708 [CrossRef]
152. Guo, M.; Abd-Rabbo, D.; Bertol, B.C.; Carew, M.; Lukhele, S.; Snell, L.M.; Xu, W.; Boukhaled, G.M.; Elsaesser, H.; Halaby, M.J. et al. Molecular, metabolic, and functional CD4 T cell paralysis in the lymph node impedes tumor control. *Cell Rep.* **2023**, *42* 113047. [CrossRef] [PubMed]
153. Sun, L.; Kienzler, J.C.; Reynoso, J.G.; Lee, A.; Shiuan, E.; Li, S.; Kim, J.; Ding, L.; Monteleone, A.J.; Owens, G.C.; et al. Immune checkpoint blockade induces distinct alterations in the microenvironments of primary and metastatic brain tumors. *J. Clin. Invest* **2023**, *133*, e169314. [CrossRef] [PubMed]

54. Simonds, E.F.; Lu, E.D.; Badillo, O.; Karimi, S.; Liu, E.V.; Tamaki, W.; Rancan, C.; Downey, K.M.; Stultz, J.; Sinha, M.; et al. Deep immune profiling reveals targetable mechanisms of immune evasion in immune checkpoint inhibitor-refractory glioblastoma. *J. Immunother Cancer* **2021**, *9*, e002181. [CrossRef]
55. Bielamowicz, K.; Fousek, K.; Byrd, T.T.; Samaha, H.; Mukherjee, M.; Aware, N.; Wu, M.F.; Orange, J.S.; Sumazin, P.; Man, T.K.; et al. Trivalent CAR T cells overcome interpatient antigenic variability in glioblastoma. *Neuro Oncol.* **2018**, *20*, 506–518. [CrossRef] [PubMed]
56. Solomon, I.; Amann, M.; Goubier, A.; Arce Vargas, F.; Zervas, D.; Qing, C.; Henry, J.Y.; Ghorani, E.; Akarca, A.U.; Marafioti, T.; et al. CD25-T(reg)-depleting antibodies preserving IL-2 signaling on effector T cells enhance effector activation and antitumor immunity. *Nat. Cancer* **2020**, *1*, 1153–1166. [CrossRef]
57. Kong, D.S.; Nam, D.H.; Kang, S.H.; Lee, J.W.; Chang, J.H.; Kim, J.H.; Lim, Y.J.; Koh, Y.C.; Chung, Y.G.; Kim, J.M.; et al. Phase III randomized trial of autologous cytokine-induced killer cell immunotherapy for newly diagnosed glioblastoma in Korea. *Oncotarget* **2017**, *8*, 7003–7013. [CrossRef]
58. Sanders, S.; Debinski, W. Challenges to Successful Implementation of the Immune Checkpoint Inhibitors for Treatment of Glioblastoma. *Int. J. Mol. Sci.* **2020**, *21*, 2759. [CrossRef]
59. Papademetriou, I.T.; Porter, T. Promising approaches to circumvent the blood-brain barrier: Progress, pitfalls and clinical prospects in brain cancer. *Ther. Deliv.* **2015**, *6*, 989–1016. [CrossRef]
60. Sonabend, A.M.; Gould, A.; Amidei, C.; Ward, R.; Schmidt, K.A.; Zhang, D.Y.; Gomez, C.; Bebawy, J.F.; Liu, B.P.; Bouchoux, G.; et al. Repeated blood-brain barrier opening with an implantable ultrasound device for delivery of albumin-bound paclitaxel in patients with recurrent glioblastoma: A phase 1 trial. *Lancet Oncol.* **2023**, *24*, 509–522. [CrossRef]
61. Liu, L.; Huh, J.R.; Shah, K. Microbiota and the gut-brain-axis: Implications for new therapeutic design in the CNS. *EBioMedicine* **2022**, *77*, 103908. [CrossRef]
62. Patrizz, A.; Dono, A.; Zorofchian, S.; Hines, G.; Takayasu, T.; Husein, N.; Otani, Y.; Arevalo, O.; Choi, H.A.; Savarraj, J.; et al. Glioma and temozolomide induced alterations in gut microbiome. *Sci. Rep.* **2020**, *10*, 21002. [CrossRef]
63. D'Alessandro, G.; Antonangeli, F.; Marrocco, F.; Porzia, A.; Lauro, C.; Santoni, A.; Limatola, C. Gut microbiota alterations affect glioma growth and innate immune cells involved in tumor immunosurveillance in mice. *Eur. J. Immunol.* **2020**, *50*, 705–711. [CrossRef] [PubMed]
64. Naghavian, R.; Faigle, W.; Oldrati, P.; Wang, J.; Toussaint, N.C.; Qiu, Y.; Medici, G.; Wacker, M.; Freudenmann, L.K.; Bonte, P.E.; et al. Microbial peptides activate tumour-infiltrating lymphocytes in glioblastoma. *Nature* **2023**, *617*, 807–817. [CrossRef] [PubMed]
65. Sivan, A.; Corrales, L.; Hubert, N.; Williams, J.B.; Aquino-Michaels, K.; Earley, Z.M.; Benyamin, F.W.; Lei, Y.M.; Jabri, B.; Alegre, M.L.; et al. Commensal Bifidobacterium promotes antitumor immunity and facilitates anti-PD-L1 efficacy. *Science* **2015**, *350*, 1084–1089. [CrossRef] [PubMed]
66. Gopalakrishnan, V.; Spencer, C.N.; Nezi, L.; Reuben, A.; Andrews, M.C.; Karpinets, T.V.; Prieto, P.A.; Vicente, D.; Hoffman, K.; Wei, S.C.; et al. Gut microbiome modulates response to anti-PD-1 immunotherapy in melanoma patients. *Science* **2018**, *359*, 97–103. [CrossRef]

Disclaimer/Publisher's Note: The statements, opinions and data contained in all publications are solely those of the individual author(s) and contributor(s) and not of MDPI and/or the editor(s). MDPI and/or the editor(s) disclaim responsibility for any injury to people or property resulting from any ideas, methods, instructions or products referred to in the content.

MDPI AG
Grosspeteranlage 5
4052 Basel
Switzerland
Tel.: +41 61 683 77 34

Cancers Editorial Office
E-mail: cancers@mdpi.com
www.mdpi.com/journal/cancers

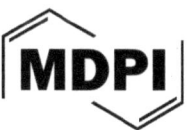

Disclaimer/Publisher's Note: The title and front matter of this reprint are at the discretion of the Guest Editors. The publisher is not responsible for their content or any associated concerns. The statements, opinions and data contained in all individual articles are solely those of the individual Editors and contributors and not of MDPI. MDPI disclaims responsibility for any injury to people or property resulting from any ideas, methods, instructions or products referred to in the content.

www.ingramcontent.com/pod-product-compliance
Lightning Source LLC
LaVergne TN
LVHW072347090526
838202LV00019B/2498